Operative Urology

Operative Urology

JOHN BLANDY
DM, MCh, FRCS, FACS
Professor of Urology in the
University of London at the
London Hospital Medical College;
Consultant Urologist,
St Peter's Hospitals;
President of the British Association
of Urological Surgeons

SECOND EDITION

Distributed in the USA and Canada by
BLACKWELL/YEAR BOOK MEDICAL PUBLISHERS • INC.

BLACKWELL SCIENTIFIC PUBLICATIONS

OXFORD LONDON EDINBURGH

BOSTON PALO ALTO MELBOURNE

© 1978, 1986 by Blackwell Scientific Publications
Editorial offices:
Osney Mead, Oxford, OX2 0EL
8 John Street, London, WC1N 2ES
23 Ainslie Place, Edinburgh, EH3 6AJ
52 Beacon Street, Boston
 Massachusetts 02108, USA
667 Lytton Avenue, Palo Alto
 California 94301, USA
107 Barry Street, Carlton
 Victoria 3053, Australia

First published 1978
Second edition 1986

Phototypeset by Oliver Burridge & Co. Ltd
Crawley, Sussex and
printed and bound in Great Britain
William Clowes Limited, Beccles and London

DISTRIBUTORS

USA
 Blackwell Mosby Book Distributors
 11830 Westline Industrial Drive
 St Louis, Missouri 63141

Canada
 Blackwell Mosby Book Distributors
 120 Melford Drive, Scarborough
 Ontario M1B 2X4

Australia
 Blackwell Scientific Publications
 (Australia) Pty Ltd
 107 Barry Street
 Carlton, Victoria 3053

British Library Cataloguing in Publication Data

Blandy, John P.
 Operative urology.—2nd ed.
 1. Genito-urinary organs—Surgery
 I. Title   II. Blandy, John P. Comparative
 urology
 617'.46059   RD571

ISBN 0-632-01194-7

Contents

Preface to second edition

In the five years since the first edition, I have been astonished to find that almost every sentence has had to be rewritten. New techniques have altered our entire attitude to surgery for stones in the kidney. The revolution in chemotherapy for cancer has entirely changed our approach to the management of cancer of the testicle and bladder. The aim of this second edition is still the same—to tell a trainee surgeon how to follow the steps of an operation and warn him what to watch out for afterwards. The introduction of endoscopic television has made it much easier for a young surgeon to learn endoscopic resection of the prostate and of bladder tumours, and the supremely difficult technique of percutaneous stone surgery is similarly made easier to learn thanks to these new teaching aids. Nevertheless, nothing matches experience in the operating room: it is still the kitchen of surgery, and the cookbook is always a pale echo of assisting and being assisted by the chef.

J.P.B.

Preface to first edition

When I was a registrar I often wished I had a book which would tell me how to do an operation, step by step, and then warn me what might go wrong afterwards. Since then there have been many changes in the style and content of urology, but it is still difficult to find a clear account of everyday operations in a form at once accessible and readable. Current journals are for obvious reasons mainly concerned with new developments and unusual problems, but just how to do quite straightforward operations is left to textbooks, and these do not seem to provide the kind of answers which are needed by the surgeon in training. Of course no cookery book ever made a chef, nor can any surgical text replace time spent in assisting and being assisted at surgical operations. Nevertheless a good recipe has value if it can help a cook avoid repeating the mistakes made by the inventor of a dish, and one of the principal aims of this book is to point out the stupid mistakes the writer has made in the past, and to warn my younger colleagues of the errors and pitfalls which experience has taught me, often at tragic cost. This book is a personal selection of surgical recipes which work in my hands: it is not intended to be a comprehensive encyclopaedia. Some operations are left out because I think better ways have been found to achieve the same ends: others are omitted because there is

no indication for them nowadays. Some are rare (notably some of the paediatric procedures) that I cannot write of them with experience. Others are too new to be recommended—notably some of the new prostheses. I have left out house-surgeon's details of pre- and post-operative care, since these are common to all surgical operations and my readers will not need to be reminded of them. In their place I have tried as far as possible to put in those little dodges and tricks which time and experience have taught me can make all the difference between an operation which is easy (and therefore safe) and one which is difficult (and therefore dangerous). For the same reason I have tried to make my drawings as clear as possible—to give a surgeon's-eye view of the essentials, rather than a true-to-life image of the operative field: they are intended to be read like a map, not an artistic landscape. I have tried to provide my registrars with a modern version of the book I wished I could have had 25 years ago. In putting it together it has been a pleasure to work with the tolerant but enthusiastic team at Blackwell Scientific Publications, and I am again happy to acknowledge my debt to Messrs Per Saugman, John Robson and Peter Danckwerts for their never-failing courtesy and skill.

J.P.B.

Chapter 1
Endoscopy

Today we take for granted that we can examine every part of the inside of the urethra and bladder with light so bright that it allows photography or television, and with lenses so sharp that the mucosae can be examined as if through a magnifying glass. Modern irrigating systems allow us to take a biopsy, crush a stone, catheterize a ureter, coagulate bleeding vessels, and cut out tumours. Flexible baskets allow stones to be removed from the ureter and, when introduced through a nephrostomy, allow the inside of the renal pelvis and calices to be examined. The flexible cystoscope bids fair to replace the rigid one, and the flexible ureteroscope already allows lesions in the ureter and renal pelvis to be seen. It was not always so, and what was visionary a mere five years ago has become commonplace today.

Urology is the oldest of all the disciplines of surgery since it began with the urethral bougie, and there is reason to suppose that gonorrhoea is as old as our species. From the bougie evolved the sound, with which until only a generation ago, stones were detected in the bladder by the unmistakable click of the instrument in the bladder. Skill with bougie and sound was for long the sure sign of the master urologist, and it is by no accident that even today the outgoing Senior Surgeon of St Peter's Hospital hands on to his successor a silver sound, the badge of his office.

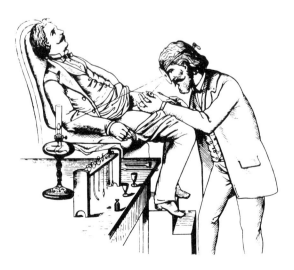

1.1. Direct viewing cystoscopy: from Grunfeld, 1881.

The sound was a clumsy method of diagnosing vesical pathology, and for conditions other than calculus, it was necessary to open the bladder via the urethra and feel round it with the finger—a procedure not to be repeated lightly. The demand for more accurate and more simple diagnosis required a means of looking at the inside of the bladder. First came a simple tube, like the auriscope, giving a limited glimpse of the opposite side of the wall of the bladder (1.1). Many direct-vision cystoscopes were constructed on this principle, and it is remarkable that despite the difficulties, our predecessors were able to catheterize ureters, and see and biopsy cancers. By 1886, von Dittel had added the incandescent Mignon lamp to Nitze's early cystoscope, and before long good irrigating systems, Albarran's deflecting lever, scissors, forceps and catheters were all added to the cystoscopic armamentarium (Blandy 1978).

After the turn of the century, the operating cystoscope changed little except in detail. My generation of surgical assistants were using instruments that Nitze would have recognized as being of his design, though perhaps a little more reliable. Then, in the early 1970s came three inventions that entirely altered the scope and character not only of cystoscopy, but of urology itself (Mitchell & Makepeace 1976).

All these inventions were due to the genius of Professor Harold Hopkins. First was the rod-lens cystoscope. Instead of mounting a row of glass lenses in a telescope tube, Hopkins used a series of glass rods and the air-spaces between them became the lenses. It was much easier to set the rods on a precise optical axis for grinding and blooming. This was a major step forward. A new order of precision was brought to the cystoscope. Ghost images and stray reflections were banished, thanks to multiple coating of the lenses. The surgeon for the first time could use in the bladder an instrument as fine and as precise as the microscope (1.2).

Hopkins' second invention was the fibre-light cable which permitted light of limitless brightness to be fed in at one end of a flexible

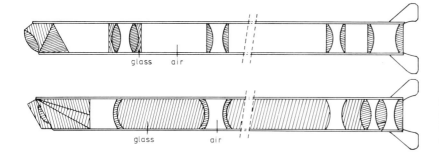

1.2. Above, diagram of conventional cystoscope telescope system; below, rod-lens system designed by Hopkins.

glass air

glass air

cable, emerging into the bladder at the other end of the cystoscope (1.3). The light was wonderfully bright: there was no Mignon lamp bulb to go out and need to be replaced just at the most critical moment of a transurethral resection (1.4).

To these two major leaps forward can be added a third—only recently adapted to urology—and again largely due to Hopkins. By using the same glass fibres, coated with glass of a different refractive index, winding them on a wheel so that when cut across at the same point on the circumference the fibres are aligned, it is possible to transmit optical images from one end of the flexible cable to the other. Today this invention has transfigured gastrointestinal and colorectal surgery. In urology we have been so content with our rigid endoscopes that we have been tardy in utilizing flexible endoscopes for the urethra, the bladder and the kidney; however, there has been a change in the last five years. Again we must acknowledge the immense debt that urology owes to its instrument-makers, and recognize that our duty to maintain contact with their advances is no less important than keeping up with advances in the recognized urological journals.

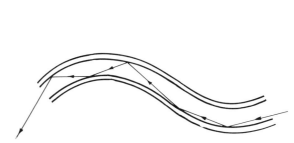

1.3. Fibre-lighting: each glass fibre is coated with glass of different refractive index, ensuring total internal reflexion whether the fibres are aligned (above) as straight lines, or (below) in curves.

The urologist's kit

Today we must recognize two types of urological endoscopy. Classical urethrocystoscopy uses rigid instruments; it is always advisable to look well at the urethra *en route* to the bladder, and when inside the bladder, it is often necessary to take a biopsy, catheterize a ureter or do something else. A complete interchangeable kit of instruments is needed. Nothing is more irritating than to have to change the light and water attachments in order to use a biopsy forceps or a resectoscope (1.5).

For rigid endoscopy all manufacturers today provide interchangeable instruments, individual items fitting each other. The minimum equipment that is needed consists of a narrow tube through which the urethra can be exam-

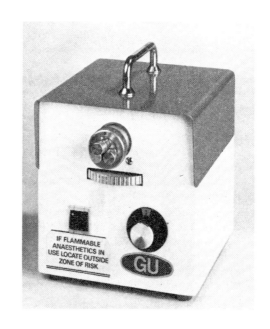

1.4. Modern light source for endoscopy (courtesy of Genito-urinary Manufacturing Co. Ltd.).

ined with a forward-looking (0°) telescope, and the bladder inspected with a right-angled (70°) telescope. If a stricture is encountered *en route* to the bladder, it is convenient to be able to cut it with an optical urethrotome introduced through the same equipment. If a suspicious area is seen in the bladder, it must be biopsied with cup forceps. If one needs to pass a catheter into a ureteric orifice, a guide with a deflecting Albarran lever should be available. If a cancer is found in the bladder, it

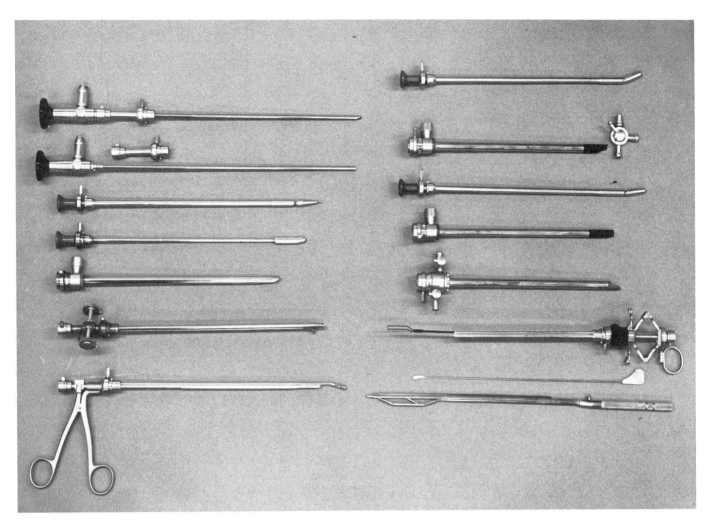

1.5. Modern interchangeable urologists 'kit': with a complete kit such as this almost any endoscopic operation can be performed without having to change light or water leads. (System designed for the author by the Genito-urinary Manufacturing Co. Ltd.)

should only be a matter of seconds to replace the cystoscope sheath by a resectoscope and remove the tumour with the cutting loop.

Because of the need to have an interchangeable kit of instruments, an important consideration arises in purchasing equipment. Today none of us lives in a Utopia where the running costs of replacing and maintaining equipment do not concern a surgeon. In a unit where there are several urologists, it is of prime importance that they agree upon the kit that is chosen, and in doing this, should give consideration no less to the availability of service and repair than to the type of instrument itself.

It is equally important to give thought to the way in which urological equipment is to be sterilized. Modern endoscopic equipment is expensive, delicate, and complicated by screws and moving parts. Liquid sterilizing agents reach these parts with great difficulty. Heat is the only truly reliable sterilizing agent, but heat will ruin some plastic parts, and the rèpeated contraction and expansion of the sheath of a Hopkins rod lens system will ruin it after

repeated sterilization by heat. Exposure to a water-bath at 70 °C will kill micro-organisms but not spores or hepatitis virus particles. Adding formaldehyde vapour to steam at this temperature, for example in a low-pressure autoclave with a formalin cycle, gives effective spore-sterilization but takes too long for it to be used between one case and another on a long list of endoscopies. Ethylene oxide gas is as good as formalin but in practice unreliable, and it requires strict quality control. Soaking instruments in glutaraldehyde solution remains our Hobson's choice, but need not be used for the majority of metal instruments which will perfectly well stand up to an autoclave.

Even more important than the sterilization of the instruments, is the sterilization of the large volumes of fluid that are needed in modern urological surgery. As soon as an incision is made in a prostate or a bladder tumour, some irrigating fluid will enter the bloodstream, so it must be sterile, free from pyrogens, and of the same pharmacological purity as any other fluid destined for intravenous injection. Unfortunately it is difficult and expensive to provide large volumes of fluid, and even when an autoclave is used, tragic examples have made hospital pharmacists wary of setting up a system for sterilizing intravenous fluids without very elaborate and expensive systems of quality control.

Today, systems that supply water from the town mains water supply are recognized to be unsafe for urological surgery. A tank is easily contaminated. A continuous filtration system with reversed osmosis to get rid of unwanted ions, and an inbuilt autoclave to sterilize the filtered water (1.6), has the potential advantage that it might be adapted to supply limitless volumes of sterile 2.0% glycine for endoscopic resection at negligible cost.

Flexible fibrescopes in urology

Fowler *et al.* (1984) have shown that the Olympus flexible endoscope designed for the purpose of examining the bile duct (the Olympus choledochoscope) can be used in routine check cystoscopy when it is necessary to examine the bladder at regular intervals after treatment for carcinoma. The instrument, which is 16 Ch, is easily and painlessly passed along the urethra, giving a clear view of the wall of the urethra *en route*. The flexibility of its terminal segment allows a view of the entire lining of the bladder. In more than a hundred endoscopies no mistakes of omission were made when flexible endoscopy was subsequently checked by conventional means (1.7).

At present the flexible cystourethroscope is in the course of being modified, and provided with biopsy and coagulation facilities. Potentially adaptable to the use of a Neodymium YAG laser, it could supplant the rigid endoscope for small recurrent bladder tumours both in follow-up and treatment.

Diathermy

Although diathermy is one of the most commonly used and important instruments in modern surgery, and without diathermy there could be no endoscopic resection, few of us know much about it. It depends upon the simple fact that electricity passing through a conductor heats it. When the pathway for the current is very wide, the heating effect is negligible. When it is small—as under the loop of the resectoscope—one may obtain almost any desired heat from mild coagulation to an arc that severs tissues as by a knife, simply by increasing the current. If direct current is used,

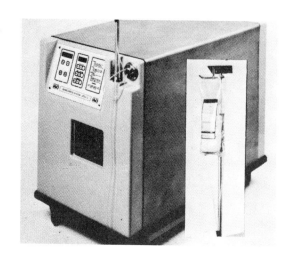

1.6. Rowater EP550 machine for supplying sterile water or glycine (courtesy of Rowater Medical Ltd.).

then of course the patient will jump each time the current is switched on or off, and an alternating current such as that obtained from the AC mains will give rise to repetitive contractions—the well known effect of Faradism—giving pain as well as sustained tetanic contraction. When the frequency of the alternating current is increased above 10 kHz (10 000 cycles per second) then there is neither pain nor muscle stimulation, and it now becomes possible to make use of the heating effects of a narrow electrode either to coagulate tissue or to cut it.

In the past, confusion arose from the notion that different wave forms produced different physical effects on the tissues. It was believed that one wave form gave cutting, and another gave coagulation. In fact, the different effects were a function of the intensity of the current, though it is true (but to a more limited extent) that the configuration of the wave form does matter in obtaining good cutting and clean coagulation. With modern diathermy machines (1.8) one may choose the wave form and voltage at will. It is more important to realize that when one is cutting under water, a very large current is passed through the tissues. Accidental contact with a small metal contact may allow current to flow to earth through a small area, and cause unwanted and dangerous heating at that contact. In urology there is a specially high risk of accidental burns. The surgeon must always be conscious of this danger: he must ensure that there is always a good *large* earth contact (so that there is hardly any significant rise in temperature under it). As more and more sophisticated monitoring equipment is used during an operation, the surgeon must always be aware of the special dangers that may arise if current finds its way back to earth, via ECG electrodes for example.

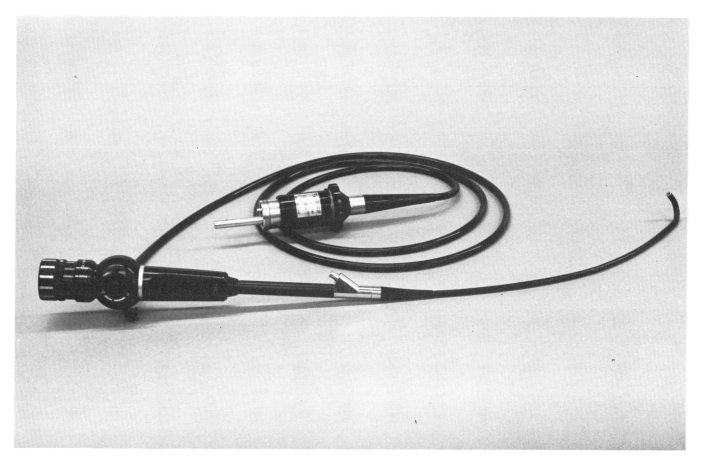

1.7. Olympus flexible choledochoscope adapted for use as a flexible urethrocystoscope (courtesy of Olympus Pty and C.G. Fowler).

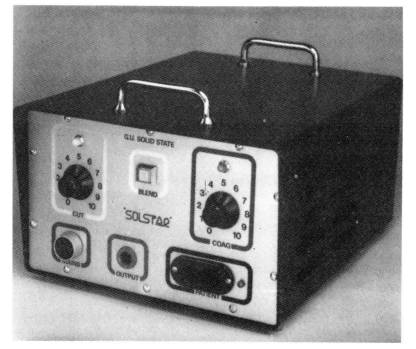

1.8. Modern solid-state diathermy machine (courtesy of the Genitourinary Manufacturing Co. Ltd.).

Preparation for endoscopy

For cystoscopy under local anaesthetic using a rigid endoscope no special precautions are needed. It is more comfortable for the patient if the bladder is not emptied before the examination. With a general anaesthetic the usual precautions are observed and food and drink avoided for six hours beforehand. A suitable premedication is given. There is no need to shave the pubes before endoscopy or transurethral resection.

Position of the patient

The patient lies flat with the legs supported on rests so that the thigh makes an angle of 10° to 20° with the horizontal (1.9). Inexperienced staff often put the patient up in the position preferred by rectal surgeons—the 'lithotomy' position. This exaggerated posture makes it difficult to inspect the trigone or catheterize the ureters, and obscures the landmarks in TUR. Worse, it may give the patient post-operative backache.

The supine position, with the legs placed apart on a suitably padded rest, is an alternative with which one should be familiar, although it does not permit adequate inspection of the anterior wall of the bladder. It may be used when the legs cannot be put up in Lloyd-Davies stirrups (1.10).

For examination of the urethra and bladder with the flexible fibrescope, the patient lies supine. There is no need for stirrups, but women must abduct their thighs to permit access to the urethra (1.11).

Preparation of the skin

One may use betadine or chlorhexidine solution to prepare the skin, using swabs held in forceps in the usual way.

Rigid endoscopy in the male

Preparation of the urethra

The urethra must be lubricated before any instrument is passed and an antiseptic such as 0.25% chlorhexidine is added to prevent infection. Commercial sterile preparations are available containing chlorhexidine and lubricant, usually with 1% lignocaine, which is a satisfactory local anaesthetic for passing rigid or flexible instruments. The gel is applied from a tube or concertina bottle with a sterilized nozzle (1.12). After putting the gel into the urethra of a male, a soft penile clamp is applied transversely just behind the glans to keep it in the urethra for a full four minutes (1.13). Never use any force in injecting the local anaesthetic, and never use lignocaine solution stronger than 1% for fear of toxicity.

Urethroscopy

Nowadays, urethroscopy always precedes passage of the cystoscope; blind passage of the cystoscope without examining the urethra has been given up.

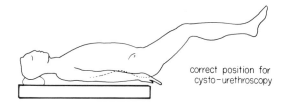

correct position for cysto-urethroscopy

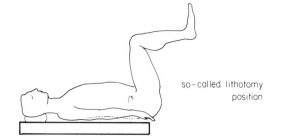

so-called lithotomy position

1.9. Above, the correct position for cystoscopy, with the thighs flexed to about 45°; below, lithotomy position often (mistakenly) used in the operating theatre.

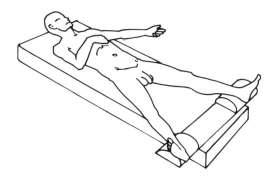

1.10. Supine position with legs apart, supported on padded board.

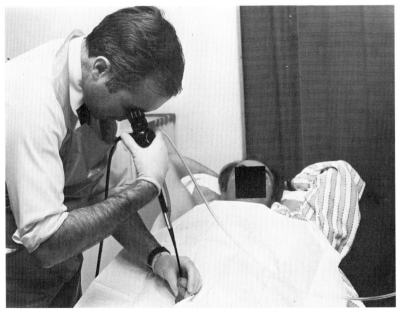

1.11. The fibre optic cystourethroscope is easily inserted into the urethra under local anaesthesia, and passed into the bladder. There is noticeably less discomfort for the patient than when using the rigid conventional instrument (courtesy of Mr C.G. Fowler and Olympus Pty).

The narrow (17 Ch) sheath and 0° telescope are placed inside the meatus and gently advanced down the urethra under direct vision as the water flows to allow clear vision. The curve of the urethra is followed, as in sigmoidoscopy or oesophagoscopy: force is never needed (1.14).

The previous instillation of lubricant and chlorhexidine causes some dilatation of the submucosal vessels of the normal anterior urethra. The openings of the urethral glands can be seen, sometimes more prominent as one approaches the bulb (1.15). The bulbar urethra becomes wider and shows helical submucosal rings like the barrel of a rifle. Follow the roof of the urethra, and swing the urethroscope down gently until the external sphincter is seen. This looks rather like the anus, occluding the lumen, but it easily dilates before the advancing endoscope. If the patient is being examined under local anaesthesia and is frightened, it may be difficult to relax the

1.12. Before passing any instrument the urethra is filled with lignocaine-chlorhexidine gel to lubricate and sterilize it.

1.13. A penile clamp is applied transversely to retain the lubricating gel.

1.15. Appearance of the anterior urethra, showing the typical pits of the para-urethral glands.

sphincter. Ask the patient to breathe in and out deeply, or pretend to urinate—this may allow the sphincter to relax and permit the instrument to slip into the prostatic urethra (1.16).

The normal prostatic urethra is usually red and granular, with exuberant frills on either side of the crest of the verumontanum. Often, little black flecks can be seen on the floor of the prostatic urethra in the vicinity of the verumontanum. Biopsy shows that these are innocent collections of lymphocytes and cystitis cystica.

The salient feature of the prostatic urethra is the verumontanum, distinguished by its central pit—the utriculus masculinus—vestige of the confluence of the Müllerian ducts. Opening on either side of the utriculus are the orifices of the ejaculatory ducts. Above the verumontanum rises the neck of the bladder and, in older men, the middle lobe of the prostate. Be very cautious when interpreting the appearance of the bladder neck. There is a very wide range of normality and appearance alone is never sufficient to diagnose obstruction.

Once past the bladder neck, the endoscope enters the bladder. The 0° telescope shows the trigone and ureteric orifices, and to study the rest of the interior of the bladder this telescope is exchanged for one with a 70°, that is nearly right-angle, view.

Cystoscopy

At cystoscopy it is possible and necessary to examine every part of the interior of the bladder. The 70° telescope is rotated, withdrawn, and deflected in order to view the anterior wall (1.17). Get used to looking at the bladder as the fluid runs in and out—this is especially useful in revealing bleeding from a Hunner's ulcer, or in showing up a small tumour just inside the internal meatus on the anterior wall. To illustrate all the normal and abnormal appearances of the bladder is beyond the scope of this or indeed any printed book, but the reader may learn much from the beautiful pictures in the atlases of Marion (1935), Ryall (1925), and Gow and Hopkins (1978). Even these do scant justice to the subtlety of colour and the fascinating variety of texture that is the daily delight of the cystoscopist. No Aladdin's cave was ever so beautiful or so full of surprises as the human bladder.

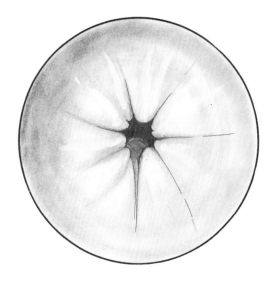

1.16. The external sphincter is easily recognized by its star-shaped appearance and its characteristic feel.

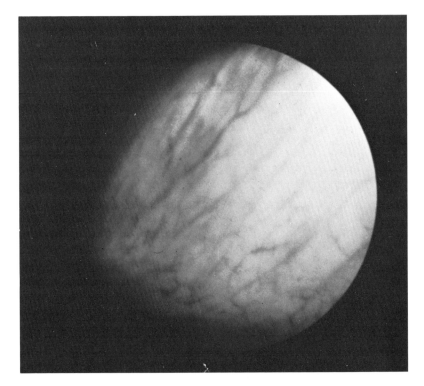

1.17. The fine vessels of the wall of the bladder.

Flexible fibrescopy

With the patient supine and his legs apart, the penis is cleansed with cetrimide, and a perforated paper sheet placed around it. Ten millilitres of 1% lignocaine gel are instilled and remain for five minutes. The flexible endoscope is advanced while sterile water flows through it, under direct vision. As the external sphincter is approached, the tip is slightly bent up, and the patient asked to pretend to void; as the sphincter relaxes the fibrescope slides

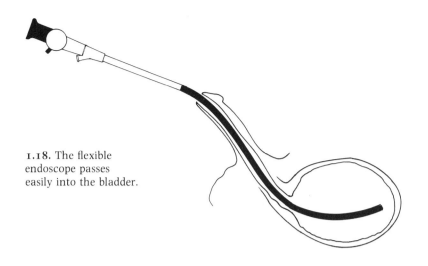

1.18. The flexible endoscope passes easily into the bladder.

into the prostatic urethra, which can be fully inspected with the flexible tip before advancing it over the middle lobe into the bladder. There the bladder is systematically inspected (1.18) and at the end, by curving the tip fully upon itself, a remarkable retrograde view of the bladder neck—or prostatic cavity—may be obtained (1.19). The operating channel of the instrument is big enough to allow passage of a biopsy forceps, ureteric catheter or diathermy electrode.

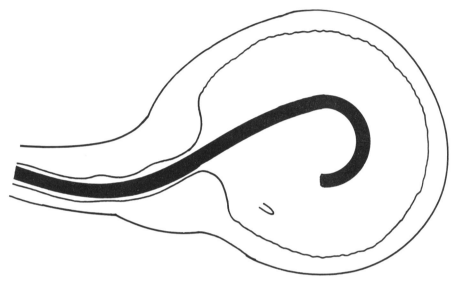

1.19. By manœuvring the flexible tip of the endoscope a unique retrograde view of the internal meatus, or the resected prostatic cavity, may be obtained.

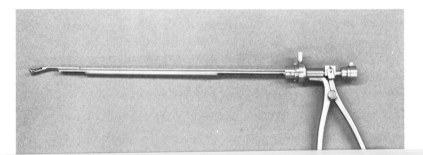

Biopsy

Whether a rigid or a flexible endoscope is used, it is often necessary to take a biopsy, and indeed one should make it a rule always to biopsy any feature that is not easily recognized. Cup forceps make it easy and safe to take

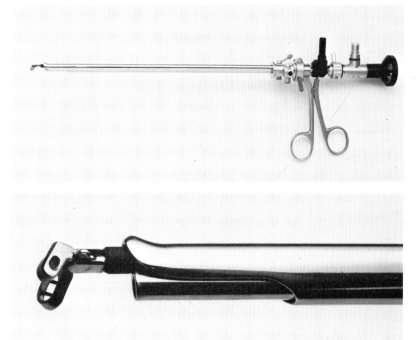

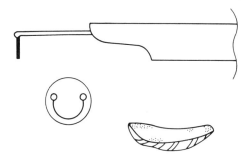

1.22. Using the resectoscope loop one may take a deep bite of tumour and bladder wall upon which to make an assessment as to its pathological (P) stage.

1.21. Tauber insulated diathermy forceps. After the biopsy has been taken, bleeding from the site can be sealed with diathermy without damage to the specimen (courtesy of Messrs Richard Wolf, UK Ltd.).

Catheterizing a ureter

Either the 30° or the 70° telescope in an operating slide with an Albarran lever (1.23) is passed down the sheath of a normal rigid endoscope. If a flexible endoscope is used, the ureteric catheter is passed down the instrument channel.

With the usual rigid instrument, to find the ureter the novice may begin by withdrawing the endoscope until the view is just cut off by the neck of the bladder at 6 o'clock in the midline posteriorly. Rotate the cystoscope through 45° and advance it for 2 cm. This will reveal (usually) one or other ureteric orifice. Its companion is found by rotating the telescope through a right angle, or by following the whitish streak that marks the hypoteneuse of the trigone (1.24).

Chromocystoscopy

If 4 ml of indigocarmine are given intravenously, after four minutes a puff of inky blue dye emerges from the ureteric orifices. This can be useful in revealing the site of a ureter that has been obscured by oedema or inflammation.

Having found the ureter a catheter may be advanced up the cystoscope until its tip emerges in the field of view. Bending it down with the Albarran lever, the tip of the catheter is placed gently in the ureteric orifice and advanced as far as necessary towards the kidney. The wire stylet is useful to stop the catheter jamming in the cystoscope, but it must be withdrawn as soon as the catheter enters the

ureter, for fear of the stiffened catheter lacerating the wall of the ureter.

A ureteric catheter often sticks about 1 cm inside the ureteric orifice. Three tricks may help it pass onwards: (1) the legs of the patient may be brought down to the horizontal position; (2) the bladder may be distended with fluid; and (3) one may remove the rubber teat from the catheterizing slide so that the ureter may be rotated between finger and thumb, allowing its tip to get away from mucosal folds

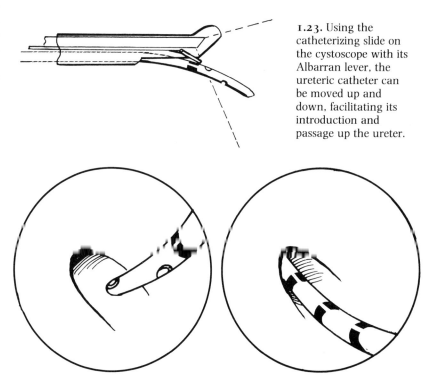

1.23. Using the catheterizing slide on the cystoscope with its Albarran lever, the ureteric catheter can be moved up and down, facilitating its introduction and passage up the ureter.

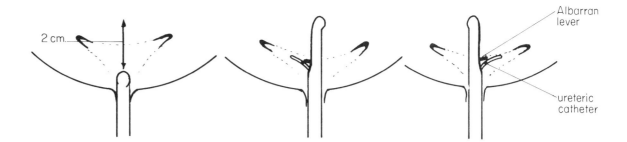

Albarran
lever

2 cm

ureteric
catheter

1.24. Finding the ureteric orifices. Above, the cystoscope is advanced 2 cm inwards from the bladder neck, and then rotated through 45° first on one side and then on the other.

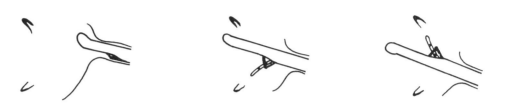

in the ureteric wall and slip upwards towards the kidney.

Centimetre marks on ureteric catheters mark how far it has entered the ureteric orifice: at 25 cm, five broad lines tell you that it has reached the kidney.

Ureterography

Today it is only necessary to pass a catheter right up to the kidney if facilities are not available for image intensification. A bulb-ended (Chevassu) catheter is usually gently lodged in the ureteric orifice (1.25), contrast injected, and the column of dye watched on the image-intensifier screen. Without this modern apparatus, a fair second-best image may be obtained by still X-ray photography if 10 to 15 ml of contrast is injected as the catheter is withdrawn.

Retrograde urography

Even less often should one need to perform classical retrograde urography, when facilities for good high-dose conventional urography are available. Nevertheless occasions still arise when it is necessary to pass a catheter right up into the renal pelvis. A film is taken when 3 ml

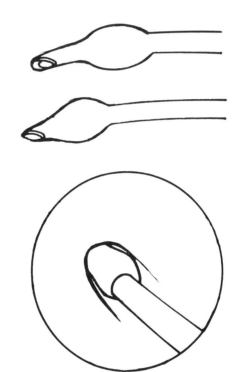

1.25. (a) Braasch- and (b) Chevassu-type bulb-ended ureteric catheters for obtaining a ureterogram. The bulb is gently jammed into the ureteric orifice (c).

rowest catheter snugly in its constricted waist (1.26).

Collecting ureteric urine

In diagnosing renal hypertension or tuberculosis, one collects urine from the ureter. The catheter is passed to 25 cm. For most purposes

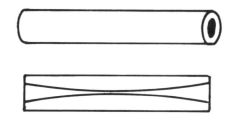

1.26. Thomson–Walker universal adapter which allows injection of contrast medium up any sized ureteric catheter (courtesy of Genitourinary Manufacturing Co. Ltd.).

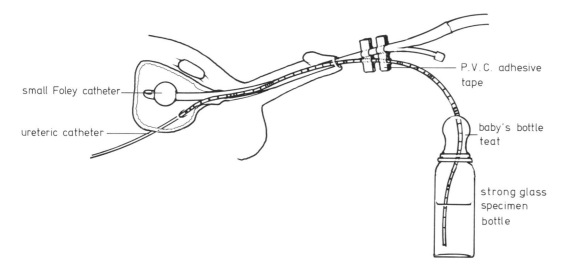

small Foley catheter

ureteric catheter

P.V.C. adhesive tape

baby's bottle teat

strong glass specimen bottle

1.27. Collecting urine from a ureteric catheter: pass a narrow Foley catheter into the bladder, blow up the balloon, and tape it to the ureteric catheter with PVC tape. Make sure the specimen bottle is a strong one—*not* a test-tube.

enough urine flows within a few minutes to collect an adequate sample for bacteriological studies. To keep the catheter in the ureter for a longer period, secure it to a small Foley catheter passed alongside the ureteric catheter with tape, leading the ureteric catheter via a baby's feeding teat to a sterile container (1.27). Bottle and catheter are taped to the thigh to prevent accidental dislodgement in the collecting period. These specimens of ureteric urine are very important and must always be collected in duplicate lest one of the bottles is broken. Do not use test-tubes; use bottles.

References

Blandy J.P. (1978) *Transurethral Resection*, 2nd edn. Pitman Medical, London.

Fowler C.G. (1984) Fibrescope urethrocystoscopy. *Brit. J. Urol.* **56**, 304.

Gow J.G. & Hopkins H.H. (1978) Handbook of Urological Endoscopy. Churchill Livingstone, Edinburgh.

Marion G. (1935) Traité d'Urologie. 13th Ed. Masson, Paris. Vol. 2.

Mitchell J.P. & Makepeace A.P.W. (1976) Optics of telescopes and fibrelighting equipment. In *Scientific Foundations of Urology*, **2** (ed. by Williams D.I. & Chisholm G.D.), p. 421. Heinemann, London.

Ryall, E.C. (1925) Operative Cystoscopy. Kimpton, London.

Chapter 2
Nephrectomy

Morris (1898) reviewed the history of the surgery of the kidney, which originated in the need to drain large perinephric abscesses that pointed in the lumbar triangle of Petit. At first it needed only a sharp knife and courage. From time to time a stone would float out on the issue of pus, and the surgeon would claim credit for a nephrolithotomy. The advent of X-rays made it possible to detect stones with certainty; later, with retrograde and intravenous urography, other structural changes could be diagnosed with precision. To operate upon such a deeply placed and vascular organ remained a difficult and dangerous enterprise until relaxant anaesthesia and blood transfusion invited the urological surgeon into the chest and made the peritoneum no longer a barrier.

Other technical advances improved the operative surgery of the kidney. First came the use of angiography, accompanied by a better understanding of the vascular anatomy of the kidney. This made it possible to perform nephrotomy and partial nephrectomy with accuracy and safety. Second, methods of preserving the kidney by cooling, arising from the needs for transplantation, allowed the surgeon ample time to operate without haste or loss of blood. Third, a technique of dealing with the cut surface of the kidney was developed by Semb (1953) and Maddern (1967) which made it possible to perform resection and reconstruction of the parenchyma without bleeding or loss of function. The fourth major technical advance was the discovery by Gil-Vernet (1965) of a bloodless plane that lay between the fat of the renal sinus and the muscular wall of the renal pelvis. This plane could be opened to display the entire intrarenal pelvis right up to the necks of the calices.

Thanks to these technical advances, nephrectomy is now a rare operation, and the method used is determined by the pathological process for which nephrectomy is indicated:

Simple nephrectomy

Indications

One reason for removing a non-malignant kidney nowadays is to prepare the patient for renal transplantation when the kidneys are known to harbour infection or seem to be responsible for severe and uncontrollable hypertension (Bennett 1976). A kidney may be so atrophied from hydronephrosis that one will not attempt to preserve it, or so hopelessly damaged from calculi that one will not try to save the kidney. Sometimes hypertension from renal artery stenosis is more appropriately dealt with by nephrectomy than by reconstruction of the artery. With malignant disease of the parenchyma, nephrectomy entails radical removal of the kidney within its surrounding package of fat and fascia, and if the malignancy arises in the urothelium, the ureter is taken *en bloc*. Because today the indications for nephrectomy are so scanty, it is rare that one embarks upon nephrectomy in an operative field that is not scarred from some previous surgical procedure.

Special precautions

Blood is seldom needed for the removal of a 'virgin' kidney but secondary nephrectomy or operation for tuberculosis or stone disease needs a very bloody mobilization indeed. Even straightforward nephrectomy may meet sudden unexpected loss of blood, so that at least two units of blood should be available.

After an operation on the kidney, patients often develop pulmonary atelectasis and pulmonary infection. Pre-operative instruction in breathing exercises and coughing may help the patient understand what is expected of him or her post-operatively. For the same reasons smoking should be forbidden, teeth extracted, and intercurrent effectively treated.

prophylactic antibiotics merely repopulate the bowel with hospital strains of bacteria to which the patient has no natural resistance, and against which there are no antibiotics.

It should go without saying, but even today it must be emphasized that the surgeon himself must make sure that he is about to operate on the correct side. Never trust your memory. Never rely on what your assistants say. Insist that the X-rays are up in the operating room. Always talk to the patient before he or she is anaesthetized. Do not be proud: one day you will make this mistake; I have.

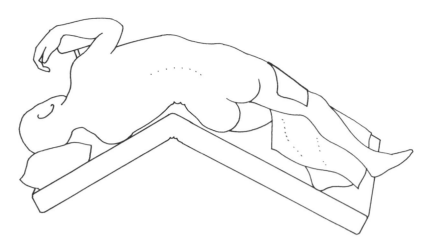

Position on the table

Place the patient in the lateral position (2.1) his back arched over a bridge, break in the table, or inflatable cushion. Have the lower thigh flexed, and place a soft pillow between the legs. Fix the diathermy earth plate to the upper thigh. Make sure that no part of the patient's skin touches metal on the table or its supports. Broad adhesive strapping is probably safer as a method of fixing the patient than any metal supports.

Anaesthetic

General anaesthesia is needed. Warn your anaesthetist that you will need profound muscular relaxation, that you need diathermy, and that you may well enter the pleura. An endotracheal tube is needed with controlled respiration.

Incision

The choice of incision is determined by the underlying pathology. If the kidney is small and not set about with adhesions, as in the contracted kidney that must be removed prior to transplantation, the vertical lumbotomy (Gil-Vernet 1965) is adequate and relatively painless, but difficult to enlarge and should not be used for a kidney of normal size, especially when difficulty is anticipated. The best all-round approach is through the 12th rib-bed. The 12th rib-tip approach gives adequate access to a small kidney and can easily be extended posteriorly if more room is needed. When the operation is likely to be difficult, make the incision along the full length of the 12th rib. One cannot emphasize too often that safety in renal surgery requires adequate access.

The 12th rib-tip approach

Begin by feeling for the tip of the 12th rib with the patient in the arched lateral position (2.2). Make a short incision down directly on to the tip of the rib, just long enough for the finger to feel through the fat to confirm that the tip which is felt is that of the 12th rather than the 11th rib—a mistake very easy to make in a fat

2.1. Standard position for nephrectomy through a loin approach.

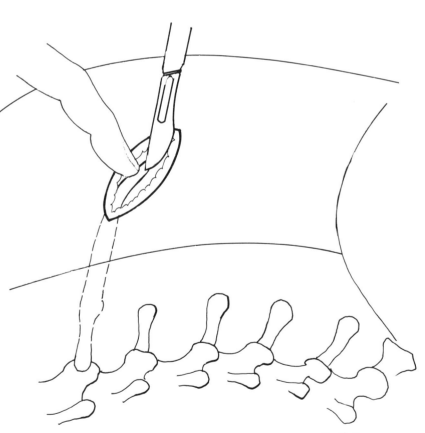

2.2. 12th rib-tip approach. Feel for the 12th rib and cut right down upon its tip (right hand)

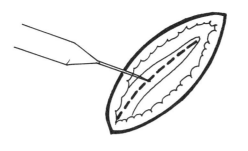
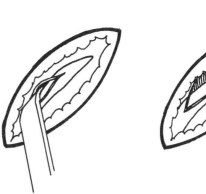

2.3. Diathermize along a line half-way between the upper and lower border of the 12th rib and strip off its periosteum from the upper border.

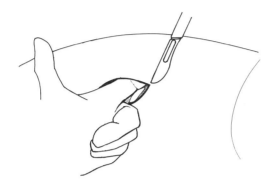

2.4. Your finger will guide you in making the anterior extension of your incision so as to avoid the subcostal neurovascular bundle (right kidney).

2.5. Carry the incision through all layers of the abdominal wall down to, but not through, the peritoneum.

external oblique
internal oblique
transversus
periosteum
lat. dorsi

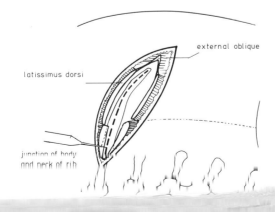

2.6. 12th rib-bed incision. Expose the whole length of the 12th rib back to the junction of the flat body and the rounded neck. Diathermize along a line half-way

latissimus dorsi
external oblique
junction of body and neck of rib

person. Enlarge this incision until it exposes the anterior 3–4 cm of the rib. With the diathermy point, coagulate a line half-way between the upper and lower borders of the rib, to seal off the periosteal vessels (2.3). Take a periosteal elevator, and strip the periosteum off the upper border of the rib for about 2 cm, until you can insert the flat blade of the elevator between the periosteum and the inner flat surface of the rib. Keeping the blade of the periosteal elevator firmly pressed up against this inner surface, slide it firmly anteriorly to the tip of the rib, peeling away the periosteum and intercostal muscles. This exposes a small gap into which the index finger can be pushed (2.4). Use the finger to separate the perirenal fat and peritoneum from the inner aspect of the abdominal muscles. One can easily feel the subcostal neurovascular bundles of the 11th and 12th rib, which act as guidelines between which the incision is now prolonged anteriorly (2.5). How far this incision is carried will be determined by the thickness of the patient's abdominal wall, the size of the kidney, and the difficulty that is anticipated in the dissection. This is an excellent approach for a small calculus in a low renal pelvis, or in the upper few inches of the ureter. If you encounter difficulty, it is easily converted into the standard 12th rib-bed incision, now to be described.

12th rib-bed incision

I prefer this incision for the majority of operations on the kidney. Begin again by feeling for the tip of the 12th rib, and cut down right upon it, confirming that it is indeed the 12th and not the 11th rib as soon as the fat has been incised. Having exposed the rib, follow it posteriorly, carrying the incision along the line of the rib through the aponeurosis until diathermy point, coagulating small muscular vessels *en route*. Coagulate a line along the length of the rib, from the boss forward to the tip, half-way between its upper and lower borders. Scrape the periosteum from the superior border of the rib, beginning at the junction of neck and flat part, at the boss. Once the blade of the elevator is in the right plane, deep to the rib, and outside the pleura and periosteum, slide it forward to strip the periosteum from the length of the upper border of the rib in a single sweep (2.7). If the blade of the elevator is in the right plane it will stay outside the pleura, which is now seen crossing the line of the rib.

Push the index finger in at the rib tip, and ease the peritoneum from the inner aspect of the abdominal wall, feeling for the guide lines of the neurovascular bundles of the 11th and 12th ribs. Now carry the incision forwards between these guidelines, cutting through the full thickness of the abdominal wall (2.8) and splitting the transversus muscle in the line of its fibres. One fairly constant vessel needs attention, communicating between the two neurovascular bundles. How far the incision must be carried will be determined by the type of operation that is being undertaken and the difficulties that are anticipated. Safety in kidney surgery means good access.

Having taken the incision forwards, the 12th rib may be easily swung downwards. This is done slowly, and care is taken to divide the thin muscular strands of diaphragm that tether the pleura to the inner aspect of the 12th rib, allowing the pleura to slide upwards (2.9). If the rib does not move down easily, it usually means that the subperiosteal plane has not been opened sufficiently far backwards to detach the costovertebral ligament: if so, strip the periosteum back another few centimetres. In very old patients the rib may be so rigid and stuck that an attempt to open up the wound will fracture it: in such a case it is better to resect a centimetre from the neck of the rib. The edges of the wound are protected with sterile towels and the wound opened with a suitable self-retaining retractor.

Vertical lumbotomy

The patient must not be placed in too exaggerated a position: the spine should be almost parallel with the table (2.10). The skin incision runs along the lateral edge of the sacrospinalis and is carried through the condensation of lumbar fascia which covers it, leading beneath the common fascial origin of the latissimus

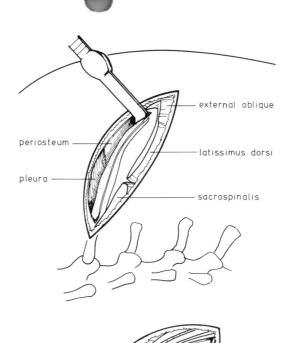

external oblique

periosteum

latissimus dorsi

pleura

sacrospinalis

2.7. Strip off the periosteum from the upper border of the rib with a periosteal elevator. Take care to avoid entering the pleura.

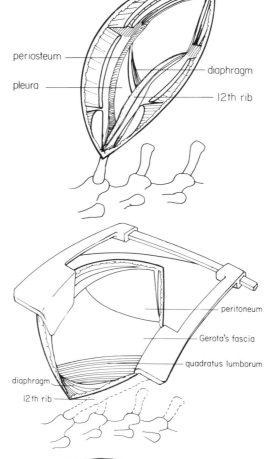

periosteum

pleura

diaphragm

12th rib

2.8. Carry the incision forwards, outside the peritoneum and avoiding the pleura.

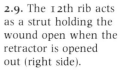

peritoneum

Gerota's fascia

quadratus lumborum

diaphragm

12th rib

2.9. The 12th rib acts as a strut holding the wound open when the retractor is opened out (right side).

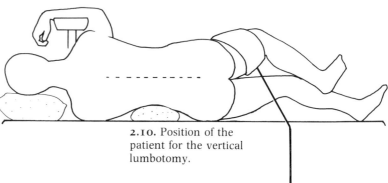

2.10. Position of the patient for the vertical lumbotomy.

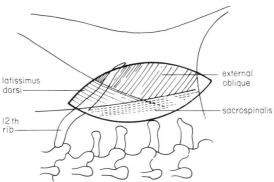

2.11. Incision for vertical lumbotomy approach to right kidney.

dorsi, the external and internal obliques, and the transversus abdominis muscles. These are retracted forwards and the deeper layer of the fascia incised again to expose the retroperitoneal fat lateral to quadratus lumborum and behind the hilum of the kidney (2.11–2.13). The 12th subcostal and iliohypogastric nerves traverse the field obliquely and must be carefully retracted. The access is restricted, and if more room is needed, one may be in difficulty, but the incision can be enlarged by resecting short segments from the neck of the 12th or

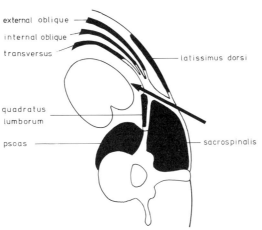
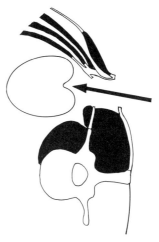

2.12 By incising the posterior layer of the lumbar fascia parallel to the outer border of sacrospinalis, all the attachments of the abdominal wall muscles are detached and can be retracted forwards, bringing you down upon the hilum of the kidney.

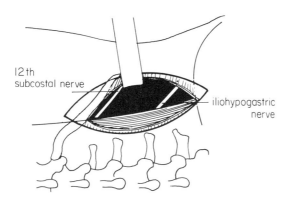

2.13. Retracting the abdominal wall muscles forwards to give access to the perirenal fat. Note that the field is traversed by the 12th subcostal and iliohypogastric nerves which must be gently retracted.

11th rib taking care not to open the pleura (2.14). If very hard pressed, the incision can be taken forward in the form of a T (Gil-Vernet *et al.* 1976).

The vertical lumbotomy is said to be less painful than oblique incisions along the line of the rib, but it crosses all Langer's lines, and gives an ugly scar.

Steps of the operation

1   Mobilization of the kidney

Whatever approach is chosen, the next step after opening the wound, is to make a deliberate incision into Gerota's fascia (2.15), stretching it with fingers to expose the kidney in its packing of fat—Zuckerkandl's fascia. This is often stiff, adherent and friable when there has been previous infection. In an easy case the fat can be peeled off the kidney with the fingers, scissors being needed only at the upper pole where the fat is always condensed and fibrous. Here and there small emissary veins should be diathermized before they are cut. After previous surgery or infection, when Zuckerkandl's fat is hard and vascular, it needs very careful dissection. The emissary veins are

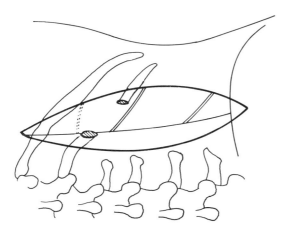

2.14. To extend the vertical lumbotomy one may resect a 1–2 cm segment from the 12th rib subperiosteally, taking care to avoid the subjacent pleura.

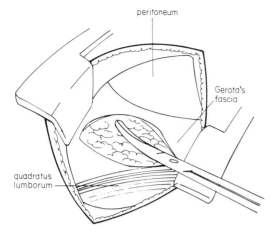

peritoneum

Gerota's fascia

quadratus lumborum

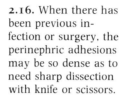

2.15. Mobilization of the right kidney. Begin by opening Gerota's fascia.

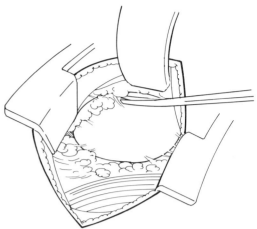

2.16. When there has been previous infection or surgery, the perinephric adhesions may be so dense as to need sharp dissection with knife or scissors.

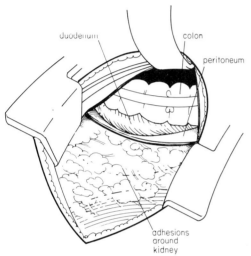

duodenum

colon

peritoneum

adhesions around kidney

2.17. When adhesions are particularly dense, and you are uncertain as to the exact whereabouts of the kidney and its pedicle, it is safer to make a deliberate opening into the peritoneum to get your bearings *before* hunting for the kidney.

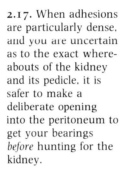

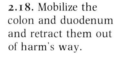

2.18. Mobilize the colon and duodenum and retract them out of harm's way.

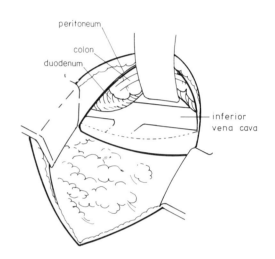

peritoneum

colon

duodenum

inferior vena cava

large, and unless great care is taken, the capsule is pulled up from the kidney, giving rise to unnecessary haemorrhage; the secret is to go slowly and gently using knife and scissors (2.16). This dissection may injure the adherent duodenum or colon, so when you anticipate such adhesions—for example when a calculus has been operated upon several times before—it is a good rule to deliberately open the peritoneum at the front of the wound (2.17) to locate the colon or duodenum; then mobilize them, and pack them well out of harm's way (2.18).

At the upper pole of the kidney take particular care not to cut a large upper pole segmental artery which may retract with the adrenal into the depths of the wound and be troublesome to secure with suture ligature. When dissecting the lower pole of the kidney, take care when separating ureter from gonadal vessels; large ovarian veins are easily torn.

2 Division of the renal vessels

Bit by bit the kidney is separated from its surrounding fat until the renal artery can be seen or felt behind the vein. Rotate the kidney forwards and dissect down on to the renal artery; it is always surrounded by fibrofatty tissue which must be dissected cleanly if the artery and vein are not to be torn. Pass a right-angled forceps round the artery to receive a ligature (2.19). Place two ligatures on the aorta side

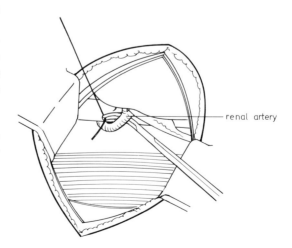

renal artery

2.19. Ligation of the right renal artery.

CHAPTER 2 / 18

of the artery before you divide it (2.20). Divide the renal vein between ligatures in the same way. Never clamp either of these vessels (2.21, 2.22).

The choice of ligature material is important when dealing with the renal vessels. With infected lesions, especially when there are stones in the kidney, non-absorbable suture material should never be used. Silk, thread or nylon are notorious for giving rise to a persistent sinus which only heals when the foreign body is removed—no easy operation. In the ordinary uninfected case use whatever ligature material you prefer. The renal artery and vein are big vessels, and you will sleep more soundly if you ligate each of them twice.

Mass ligature

One should always try hard to ligate artery and vein separately, for mass ligature has been followed by arteriovenous fistula. This is a very rare condition, and from time to time every surgeon will encounter a renal pedicle so obscured by fibrous tissue that the hazards of attempting to dissect artery from vein far

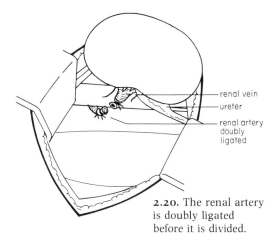

2.20. The renal artery is doubly ligated before it is divided.

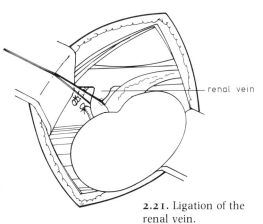

2.21. Ligation of the renal vein.

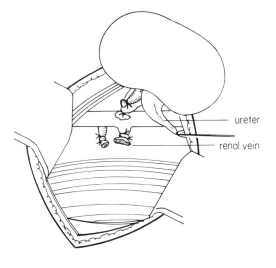

2.22. The right renal vein is doubly tied and divided. The ureter is ligated with catgut.

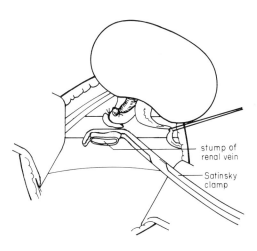

2.23. When the renal vein is very short, place a Satinsky arterial clamp on the side of the cava before dividing the vein.

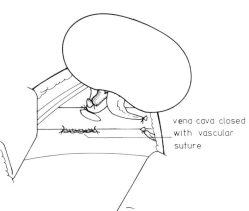

2.24. Oversewing the right renal vein flush with the cava.

outweigh the risk of causing an arteriovenous fistula. Commonsense and safety should be your watchwords.

A very short renal vein

Occasionally the renal vein is very short on the right side. Here it may be safer to apply an angled DeBakey or Satinsky clamp (2.23) at the junction of renal vein and vena cava, cutting the vein to leave a cuff which can be sewn over with vascular sutures of silk or Tevdek (2.24).

3 Division of the ureter

In a simple nephrectomy the ureter may be divided at any convenient distance down from the kidney (2.24). Ligate the ureter with catgut rather than non-absorbable material in view of the (remote) risk of calculus formation should urine reflux up the ureteric stump.

Operative hazards

As the kidney is being exposed it is easy to injure the pleura when stripping periosteum and diaphragm from the superior edge of the 12th rib. This is seldom of any importance, but one must take care to close the pleura after expelling the air from the pleural cavity at the end of the operation. A simple way to do this is to leave a small rubber catheter with one end under a bowl of water while the wound is closed around it (2.25). When the last skin sutures are about to be tied, the anaesthetist inflates the lung, expelling the last bubbles of air as the tube is withdrawn. The wound drain in such patients should be connected to standard underwater sealed drainage, as in any thoracic operation, to stop air being drawn into the lung from the wound drain. A plain radiograph of the chest is taken a few hours post-operatively, and on the following day, to make sure that no more than a trivial pneumothorax remains.

Occasionally, if the pleura has been opened, and the lung retracts during the operation, an old pleural adhesion may tear the lung parenchyma, and a tension pneumothorax may occur soon after the end of the operation. If such a torn lung parenchyma is recognized during the operation, it is wise to leave in a pair of apical and basal chest drains connected to underwater seals and leave them until the lung is fully expanded and adherent.

Viscera may be injured during the mobilization of the kidney. On the right side the colon or duodenum are at risk, and on the left the colon and duodenojejunal flexure. To avoid damaging them, the peritoneum should always be deliberately opened at the beginning of the operation when severe adhesions are anticipated. The adrenal gland is easily torn in a difficult dissection of the kidney, and bleeds freely from its soft centre. A suture ligature is used to control this bleeding. On the left side an adherent spleen may be injured, and very occasionally may have to be removed, though small tears can be safely repaired with a little gelfoam and a wisp of omentum. On the left side too, the pancreas may be injured if retraction is too forcible.

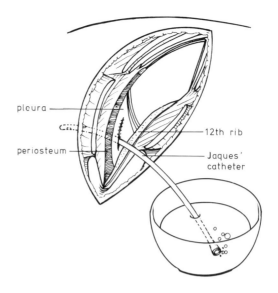

pleura

periosteum

12th rib

Jaques' catheter

2.25 If the pleura has been opened leave a small Jaques' catheter *in situ* until the skin is closed to allow all the air in the pleural cavity to be expelled.

Operative haemorrhage

Every surgeon of experience will tell his favourite horror story about haemorrhage during a kidney operation, and if you have not encountered it, you are either wanting in experience or unusually fortunate. Sooner or later you will get a tear in the vena cava. The bleeding is immense, daunting, and terrifying. The first essential is not to panic. The old rule is still a good one: put in a pack, and wait ten minutes by the clock. This does, however, need determination and patience: no interval of time passes so slowly as ten minutes when your finger is pressing a pack into a hole in the vena cava. The secret is to make good use of every one of those minutes. Ask your scrub nurse to have ready a Satinsky or DeBakey clamp and vascular sutures, and if they are not at hand, to have them sent for. See to it that a second sucker is connected and working properly. Make sure that blood is not merely cross-matched and in the hospital, but insist that it is brought to the operating room. Inform your anaesthetic colleague of the position, and make sure that he has time to check that his intravenous drip is running well, and if not, to set up another so that a massive transfusion of blood may be given in a hurry.

In practice, there has usually been a considerable loss of blood during the difficult dissection that has preceded making a hole in the cava, for this seldom happens in an easy case: hence it may be prudent to delay your next move until the patient's blood loss has been restored and his condition is once more stable. Making sure of all these points gives you and your assistants plenty of work to do in the ten minutes, for only when everything is ready, should you think of taking out the pack. The longer you procrastinate the easier will it become.

Then comes the moment of truth. Get your assistant to replace your hand with his. Irrigate and suck out the wound until you can see exactly what you are doing. Arm yourself with a vascular suture. Slowly begin to peel away the pack. The usual accidental hole in the cava is a short tear where a lumbar vein has been avulsed, or where an adrenal vein has torn from the cava. As soon as the hole is seen, and blood begins to well up, insert the vascular suture. Tie it, and have one end held in forceps. Slowly peel away another centimetre of the edge of the pack, exposing a little more of the rent, and put in another two or three sutures, pulling them up firmly again. Continue until the pack is all out and the hole sewn up.

Closing the wound

When the kidney is small and uninfected, there is no need to drain the wound, but if a large cavity is left, with rigid walls, serum is bound to collect and should be drained. A silicone rubber tube is led to a closed drainage system through a separate stab wound away from the incision. Since most patients spend their first few days reclining in bed, the dependent position for the drain is at the lower and anterior end of the wound where it is comfortable and clear of the pillows.

Have the table unbroken. Where the muscle layers are well defined, close the wound in layers (2.26). In the 12th rib incision, where the periosteum is stripped from the upper edge of the rib, it is easy to find the tough white strip of periosteum, but the inferior edge of this layer is formed by the fascia covering the external oblique muscle in the anterior part of the wound, and the sacrospinalis muscle in the posterior part (2.27). If the pleura has been opened, precautions are taken to expel air before the wound is closed, and the wound drain, if any, is connected to an underwater drainage bottle. In operations where previous exploration of the kidney has been performed, the muscle layers are obscured by scarring, and it is usual to close the wound with a series of interrupted sutures that take in all layers. They are held in forceps, pulled up together, and tied only when they have all been inserted. Never use non-absorbable sutures to close the infected case; even nylon may give rise to a persistent sinus. Catgut is perfectly safe, and with the rib-bed approach, late herniation is almost unknown.

Post-operative care and complications

1 Pulmonary

In the immediate post-operative period, if the pleura has been opened there is often a small pneumothorax. If it is small and shallow, nothing needs to be done about it. If the lung is torn and the pleura not drained properly, a tension pneumothorax may cause respiratory distress, cyanosis, and even death. In an emergency, thrust a needle into the second intercostal space to let out the air under pressure. Follow this at once by inserting an intercostal pleural drain connected to an underwater sealed bottle. Even without a breach in the pleura, pain inhibits the patient from coughing, and sputum is retained leading to atelectasis and infection. Injection of a

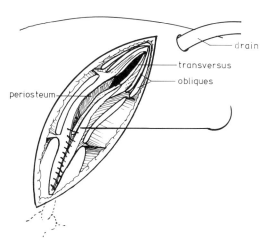

2.26. Closure of the 12th rib-bed incision in layers: the periosteum which was stripped off is sutured to the fascia and periosteum along the 12th rib, and continued forwards to take up the transversus and its fascia, in the first layer.

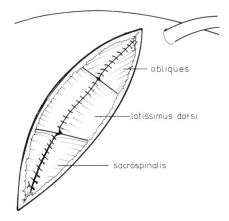

2.27. The external and internal oblique may be closed in a single layer along with latissimus dorsi and the sacrospinalis.

few ml of 1% marcaine may render the first few hours pain-free after operation, but despite this adequate analgesia is needed as well for breathing and coughing. Bronchoscopy is rarely needed nowadays but it can be a life saving manoeuvre, and should not be forgotten if the collapsed lung fails to re-expand.

A pleural effusion may follow haemorrhage into the pleura at the time of incision or may follow atelectasis and pneumonitis. The effusion is usually sterile, but a large volume may cause distress and call for aspiration.

2 Haemorrhage

Reactionary haemorrhage within the first twenty-four hours of the operation is almost never due to the ligature coming off the renal pedicle, despite the nightmares of the surgeon. More often it comes from a vessel in the muscles divided in the incision. There are signs of internal bleeding and blood on the dressing. Firm pressure on the wound often stops it; otherwise the patient is returned to the operating theatre, the lost blood is replaced by transfusion, and the wound is reopened and the offending vessel suture-ligated. In such circumstances, mercifully uncommon, I have never been able to refrain from checking the renal pedicle, but it has always been perfectly dry.

Secondary haemorrhage used to be a much feared complication in days when nephrectomy was performed with clamp and mass ligature for renal carbuncle or pyonephrosis. I have never seen this complication in the past thirty years.

3 Complications in the wound

Infection is not a particular feature of nephrectomy, nor do nephrectomy incisions become infected especially often. It is detected and treated along the usual lines and it seems most often to arise in a haematoma in the wound which does not make itself apparent until some eight to ten days after operation, just when the patient is about to go home.

A persistent wound *sinus* was notorious a few decades ago when many nephrectomies were performed for tuberculosis: today it is very rare, but may still be seen when nephrectomy performed for an infected stone or a pyonephrosis is unwisely closed with non-absorbable sutures, or when in similar circumstances the pedicle has been tied with non-absorbable material. From time to time, inexperienced surgeons develop a craze for the latest suture material guaranteed by the manufacturer never to give rise to sinuses.

Wound dehiscence is rare in loin incisions unless the patient is very anaemic, uraemic, or debilitated. In such patients one should consider using the vertical lumbotomy, whose design virtually excludes dehiscence.

As with all abdominal incisions, deep dehiscence may pass unnoticed but failure of union of the deeper layers of the wound may lead to ventral hernia weeks later. Such a bulge was seen more often when part of the rib was resected as a routine, but today it is virtually eliminated by the 12th rib-bed and rib-tip approach.

Unhappily, a diffuse bulge of the abdominal wall, without a discrete neck and caused not by deep dehiscence of the wound but by denervation of the abdominal muscles, is still seen from time to time. Care taken to make the incision between the guide-lines of the 11th and 12th neurovascular bundles ought to avoid damage to the innervation of the abdominal wall. In cases where there is a definite sac, repair of the hernia is possible, but there is no treatment other than the provision of a suitable corset for a diffuse bulge.

Pain in the nephrectomy incision is exceedingly common even when great care has been taken not to injure the subcostal nerves when making or closing the incision. There is no simple remedy for it, and infiltration with local anaesthesia or neurolysis usually fails to stop the pain, as with so many other post-operative neuralgias.

Secondary and difficult nephrectomy for benign conditions

If calculi have been left *in situ* or when pyonephrosis or perinephric abscesses have had to be drained, the nephrectomy is made difficult by adhesions or xanthogranuloma. Dissection may well need the knife, for the kidney may be surrounded by a shell as dense as cartilage from which may issue a rabbit warren of sinuses and fistulae. Sometimes a persistent sinus is caused by the use of non-absorbable ligature material at a previous infected nephrectomy, by calculi, or tuberculosis. In all these cases extra care is needed.

Special precautions

For such difficult secondary nephrectomies, four to six units of blood should be made ready; the patient's bowel must be prepared by enemas and antibiotics in case the colon or duodenum is injured.

Position

Usually the patient is in the lateral position. Where the loin has been entered many times before, an anterior approach as used for carcinoma of the kidney, may be more easy and therefore more safe, since it allows the structures at most risk—the bowel, spleen, and pancreas—to be set aside early in the operation, and the great vessels may be dealt with before mobilizing the kidney.

Incision

Wide exposure is the key to safety in these difficult and dangerous operations. Use a long 12th rib-bed incision in most cases, or if the 12th rib is short, use the same manoeuvre through the bed of the 11th rib, opening the pleura if need be as a deliberate step. Always be prepared to consider the anterior transabdominal approach.

Steps of the operation

Mobilization of the kidney

Often one encounters a solid wall of scar tissue as soon as the skin and muscles have been divided. It may be impossible to see where to separate kidney from rib. The trick is to begin the dissection anteriorly, entering normal tissue after opening the peritoneum and making sure where the colon is situated. Indeed the most important steps in the dissection are directed to safeguard the colon and duodenum. Never hurry over this part of the dissection: take your time.

Once the colon and bowel are safe, the next care is to identify and mobilize the duodenum or duodenojejunal flexure and spleen on the left. In some patients you may have to spend time liberating the gall bladder and liver before the right kidney is safely exposed.

Only when these important viscera have been made secure is it safe to return to the kidney. Slowly dissect the mass from the diaphragm and pleura, dividing the slip of diaphragm which tethers the pleura. Gradually open up the wound, bit by bit, increasing the exposure as each new centimetre of rib is cleared, so that you are led slowly but steadily behind the kidney where, usually, a clean plane of cleavage is found either in front of, or more usually behind, the fascia covering the psoas muscle. Begin now to clear the entire surface of the kidney by a combination of sharp and blunt dissection—often a very tedious and slow process. From time to time you may wish to stop and consider the alternative, if more bloody, procedure of subcapsular nephrectomy.

Subcapsular nephrectomy

When adhesions around the kidney are exceptionally dense, a deliberate incision may be made through the thickened capsule to expose the parenchyma (2.28). Slide the scissors under the capsule and slit it along the convex border of the kidney. Use a finger (2.29) to peel the capsule from the cortex until the bulk of the kidney emerges from its shell. In doing this, several hard white scars have to be divided, where capsule and parenchyma are attached. Also large capsular veins must be

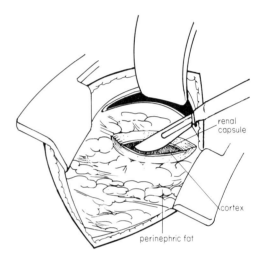

2.28. Subcapsular nephrectomy: an incision is made through the thickened fibrofatty tissue around the kidney right down and through the capsule until you come across the naked renal parenchyma.

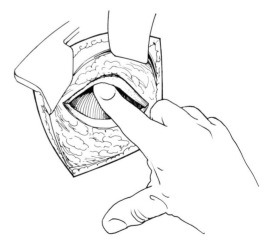

2.29. The capsule is stripped off the renal parenchyma with the finger, delivering the kidney.

divided. Hence this dissection is always bloody, and it behoves one not to be too slow in doing it. The loss of blood from the denuded parenchyma will not cease until the pedicle is secured.

When the main bulk of the kidney has been delivered, like a banana from its skin, it is necessary to cut through the reflected capsule in order to reach the renal artery and vein. In practice it is only possible to approach the pedicle from in front. Carefully incise the capsule (2.30) just deep enough to enter the perirenal fat which is unexpectedly thick, firm, and white. With right-angled forceps, helped by scissors, pass a 2-chromic catgut ligature right around the entire renal pedicle so as to include the artery and vein *en masse* (2.31). You may be lucky enough to separate artery from vein, but usually the tissue in the renal hilum is so dense that it is only possible to get a mass ligature of catgut around all the main vessels. Once this encircling ligature has been tied, the bleeding will stop, but the ligature will have included a very thick lump of tissue in its grasp, and cannot be relied upon by itself. The pedicle is then divided by cutting through renal parenchyma well away from the encircling ligature (2.32). Make this incision bit by bit, securing each individual branch of the renal vein and artery as it is cut across. Finally remove the kidney, leaving the main part of its capsule *in situ* (2.33). Always leave a drain after subcapsular nephrectomy. If the peritoneum has been opened, close it, but do not drain it. Use catgut throughout in view of the risk of persistent sinuses from non-absorbable suture material.

Wounds opened several times before should be closed in a single layer of interrupted, through-and-through catgut sutures placed first, held in forceps, and tied after the table has been unbroken.

Operative hazards

In addition to all the usual risks of nephrectomy, secondary nephrectomy carries the special dangers of injury to the bowel hence the precaution of first opening the peritoneum. A hole in the small bowel should be carefully repaired in the transverse axis of the intestine and left alone. Small holes in the colon may be reliably closed in the same way, but patched over with a lump of omentum. Large defects in the colon should be brought out as a colostomy, to be repaired later on. Better by far to have the problem of explaining a colostomy than a dead patient.

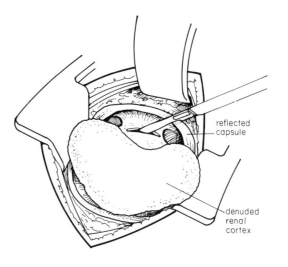

2.30. After shelling out the kidney, you must deliberately incise through the reflected capsule in order to reach the renal artery and vein.

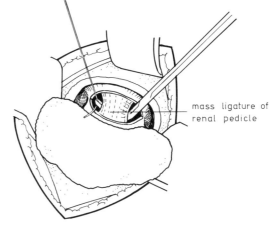

2.31. A thick catgut ligature is used to tie the pedicle *en masse*.

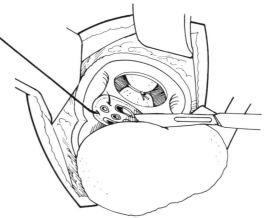

2.32. Having tied the pedicle, the kidney is cut off well clear of the mass ligature, your knife going through the branches of the artery and vein in the hilum, and through the renal pelvis, making a good big pedicle. Each branch is suture-ligated as you cut it across.

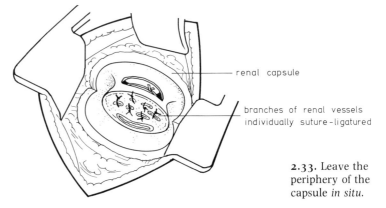

2.33. Leave the periphery of the capsule *in situ*.

If the tail of the pancreas is injured, it may be removed, taking care to ligate the pancreatic duct and drain the raw surface. Accidental injury to the spleen, when it is only a small laceration, does not always call for splenectomy: a patch of Gelfoam or Oxycel supported by omentum is often all that is required.

One other danger awaits even the most experienced surgeon. On several occasions I have not recognized xanthogranulomatous pyelonephritis in spite of considerable experience of the condition. Its hard yellow consistence exactly mimics invasive carcinoma of the renal parenchyma. Even a frozen section may be misleading, for the lipid-filled macrophages of xanthogranuloma look very much like clear-celled renal adenocarcinoma. If you do not want to fall into the same trap, be particularly suspicious of xanthogranuloma when there is a hard mass accompanying a calculus, especially when the bowel is attached. It is true that rather radical resection of xanthogranuloma is the only way to cure it, but it does not require such a radical *en-bloc* resection as does cancer.

Nephrectomy for carcinoma of the kidney

Indications

Even when there are distant metastases a patient with renal cell carcinoma has his best (and only) chance of cure if the primary tumour can be removed. Neither cavography nor angiography tell for certain that the tumour is inoperable: the critical question is whether or not it is possible to get the growth from the aorta and the vena cava, and this can only be determined at operation.

Special precautions

An angiogram can be of value at the time of operation in warning of the existence and situation of multiple renal arteries, but this alone does not justify the investigation. If there is some good reason to embolize the renal artery before nephrectomy, for example if the tumour is unusually large and vascular, or if one is hoping to make use of the immunotherapeutic advantage (Swanson *et al.* 1979) that may follow embolization, then it is sensible to combine embolization with the diagnostic angiogram. However for routine nephrectomy for most renal cell carcinomas, I (and many other surgeons) have found pre-operative embolization of the renal artery painful for the patient, wasteful of time in hospital, and of no advantage at the time of operation; often the healthy renal parenchyma is rendered avascular, not the carcinoma, and it is still necessary to secure the renal artery first. Embolization was a fashionable preliminary a few years ago: today it is almost given up (Wesolowski *et al.* 1979).

In children with Wilms' tumour, nephrectomy is part of a planned procedure combined with chemotherapy, in which appropriate doses of D-Actinomycin and Vincristine are given before and after operation. In transitional cell carcinoma of the kidney, if the biopsy and cytology of the tumour show that it is poorly differentiated, there is sound reason to give a full course of irradiation to the kidney before nephrectomy (Babaian & Johnson 1980).

Blood loss can be considerable during a nephrectomy for cancer and four units should be available.

In children, and in very large tumours in adults, it may be necessary to resect adherent intestine, so that the colon should be prepared in the routine way.

Approach to the kidney

The anterior transabdominal approach is the best, using an oblique horizontal incision in the usual rather stout patient, or a long paramedian in the thin one. For very large tumours arising in the upper pole a thoraco-abdominal incision may give better access, particularly if it is necessary to resect part of the liver.

Anterior approach

The patient is supine with a small sandbag or cushion under the loin on the side of the tumour (2.34). In the usual rather broad

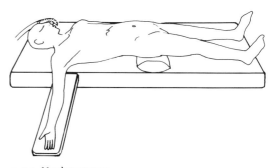

2.34. Nephrectomy for carcinoma of the kidney: position for the anterior approach.

patient, an obliquely horizontal incision (2.35) starts from the tip of the 11th or 12th rib and is carried right across both bellies of the rectus abdominis muscle. Lift up the linea alba with two pairs of forceps (2.36), and enter the peritoneal cavity on one or other side of the falciform ligament which is then divided between ligatures (2.37). With the fingers of one hand lift up the belly of the rectus abdominis, first on one side and then on the other. Divide its muscle fibres with the diathermy, coagulating the smaller vessels as you go, but ligating the superior epigastric vessels. Cut right across both recti, and carry the incision through all layers of the abdominal wall towards the tip of the 12th rib, cutting and coagulating as you go.

In a long thin patient, a midline or paramedian incision is made in the classical way (2.38).

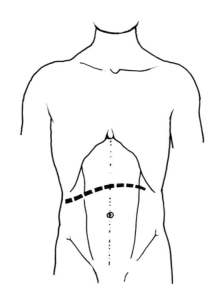

2.35. Incision for the anterior transabdominal approach to the right kidney.

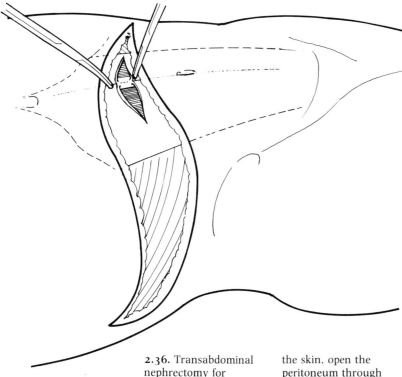

2.36. Transabdominal nephrectomy for carcinoma. Right kidney. After dividing the skin, open the peritoneum through the linea alba in the midline.

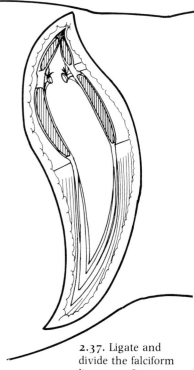

2.37. Ligate and divide the falciform ligament. Cut across both bellies of the rectus abdominis muscle, and continue the incision through all layers laterally.

Thoracoabdominal approach

The patient lies on the table in the 'half-lateral' position, the back rolled over somewhat towards the surgeon (2.39). The pelvis and chest are secured with strapping to the table. The upper thigh is slightly flexed, but not so much as to interfere with prolongation of the incision down into the abdomen. The line of the incision should be along the 9th or 10th rib (2.40) but, having marked the position of the rib, begin by making the abdominal part of the incision first (2.41) continuing the line of the rib down to or beyond the umbilicus. This will allow you to examine the tumour mass and its attachment to the cava and aorta, and decide whether or not the growth is operable.

Having decided that the growth is worth trying to remove, the incision is completed along the course of the 9th or 10th ribs

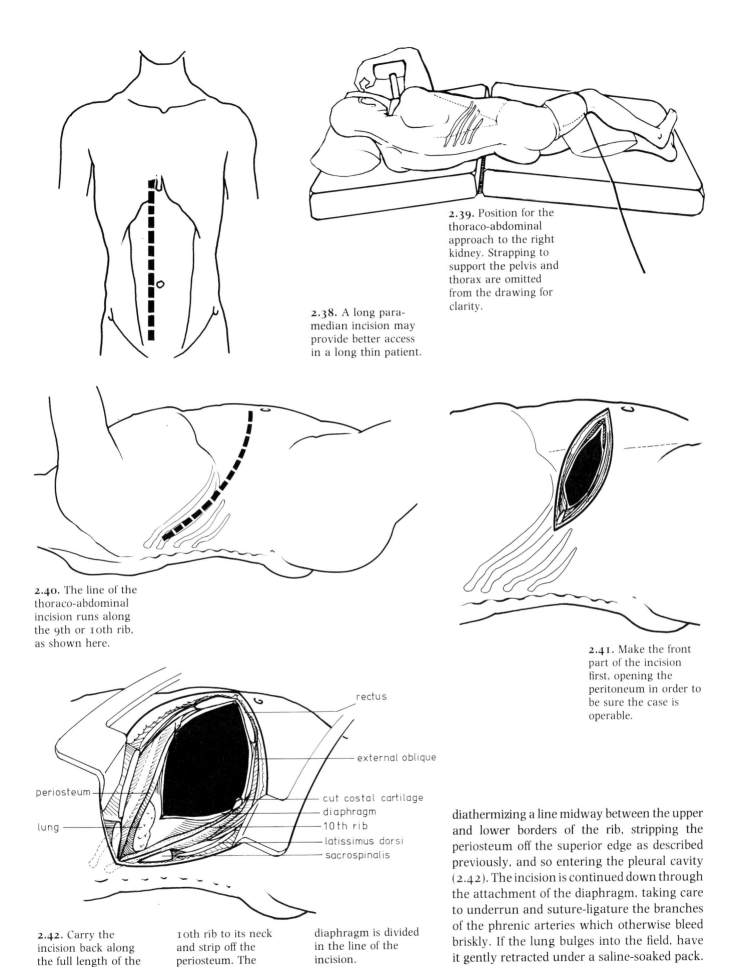

2.38. A long para-median incision may provide better access in a long thin patient.

2.39. Position for the thoraco-abdominal approach to the right kidney. Strapping to support the pelvis and thorax are omitted from the drawing for clarity.

2.40. The line of the thoraco-abdominal incision runs along the 9th or 10th rib, as shown here.

2.41. Make the front part of the incision first, opening the peritoneum in order to be sure the case is operable.

rectus

external oblique

periosteum

cut costal cartilage
diaphragm
10th rib
latissimus dorsi
sacrospinalis

lung

2.42. Carry the incision back along the full length of the 10th rib to its neck and strip off the periosteum. The diaphragm is divided in the line of the incision.

diathermizing a line midway between the upper and lower borders of the rib, stripping the periosteum off the superior edge as described previously, and so entering the pleural cavity (2.42). The incision is continued down through the attachment of the diaphragm, taking care to underrun and suture-ligature the branches of the phrenic arteries which otherwise bleed briskly. If the lung bulges into the field, have it gently retracted under a saline-soaked pack.

Steps of the operation

Display the renal vessels

The first object of the operation is to tie the renal artery in continuity, and so cut off the blood supply which otherwise swells and distends the innumerable collateral veins which are always present in the fat around the kidney with cancer.

On the right side begin by dividing the peritoneal reflexion over the lateral aspect of the ascending colon (2.43), freeing the colon and the right hepatocolic ligament so that the bowel is displaced medially (2.44). The lateral aspect of the duodenum is similarly mobilized and reflected medially, having due regard for the common bile duct which may well be displayed at this stage. This exposes the inferior vena cava, covered with thin fibrofatty tissue, and usually obscured by a tangle of lymph nodes (2.45).

On the left side the dissection is similar: first the descending colon is swept medially (2.46) and then the duodenojejunal flexure is mobilized, taking care not to injure the spleen or tail of the pancreas (2.47). The spleno-colic ligament is divided between ligatures. When the tumour is very large and invades the left mesocolon, it is safer to approach the pedicle just lateral to the duodenojejunal flexure (2.48) by incising the peritoneum along the lateral as-

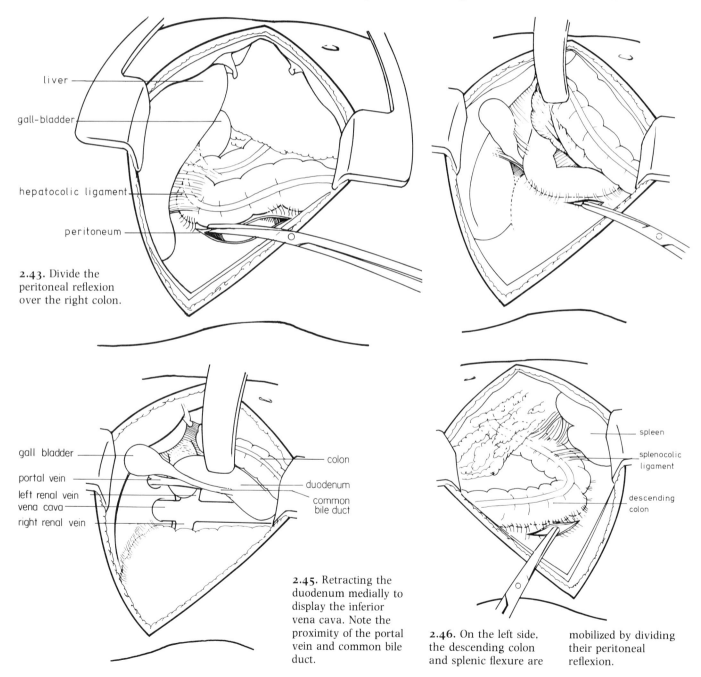

2.43. Divide the peritoneal reflexion over the right colon.

2.44. Having divided the hepatocolic ligament and peritoneal reflexion the colon is retracted medially, and the duodenum is then similarly mobilized.

2.45. Retracting the duodenum medially to display the inferior vena cava. Note the proximity of the portal vein and common bile duct.

2.46. On the left side, the descending colon and splenic flexure are mobilized by dividing their peritoneal reflexion.

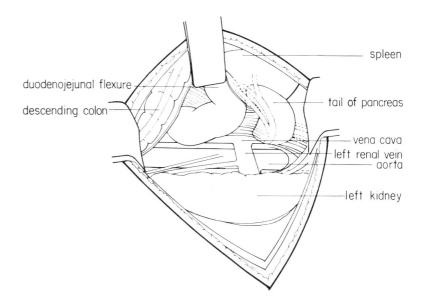

spleen

duodenojejunal flexure

descending colon

tail of pancreas

vena cava
left renal vein
aorta

left kidney

2.47. Left side: mobilize the duodenum medially to display the aorta and renal vessels.

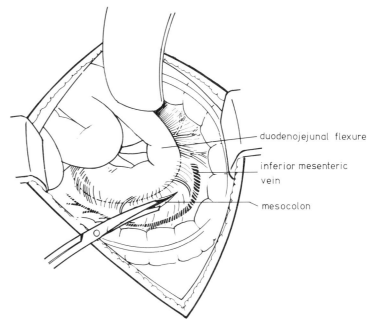

duodenojejunal flexure

inferior mesenteric vein

mesocolon

2.48. If it seems that the tumour may be invading the colon or mesocolon, on the left side, you can approach the vessels by dividing the peritoneal reflexion over the lateral aspect of the duodenum. The inferior mesenteric vein will need to be retracted or divided between ligatures.

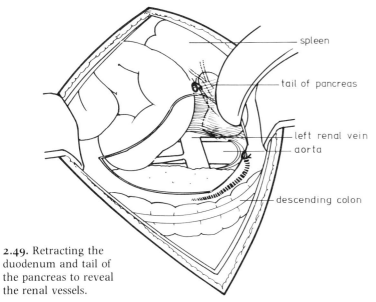

spleen

tail of pancreas

left renal vein
aorta

descending colon

2.49. Retracting the duodenum and tail of the pancreas to reveal the renal vessels.

pect of the duodenum, and displacing it medially (2.49). Either displace the inferior mesenteric vein upwards, or deliberately divide it between ligatures: do not tear it, or the field will be obscured by a troublesome haematoma. When retracting the duodenum upwards and medially, it is necessary to be gentle, since the retractor will squeeze the tail of the pancreas, but it does not take much retraction to give an adequate view of the left renal vein and the aorta.

Divide the renal vessels

On the right side the renal vein may contain tumour and must be handled with care. Sometimes a lump of growth is visible wobbling in the stream of blood within the renal vein and cava. Careless manipulation may dislodge a malignant embolism. If no obvious tumour is present, the first step is to get access to the renal artery: Dissect the connective tissue sheath off the renal vein and cava. A right-angled forceps is gently insinuated behind the renal vein (2.50) until the tips emerge and seize a strong silk or thread ligature which is used to retract the vein at this stage while a search is made for artery. The renal artery is found behind and sometimes a little superior to the vein. A finger tip often feels its pulsations before it can be seen clearly. Dissect away the tough fibrofatty tissue that always ensheaths the artery until its wall is clearly seen. Pass a right-angled forceps around the renal artery to grasp a ligature and tie the artery in continuity (2.51).

If an angiogram has been performed, this will have shown whether there is more than one main renal artery, and these are similarly sought and ligated. Only when all the blood has been stopped from entering the kidney should the renal vein be ligated. It is of course easier, and must seem very tempting to the inexperienced surgeon, to ligate the renal vein first, and indeed it may have the theoretical advantage that tumour cells are prevented from entering the circulation. But be warned: if you tie the renal vein first you will regret it. The field of operation becomes a congested nightmare: every capillary swells up and bleeds, and it becomes impossible to find any anatomical landmark. Only when the main renal arteries have been secured is vision restored, and by then many units of blood may have been lost.

When the arteries have all been ligated, the renal vein is trebly ligated and divided, always leaving two strong ligatures on the cava side of the vein (2.52). If the renal vein is very short, place a Satinsky or DeBakey clamp along the side of the cava and after dividing the vein, close it with a 4-0 vascular suture.

Once the renal vein is secured, the next step is to dissect out and divide between ligatures the renal artery and accessory arteries. This is performed in a relatively bloodless field, and in making this dissection, all the fibrofatty and lymphatic tissue is swept off the lateral wall of the vena cava or aorta towards the tumour.

If an obvious lump of tumour is found in the renal vein, protruding into the lumen of the cava, a more complete dissection is needed before manipulating the renal vein for fear of dislodging a tumour embolism. The first essential is to secure the right renal artery. In such

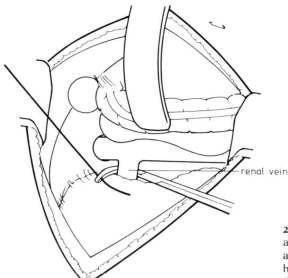

2.50. Right side: Pass a stout ligature around the renal vein but do not tie it at this stage.

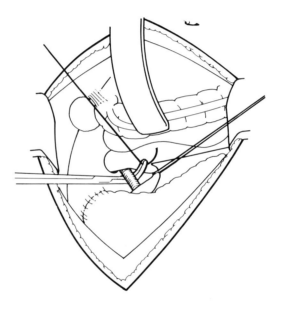

2.51. Lift up the renal vein and pass a ligature around the renal artery (right side). Tie the artery in continuity.

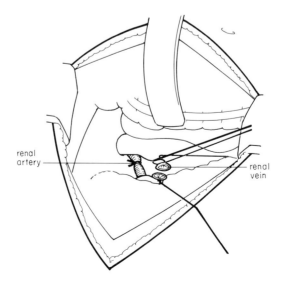

2.52. Only when the artery has been ligated should you doubly ligate and divide the renal vein (right side).

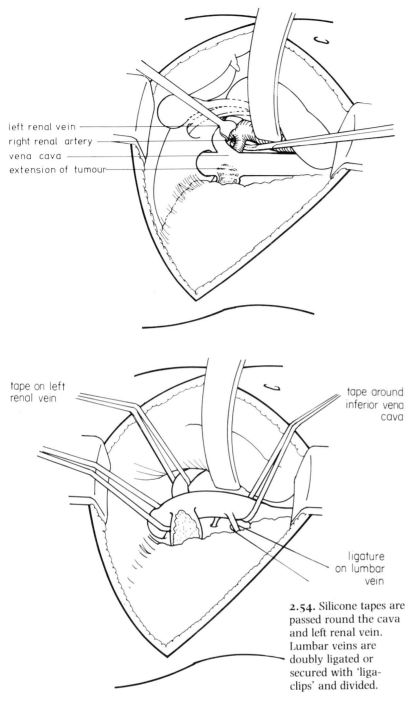

left renal vein ──
right renal artery ──
vena cava ──
extension of tumour──

2.53. When you find extension of tumour in the right renal vein, the right artery is approached by retracting the left renal vein, and passing a right-angled forceps round the right renal artery on the right side of the aorta. The artery is tied in continuity.

tape on left renal vein

tape around inferior vena cava

ligature on lumbar vein

2.54. Silicone tapes are passed round the cava and left renal vein. Lumbar veins are doubly ligated or secured with 'liga-clips' and divided.

cases it must be tied in the space between aorta and cava. This is reached by lifting up the duodenum and head of the pancreas, following the line of the left renal vein in front of the aorta. The left renal vein is gently retracted upwards, and a dissection is now made between the adjacent aorta and cava until the right renal artery can first be felt with the finger-tip, and later shown by gentle retraction. A ligature is passed around the right renal artery using right-angled forceps and the artery is ligated in continuity (2.53). The rest of the operation is relatively easy.

First, all the blood running into the cava must be cut off before it is opened. The left renal vein is occluded with a Rummel tourniquet. The vena cava is gently rolled medially, and the lumbar veins entering it from behind are each doubly ligated and divided (2.54). An aortic clamp is used to pass a tape around the inferior vena cava well down from the renal vein and another one above the junction of the renal vein and cava.

Many vascular clamps are available for occluding the cava, but the homely Rummel tourniquet is safer, and can always be fashioned on the spot from silastic arterial sling and rubber tubing (2.55). Once the tapes are all in position, the wall of the cava may be incised well clear of the lump of tumour (2.56). The blood is sucked out, and it is now possible to see in a bloodless field exactly how much of the wall of the cava has been invaded by the growth. Usually the tumour extension lies free within the lumen of the cava, but if it is invading its wall, part of the cava must be removed.

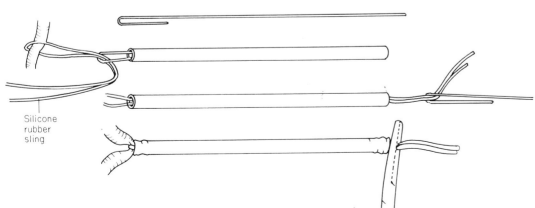

Silicone rubber sling

2.55. A Rummel tourniquet is easily made by drawing a silicone rubber sling through a rubber tube.

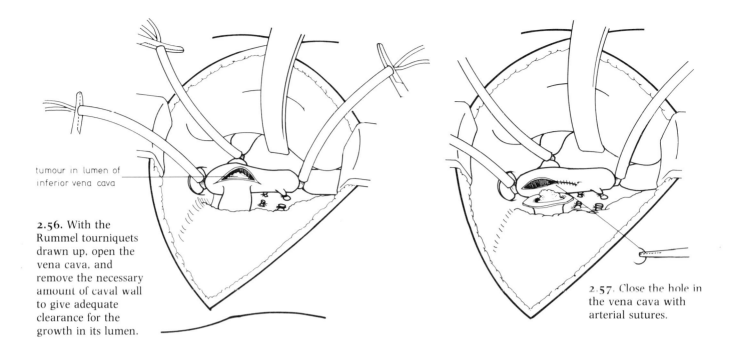

tumour in lumen of inferior vena cava

2.56. With the Rummel tourniquets drawn up, open the vena cava, and remove the necessary amount of caval wall to give adequate clearance for the growth in its lumen.

2.57. Close the hole in the vena cava with arterial sutures.

Gently retracting the mass of tumour and the tumour thrombus, the clear edges of the vena cava are irrigated with heparinized saline and closed with 4-o Tevdek or arterial silk (2.57). The lumen is flooded with heparinized saline just before the last suture is drawn up and tied. The tapes are released one after the other, and a small swab is applied to the suture line for three to four minutes. Very occasionally a recovery suture is needed to close off the vena cava.

Occasionally it is quite clear that there is only a small mobile extension of tumour into the cava, and in such cases a curved Satinsky clamp may be applied to the side of the cava (2.58) and the tumour extension and renal vein removed without having to obstruct the return of blood to the heart. It is wise even in these cases, however, to have slings with Rummel tourniquets ready, for the best vascular clamps have been known to slip off, and the vena cava is easily torn. Whatever method is used to deal with the renal vein, the renal artery should be ligated in continuity as the first step. It is now doubly ligated and divided as described above.

Mobilize and remove the kidney

The main object of dividing the renal vessels early in the operation is to prevent unnecessary loss of blood, but it also helps prevent dislodgement of tumour emboli, for by using the anterior transperitoneal approach there is no need to handle the main mass of the tumour until after the vessels have been divided.

Start to mobilize the kidney by continuing the plane of dissection along the right side of

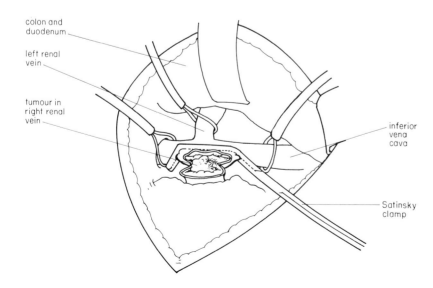

colon and duodenum

left renal vein

tumour in right renal vein

inferior vena cava

Satinsky clamp

2.58. A Satinsky clamp is applied to the vena cava. Note that Rummel tourniquets are placed in readiness.

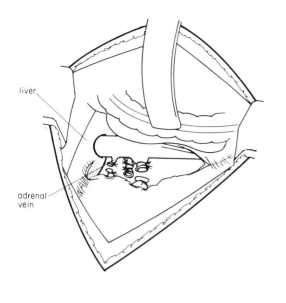

2.59. Dissect the mass of tumour, enclosed in its fascia and fat, away from the side of the vena cava, making sure you secure even the smallest adrenal vein.

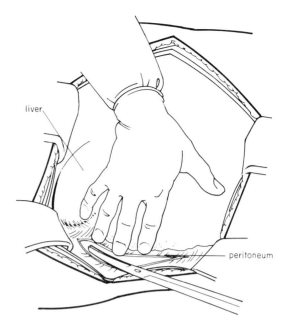

2.60. Have the mass retracted medially as you divide the peritoneum over the lateral aspect of the kidney.

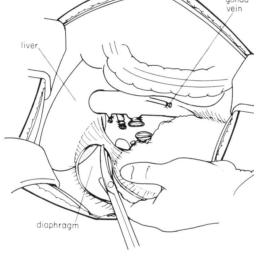

2.61. Pull the mass downwards and divide adhesions tethering the kidney to the underside of the diaphragm and the liver. Divide the gonadal vessels if they have not already been dealt with.

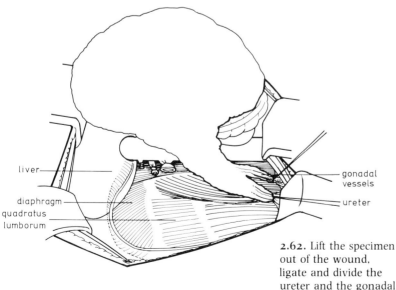

2.62. Lift the specimen out of the wound, ligate and divide the ureter and the gonadal vessels in the lowest part of the wound.

the vena cava, dissecting the fibrous tissue and lymph nodes laterally, and laying the cava bare. As this plane is cleared upwards, the adrenal vein is found and carefully divided between ligatures (2.59). Any clumsiness in this dissection may tear a lumbar vein or a small tributary of the cava and cause furious bleeding; each one, no matter how small, must be carefully ligated or secured with a ligaclip.

On the left side the dissection proceeds in the same way, the lateral aspect of the aorta being dissected cleanly, and the adrenal and gonadal veins divided between ligatures to expose a good long length of renal vein.

In this way the whole block of tissue, comprising kidney tumour adrenal and fibrofatty tissue, with all the lymph nodes along the side of the aorta or the cava, is displaced laterally.

Now divide the peritoneal reflexion over the lateral aspect of the kidney (2.60) keeping outside Gerota's fascia. This leads directly down to the diaphragm. The plane is easy to open up with fingers or scissors, but take care to ligate the little tributary veins emerging from the diaphragm. Scoop out the tumour mass in the hollow of your hand (2.61), taking care not to damage the spleen on the left side, or the liver on the right. It only remains to divide the inferior attachments of the mass—a thick fold of peritoneum ensheathing the gonadal vessels and the ureter. The ureter is divided a convenient distance down from the kidney, a little above the pelvic brim (2.62).

The specimen consists of kidney, tumour, adrenal, perinephric fat, Gerota's fascia, and all the lymph nodes along the side of the aorta or the cava. If there is some oozing after the mass has been removed, pack the wound for four minutes. Often a few small vessels that ooze from the underside of the diaphragm need to be diathermized or clipped. Any lymph nodes left behind on the side of the aorta or cava are now removed. If it seems that any tumour has been left behind, mark it with a ligaclip for subsequent radiotherapy.

Closure of the wound

The *paramedian* incision is closed in the usual way: my preference is for non-absorbable figure-of-eight nylon sutures for the anterior rectus sheath as a precaution against dehiscence. The more usual *transverse* anterior incision may be safely closed with o-chromic catgut in layers, since wound dehiscence is almost unknown with this incision. There is no need to drain the cavity and no need to 'reperitonealize' the defect left by removal of the lump.

In closing the *thoracoabdominal* incision, non-absorbable sutures are used for the diaphragm. An apical and basal chest drain are connected to underwater sealed bottles. The adjacent ribs are approximated and sewn together with heavy catgut sutures passed through drill holes in the lower rib and over the upper edge of the upper one. The muscular layers of the chest are closed with continuous catgut. The abdominal part of the incision may be reinforced with a few nylon sutures to the rectus sheath. If for any reason it seems wise to drain the space left behind, the drain should be connected to an underwater seal.

The chest drains usually come out after forty-eight hours if chest radiographs show satisfactory expansion of the lung and no collection of fluid in the pleural cavity, and if the drains have stopped swinging.

Operative hazards

In addition to the difficulties described when there is tumour in the lumen of the vena cava, in practice it may be difficult to make a clean dissection between the upper pole of the kidney and the diaphragm, and this is more easy if a thoraco-abdominal approach is used. If the tumour invades the fascia overlying psoas, it is necessary to shave off the front of the psoas muscle *en bloc* with the kidney—especially in Wilms' tumours in children—and in doing this it is necessary to spend time underrunning many small lumbar vessels.

Another special hazard of the relatively enormous tumours encountered in children is the distortion of the vena cava that occurs when it is compressed from side to side and stretched over the tumour like a thin ribbon— so thin that it is hard to imagine that it can be the cava (2.63). When this happens it is dreadfully easy to mistake the opposite renal vein for the vena cava, and divide cava and contralateral vein in one single and irremediable stroke.

In Wilms' tumour the bowel is often invaded, but since in any large tumour at any age one must be ready to resect colon if it is adherent, it is always wise, when in doubt, to make sure that the bowel is prepared.

Wilms' tumours are bilateral in about 10% of cases, so one should always examine the other kidney at the time of operation. If contralateral tumour is found, it is biopsied and, if appropriate, a partial nephrectomy performed. With such treatment, combined with radiotherapy and chemotherapy, prolonged survival may be achieved, but it is necessary that the existence of the contralateral tumour should be discovered. (Swanson & Borges 1983.)

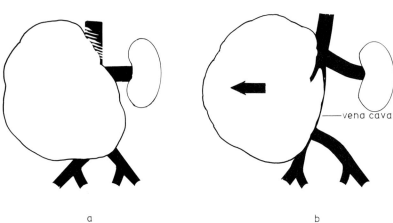

a   b

2.63. In a child with a Wilms' tumour the 'renal vein' which seems to emerge from the kidney (a) may in fact be the vein on the other side, the true anatomy (b) being obscured by compression and distortion of the cava and the vein emerging from the tumour.

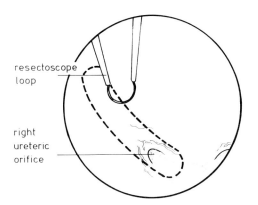

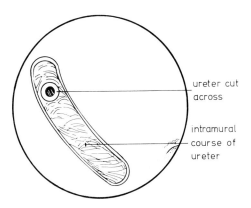

resectoscope loop

right ureteric orifice

ureter cut across

intramural course of ureter

2.64. Semple's 'pluck' nephro-ureterectomy. First step, resect the right ureteric orifice and intramural ureter transurethrally.

Nephroureterectomy

For the refluxing megaureter and scarred kidney

Semple's operation for the lower end of the ureter deserves to be better known. The lower end of the ureter and its intramural portion are removed with the resectoscope (2.64). It is easy to see the intramural part of the ureter and resect it until fat is clearly seen. Haemostasis must be exact and careful. Then the bladder is drained with a catheter.

Having finished this part of the operation, the patient's legs are brought down from the cystoscopy position, and an anterior approach to the kidney made through a shortened version of the transperitoneal approach described above. Alternatively, the patient is turned into the lateral kidney position, and a 12th rib-tip incision made as usual.

Nephrectomy is performed in the usual way, but the ureter is not divided. Instead, as the kidney is drawn out of the wound and the ureter is liberated from its flimsy attachments between finger and thumb, separating it from the back of the peritoneum and taking care not to tear the gonadal vessels, it is followed down into the pelvis until the place where it crosses the bifurcation of the common iliac artery is distinctly felt. Here extra caution is exercised to make sure the ureter is gently separated with fingers from the vessels, and with a little traction the ureter is followed right down to its entry into the bladder (2.65). Now it comes away in the hand. Check that any bleeding from the gonadal vessels has been controlled and close the wound with a drain leading down behind the peritoneum. This method may seem blind and rough, but it is very simple, and has the great advantage that there is no need for an additional incision

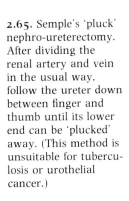

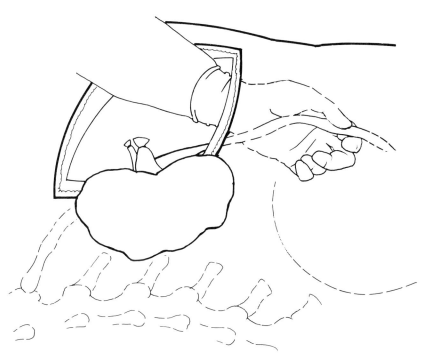

2.65. Semple's 'pluck' nephro-ureterectomy. After dividing the renal artery and vein in the usual way, follow the ureter down between finger and thumb until its lower end can be 'plucked' away. (This method is unsuitable for tuberculosis or urothelial cancer.)

in the lower abdomen, and no need to deliberately open and close the bladder. I have used it consistently without any complications in the last seven years.

For the tuberculous kidney and ureter

Today there is no need to remove the lower end of the ureter in the ordinary straightforward case of tuberculosis. Recurrence is almost never seen in the stump of ureter left behind after nephrectomy, provided that the patient has been given a full course of treatment for tuberculosis. It may, however, be required if the ureter itself is badly scarred, calcified, or involved in active disease. In such patients the ureter may be very adherent to the iliac vessels, and Semple's pluck operation is dangerous. Instead, after nephrectomy has been performed through an anterior approach, the wound is left open (2.66). A second (Pfannenstiel) incision is now made, and the ureter carefully separated from the common iliac vessels (2.67) after dividing the superior vesical vessels between ligatures. Be sure always to use absorbable catgut ligatures in these operations—persistent sinuses are notorious after operations for tuberculosis. The ureter in tuberculosis may be as thick as a finger, and exceedingly adherent to surrounding tissues, including the vena cava. While the dissection is continued in the pelvis through the second incision, if the ureter seems to be dangerously stuck to the common iliac vessels, make sure they are taped above and below the danger area before proceeding with the dissection. If the vessel is opened, it is only a moment's work to pull up the Rummel tourniquets, control bleeding, and, after separating the ureter, close the tear in the artery.

Following down the ureter in a woman leads the surgeon into Mackenrodt's ligament which must be deliberately incised using right-angled forceps and scissors or knife. On reaching the bladder, the ureter is tented up, cut across, and ligated. In tuberculosis there is no need to excise an ellipse of bladder as one must do for cancer of the lower third of the ureter (2.68).

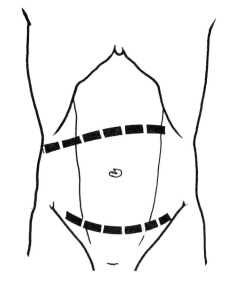

2.66. Incisions for removing kidney and ureter in tuberculosis or cancer. The patient is supine.

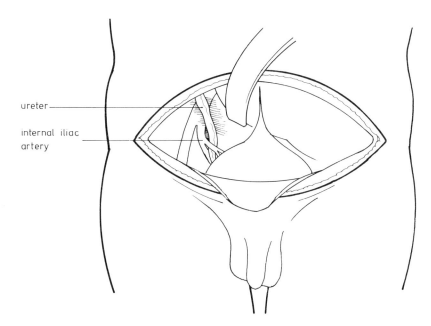

ureter

internal iliac artery

2.67. In tuberculosis the main hazard is where the ureter crosses the bifurcation of the common iliac artery. The wall of the artery may be densely adherent to the ureter and the dissection must be carried out under direct vision.

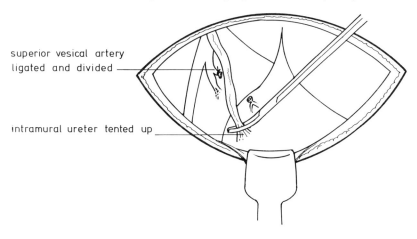

superior vesical artery ligated and divided

intramural ureter tented up

2.68. The ureter is freed from its adhesions, and by division of the superior vesical artery, the intramural ureter can be divided after it has been tented up. There is no need to make a separate opening in the bladder in tuberculosis.

For transitional cell carcinoma of the kidney or ureter

In recent years there has been a change in the approach to transitional cell carcinoma of the kidney and ureter. For several years there have been two opposing views: on the one hand it was felt that all these tumours must be treated radically, by *en bloc* excision of the kidney and ureter together with a cuff of bladder; on the other hand some surgeons were reporting good results from very conservative operations in which as much of the kidney and ureter as possible were preserved. The discrepancy has only been resolved recently, when it has been shown that the difference in results depends upon differences in the *Grade* of the tumour. Bad results follow conservative operations if the tumour is undifferentiated. Indeed, in less than well differentiated tumours, any resection is inadequate, and ought to be combined with adjuvant radiotherapy (Babaian & Johnson 1980). On the other hand, if the tumour is well differentiated, then one should whenever possible, attempt to preserve all of the urinary tract that is not affected by tumour (Mills & Vaughan 1983).

Hence an essential preliminary to intelligent treatment of upper tract urothelial cancer is obtaining information about tumour Grade. Ideally a brush biopsy of the tumour should be obtained but failing that, cytological examination of urine from the vicinity of the tumour may give good evidence of its Grade. In patients with high grade (G3) tumours, a pre-operative course of radiotherapy is indicated.

Nephroureterectomy is then performed after the completion of radiotherapy. There is good evidence that this nephroureterectomy ought to take all the tissues outside Gerota's fascia. Therefore an anterior transperitoneal approach for the nephrectomy part of the operation is indicated, the steps being exactly as those described for renal cell carcinoma above.

If an oblique anterior incision has been used for the nephrectomy, then a second transverse incision is made for the removal of the ureter, using the Pfannenstiel approach. If the nephrectomy is being performed through a paramedian incision, then this is continued right down to the symphysis pubis: the choice of incision is governed by the size and shape of the patient.

The dissection of the ureter towards the bladder follows the rules described above for tuberculosis. First, the superior vesical pedicle is divided between ligatures to liberate the ureter and allow the bladder to be retracted medially, as the ureter is dissected with its surrounding tissues towards the bladder. Great care must be taken in this dissection to secure even seemingly trivial veins in the pelvis, otherwise there can be tremendous and daunting bleeding, which makes the dissection difficult to follow.

In a male the vas deferens arches over the ureter to enter the seminal vesicle behind the bladder and may be coagulated and divided

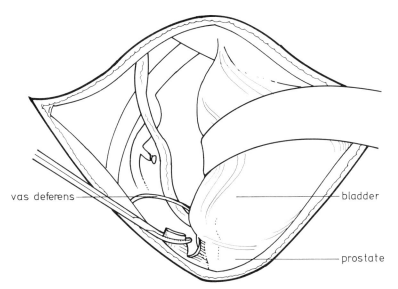

vas deferens — bladder

— prostate

2.69. Nephroureterectomy for urothelial carcinoma: mobilize the right side of the bladder by dividing the superior vesical vessels and the fibrous tissue tethering the lateral aspect of the trigone and prostate. The vas deferens may have to be divided to liberate the ureter.

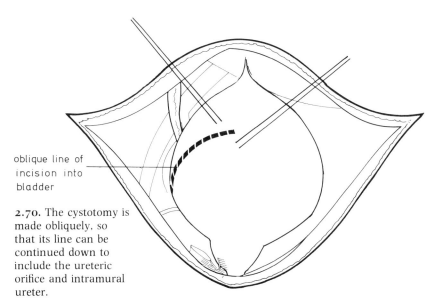

oblique line of incision into bladder

2.70. The cystotomy is made obliquely, so that its line can be continued down to include the ureteric orifice and intramural ureter.

to set the ureter free. The ureter is followed down behind the bladder, and a plane of cleavage is opened up under the trigone, in front of Denonvilliers' fascia. A stiff band of fascia (2.69) must be divided on the lateral aspect of the ureter at this stage, and a vessel running in it must be ligated, but when this is cut, the side of the bladder and trigone may be rolled up.

Now a formal cystostomy is made between stay sutures (2.70) starting at the upper end of the ellipse that you plan to remove. A diathermy needle is used to make this elliptical incision, so that small bleeding vessels can be coagulated as the incision progresses inch by inch. Once the bladder has been opened, a ureteric catheter is slipped into the opposite (good) ureter to protect it (2.71). The trigone is easily distorted during the subsequent dis-

section, and it is all too easy to catch the good ureteric orifice when closing the bladder.

A finger is placed under the trigone to lift it up as the ellipse is completed (2.72). A centimetre of healthy bladder is taken all around the ureteric orifice. After lifting out the ellipse of bladder and the ureter together with the specimen, close the defect in the bladder in one or two layers with continuous 3-0 chromic catgut. A Foley catheter is left in the bladder and the wounds are closed with catgut (2.73), with a drain to the suture line. The drain may be removed on the fourth day and the Foley catheter on the eighth.

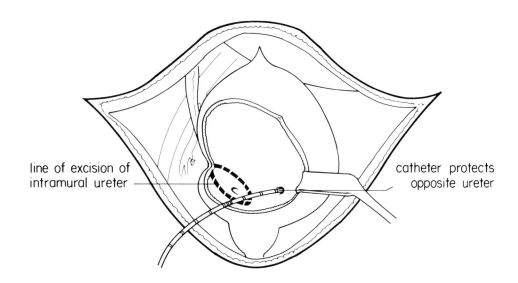

line of excision of intramural ureter

catheter protects opposite ureter

2.71. Protect the opposite ureteric orifice by means of a catheter. Mark out the ellipse of bladder wall and trigone to be taken along with the ureteric orifice.

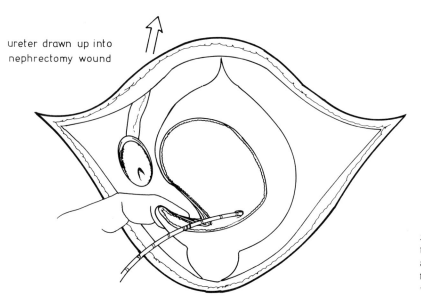

ureter drawn up into nephrectomy wound

2.72. A finger behind the trigone lifts it up and makes excision of the ellipse of bladder wall much easier.

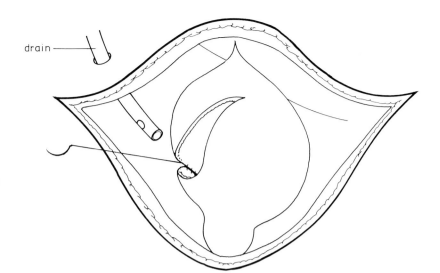

drain

2.73. The defect in the trigone and bladder wall is closed with continuous catgut. A drain is placed down to the bed of the ureter.

Hazards of nephroureterectomy

In addition to the post-operative complications of any abdominal operation, a special hazard of nephroureterectomy arises from damage to the common and internal iliac vessels. It can be avoided by following the cardinal rules: never cut where you cannot see, and always insist on good exposure.

References

Babaian R.J. & Johnson D.E. (1980) Primary carcinoma of the ureter. *J. Urol* **123**, 357.

Bennett W.M. (1976) Cost benefit ratio of post-transplant bilateral nephrectomy. *J.A.M.A.* **235**, 1703.

Gil-Vernet J.M. (1965) New surgical concepts in removing renal calculi. *Urol. Internat.* **20**, 255.

Gil-Vernet J.M., Carretero P., Ballesteros J.J. & Figuls J. (1976) A new approach to the kidney in kyphoscoliosis. *European Urology*, **2**, 105.

Maddern J.P. (1967) Surgery of the staghorn calculus. *Brit. J. Urol.* **39**, 323.

Mills C. & Vaughan E.D. (1983) Carcinoma of the ureter: natural history management and 5 year survival. *J. Urol.* **129**, 275.

Morris H. (1898) *On the origin and progress of Renal Surgery.* Cassell, London.

Parry J.W., Walmsley B.H., Abercrombie G.F. and O'Donohue N. (1983) The 'rip and pluck' nephro-ureterectomy: a review. *Brit J. Urol.*

Semb C. (1953) The selective principle in the treatment of renal tuberculosis. Acta Chin Scand. **110**, 42.

Swanson D.A. & Borges P.M. (1983) Complications of transabdominal radical nephrectomy for renal cell carcinoma. *J. Urol.* **129**, 704.

Swanson D.A., Bracken R.B., Johnson D.E. & Wallace S. (1979) Combination renal artery occlusion, nephrectomy, and progestin therapy for metastatic renal cell carcinoma. *Proceedings Societe Internationale d'urologie*, **2**, 148.

Wesolowski S., Malanowska S., Malewski A. & Czaplicki M. (1979) Spinal cord damage as a complication of renal artery embolization in patients with renal carcinoma. *Proc. Societe International d'urologie*, **2**, 134.

Chapter 3
Operations for stones in the kidney

Stones that are too large to go safely down the ureter should be removed, unless they are safely lodged in an outlying calix and unlikely to cause trouble. Occasionally a small, unobstructing stone in an outlying calix gives rise to so much genuine pain, that it demands to be removed. There are some exceptions to these general rules: if stones are soluble, for example some cystine stones and some urate stones, then it is legitimate to offer the patient a trial of forced fluids with alkalinization of the urine and perhaps the addition of penicillamine.

At the time of writing two revolutionary methods of dealing with urinary calculi have taken the world of urology by storm. Of these the most exciting and imaginative is the shock wave method (Chaussy *et al.* 1980, 1982). Using a very sophisticated system of radiological positioning, the patient's stone is made to lie exactly at the second focus of an ellipsoidal mirror (3.1). The patient is placed in a water-bath. A powerful spark is let off at the first focus of the ellipsoid, and the shock wave

transmitted through the water and the soft tissues of the body to produce a similar shock that disintegrates the stone. The system is expensive to build, install and run, but it avoids any need for surgical intervention. The fragmented stone is shattered into tiny particles of a size that pass easily down the ureter.

The second revolutionary technique has an older history. Many surgeons have succeeded in extracting small stones through a nephrostomy tube. This principle has been adapted to the modern technique of percutaneous nephrolithotomy (Alken *et al.* 1981; Wickham & Kellett 1981).

Percutaneous nephrolithotomy

Under local anaesthesia a fine needle is passed through the skin into the renal pelvis (3.2). A little contrast is injected and the kidney screened in two planes, while the anatomy of the renal pelvis is carefully observed in relation to the position of the stone. A flexible guide-wire is then passed through the needle, the

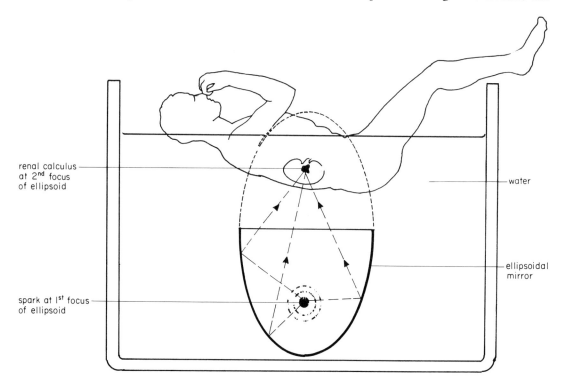

renal calculus at 2nd focus of ellipsoid

water

spark at 1st focus of ellipsoid

ellipsoidal mirror

3.1. Dornier shock wave system of fragmenting stones within the renal pelvis. A powerful spark is discharged at the first focus of an ellipsoidal mirror. The shock waves pass through the water-bath to concentrate at the second focus of the ellipse, where the stone is carefully sited using cross-beams of X-rays.

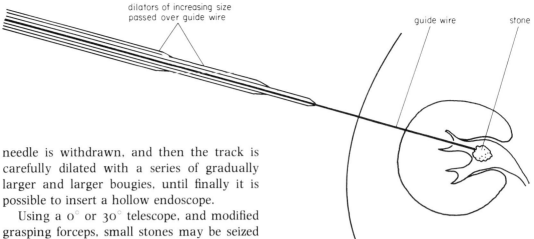

3.2. A guide wire is passed to the stone in the kidney under image-intensifier control. Over the guide wire dilators are passed.

needle is withdrawn, and then the track is carefully dilated with a series of gradually larger and larger bougies, until finally it is possible to insert a hollow endoscope.

Using a 0° or 30° telescope, and modified grasping forceps, small stones may be seized and withdrawn through the hollow endoscopic tube. If they are lost, one may insert a flexible endoscope and search through the renal pelvis. If the stones are too large to be removed through the lumen of the endoscope, they may be broken up with the assistance of an ultrasound probe (3.3). Essentially, the ultrasound disintegrator is a hollow cylinder with teeth at its end, which oscillates at ultrasonic frequency, shattering and grinding the stone into fragments. A continuous stream of water aspirates the fragments up the lumen of the nephroscope.

The advantages of this method are obvious: the patient suffers no prolonged morbidity from a large incision to expose the kidney, and may leave the hospital within a few days when all goes well. But the method is exceedingly difficult to learn and takes many hours, during which patient and surgeon are exposed to high levels of radiation and possible ultrasonic damage to the internal ear. At the time of writing this exciting new technique is still too new to have been evaluated fully, and the reader is warned against believing all that he

reads. Haemorrhage, septicaemia, the TUR syndrome, and the need for frequent repeat percutaneous endoscopic procedures are all reported by those with experience of the method.

Pyelolithotomy

Special preparations

A recent radiograph must always be present in the operating theatre before the operation begins. For any stone that is small enough to move around within the collecting system a plain radiograph must be taken *en route* between ward and operating theatre. When stones are large and branched, or when several stones need to be removed, radiographs may be needed on the table and appropriate X-ray films must be sterilized ahead of time. If the renal parenchyma is thick and healthy, and outlying portions of stone may need a nephrotomy incision to reach them,

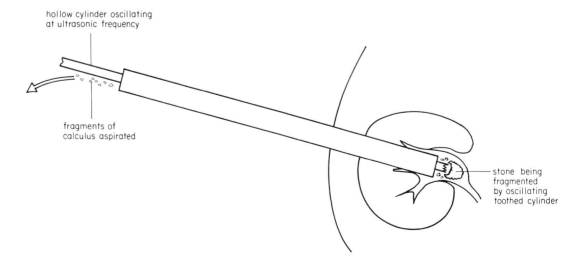

hollow cylinder oscillating
at ultrasonic frequency

fragments of
calculus aspirated

stone being
fragmented
by oscillating
toothed cylinder

3.3. The stone is fragmented by the oscillating toothed cylinder passed down the nephroscope tube.

preparations should be made to be able to cool the kidney as and when required. This does not need elaborate or expensive apparatus: sterile ice slush or cooling coils and unsterile ice are all that are required, but they do need to be thought of in advance.

Position on the table

The patient is placed in the lateral position, rolling if anything slightly forwards.

Incision

For a small stone in an accessible renal pelvis, the 12th rib-tip approach is excellent (page 14). One may use the vertical lumbotomy except when the incision may need to be enlarged. For most purposes the full length 12th rib-bed approach is best.

Small calculus in the renal pelvis– pyelolithotomy

Here a simple pyelolithotomy is all that is required (3.4). Make the appropriate incision; retract the wound edges; open Gerota's fascia, and feel for the stone. Often a stone in a renal pelvis is easily felt with the finger (3.5). Do not mobilize the kidney fully, or make a meal out of what should be a quick and easy operation. Having felt the stone, roll the kidney forwards a little and dissect the fat from the edge of the kidney until the muscle of the renal pelvis is exposed. Clear it of overlying fat; put in two stay sutures of 4-0 plain catgut; incise directly on to the stone (3.6). The stone must be freed from the soft inner mucosa of the renal pelvis, which is often oedematous and adherent to the rough outside of the calculus (3.7). Lift out the stone. Irrigate the renal pelvis. You need

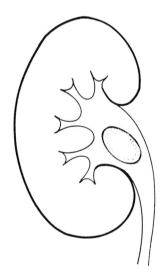

3.4. Pyelolithotomy for small calculus in the renal pelvis.

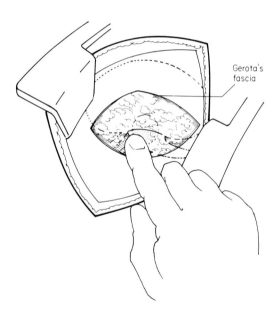

3.5. A small stone can often be felt with the finger as soon as Gerota's fascia has been incised.

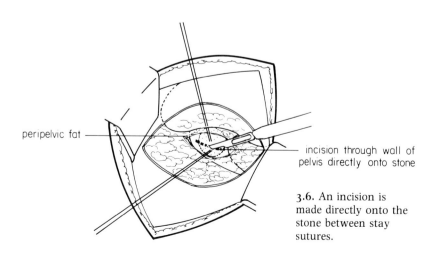

3.6. An incision is made directly onto the stone between stay sutures.

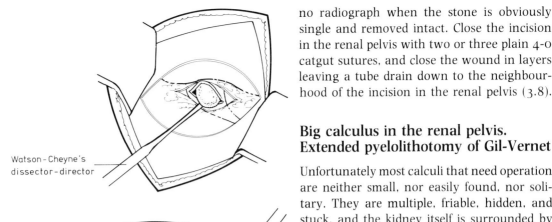

3.7. The calculus is freed from the adherent pelvic mucosa and removed.

Watson-Cheyne's dissector-director

3.8. The pelvis is closed and a drain led down to it.

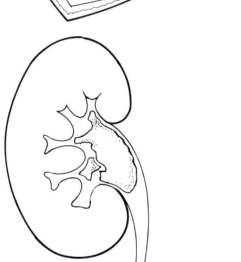

3.9. Large calculus in the renal pelvis.

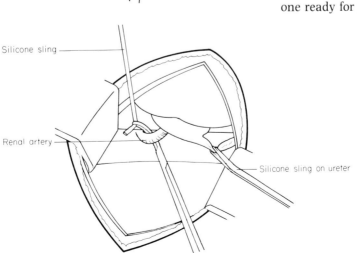

Silicone sling

Renal artery

Silicone sling on ureter

3.10. A Silicone rubber sling is passed around the renal artery, and a second one around the ureter.

no radiograph when the stone is obviously single and removed intact. Close the incision in the renal pelvis with two or three plain 4-0 catgut sutures, and close the wound in layers leaving a tube drain down to the neighbourhood of the incision in the renal pelvis (3.8).

Big calculus in the renal pelvis. Extended pyelolithotomy of Gil-Vernet

Unfortunately most calculi that need operation are neither small, nor easily found, nor solitary. They are multiple, friable, hidden, and stuck, and the kidney itself is surrounded by dense adhesions resulting from previous infection or surgery (3.9).

Start off by making an incision right along the length of the 12th rib-bed. Good access is the first step to safety. Mobilize the kidney completely, being prepared to spend time dividing adhesions. In a patient operated on before, open the peritoneum early on in the dissection so that you know just where the colon and duodenum are situated and can retract them out of harm's way.

As you begin to mobilize the lower pole of the kidney, feel for the ureter. Pass a silicone sling around it to prevent small fragments of stone slipping down the ureter during later manipulations.

Now turn the kidney forwards and feel for the pulsations of the renal artery with a forefinger, remembering that it lies well down towards the midline, concealed by dense fibrofatty tissue. When the renal artery has been felt by its pulsations, it is necessary to expose it by dissecting away the sleeve of investing fibrous tissue that always conceals it. Once the artery has been clearly exposed, a right-angled forceps is passed round it to seize a silicone rubber sling (3.10). Now try an arterial clamp for size: make sure that your scrub nurse has one ready for you.

Mobilize the kidney completely from all its adhesions. A radiograph of the kidney must be taken at the end of the procedure and cannot be obtained unless the kidney is fully mobilized.

The bloodless plane of Gil-Vernet (1964) lies between the connective tissue of the renal sinus and the renal pelvis. Start the dissection a little distance from the edge of the kidney (Blandy & Tresidder 1967). Thrust in the dissecting scissors and open them gently to display the plane of cleavage between the muscle of the renal pelvis and the fat of the renal sinus (3.11). Gil-Vernet's plane lies under the adventitia that covers the renal pelvis just like a major artery (3.12). Sometimes the tissues are particularly dense around the border of the

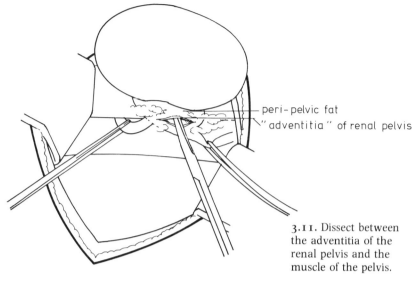

peri-pelvic fat
"adventitia" of renal pelvis

3.11. Dissect between the adventitia of the renal pelvis and the muscle of the pelvis.

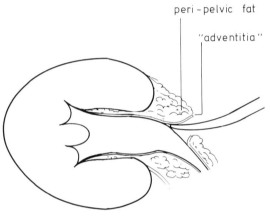

peri-pelvic fat

"adventitia"

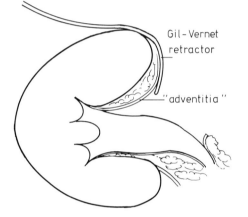

Gil-Vernet retractor

"adventitia"

3.12. The plane of Gil-Vernet lies between the muscle of the pelvis and connective tissue adventitia around it.

kidney. In such a case, find the ureter and follow the plane between ureter and adventitia right up into the renal sinus.

Gil-Vernet's plane of cleavage can sometimes be extended right out to the necks of the calices (3.13). How far this plane should be followed will be governed by the shape and situation of the branches of the staghorn calculus, and the degree to which the pelvis is enveloped by the renal parenchyma. When the pelvis is small, and only a limited dissection is necessary, insert two stay sutures and cut down on to the stone. If the pelvis is well displayed and the stone is bulky you need no stay sutures: merely let the knife grate on the stone. The incision in the renal pelvis should run parallel to the border of the kidney. It should not cross the pelviureteric junction. It may be extended up to and through the neck of the superior or inferior major calix, according to the shape of the calculus (3.14).

Many stones are firm and slippery, especially those caused by some metabolic disorder, for example cystinuria or uric acid stone disease.

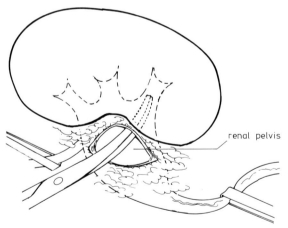

renal pelvis

3.13. The plane is extended out towards the necks of the calices.

Others are crumbly, rough, and adherent to the lining of the pelvis and calices, especially those due to infection. A smooth stone is easily lifted out. Crumbly stones must be teased away from the mucosa with the flat blade of the Watson–Cheyne dissector (3.15, 3.16). When all the stones have been removed, irrigate the pelvis thoroughly with saline in a Dakin's syringe.

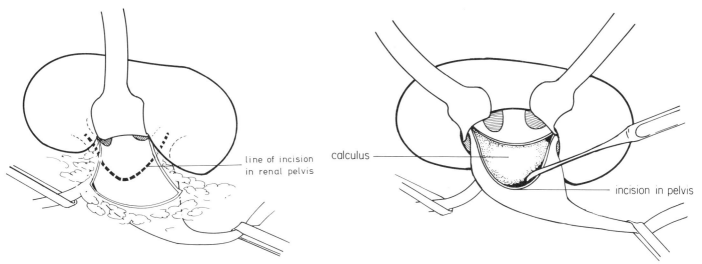

3.14. The parenchyma is retracted to reveal the pelvis and calices.

line of incision
in renal pelvis

calculus

incision in pelvis

3.15. The stone is freed from the adherent pelvis.

It is not so easy, in practice, to be sure that all the stones have been removed. The most simple, and most practicable adjuvant at this stage is to insert a finger and feel directly between finger and thumb for stones in outlying calices. If the renal parenchyma is very thin, this is easy and reliable. If the parenchyma is thick or oedematous and scarred, it is easy to miss small outlying fragments of stone.

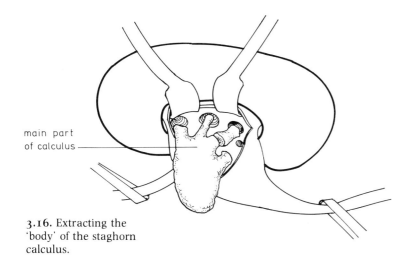

main part
of calculus

3.16. Extracting the 'body' of the staghorn calculus.

Operative nephroscopy

Many nephroscopes have been devised that permit the surgeon to peer into the outlying calices to seek small fragments of stone. They fall into two categories. Rigid right-angled nephroscopes (3.17) have the advantage of being equipped with good irrigating facilities and forceps that allow small fragments to be extracted. Flexible fibre-optic instruments take a little skill to learn how to use, are provided with excellent irrigating systems, and give a remarkable view of the interior of the calices (3.18).

Operative ultrasound detection of calculi

The happy coincidence of Lytton's interest in renal calculi, and a mature, ex-submarine-commander medical student, led to the development of ultrasound as a way of detecting small fragments of stone within the kidney (Cook & Lytton 1977). Subsequently this method of searching for and locating small

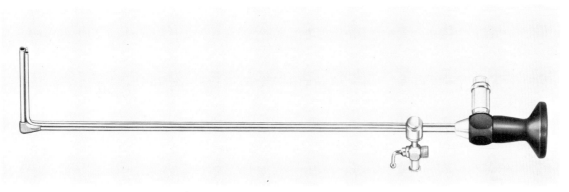

3.17. Rigid nephroscope (courtesy of Messrs Rimmer Brothers, UK Agents for Karl Storz A.G.).

outlying bits of stone has been developed into a fine art by Alken *et al.* (1981) in Mainz. A small hand-held ultrasound probe, previously sterilized, is applied to the surface of the kidney. Stones are detected by their image on the sonar screen—a typical reflection from the stone, and an even more typical sonic shadow behind the stone. The apparatus is expensive, and the skill to use it effectively not easily acquired, but the method is an undoubted advance.

Peroperative use of ultrasound probe

With the advent of the ultrasound lithotriptor a new instrument has been added to the armamentarium of the surgeon embarking on removal of staghorn calculi from the kidney. Once a small outlying calculus has been located in a peripheral calix, it may be difficult to extract it with a forceps, but the stone can be shattered by the teeth of a cylindrical probe that oscillates at ultrasonic frequency, and the fragments then aspirated in a stream of water. The calix can be completely cleared of stone and the renal parenchyma left entirely undamaged. The technique is very similar to the method employed in percutaneous stone removal (page 40).

Operative X-rays

Once the surgeon is 'sure' that all the bits of stone have been removed from the kidney, an

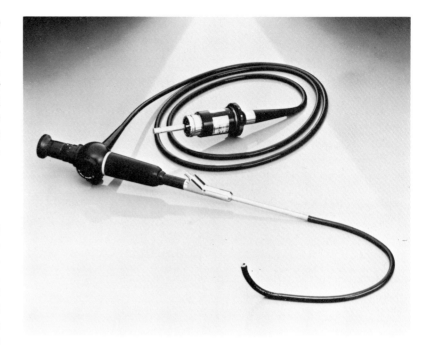

X-ray is taken *in situ*. Special kidney films with a pair of plates in each packet, each of different sensitivity, are placed behind the kidney. The kidney is held up, for convenience, in a sleeve of 'Netelast' (Wickham 1975), to which a few ligaclips are attached to give reference points for localization of the stone fragments, if any, that remain behind (3.19). Use a tube–film distance of about 75 cm, and an exposure of 50 mAS, 60 kV. The respiration is suspended.

3.18. Modified Olympus choledochonephroscope adapted for examination of the interior of the kidney (courtesy of Messrs Keymed, UK Agents for Olympus Optical Instruments).

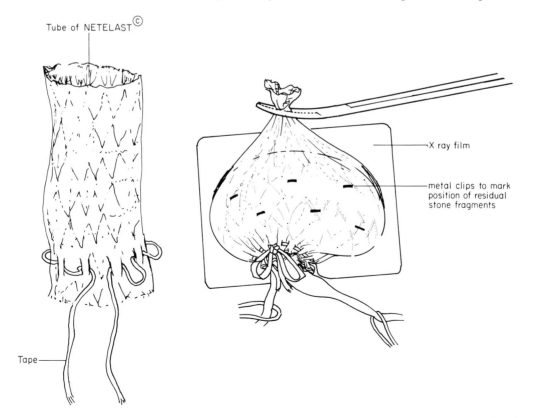

Tube of NETELAST©

Tape

X ray film

metal clips to mark position of residual stone fragments

3.19. Wickham's method of holding kidney in wound for radiography *in situ*. 'Netelast' (C) tubing is used to hold the kidney against an X-ray plate in the wound. Metal ligaclips are attached to the Netelast to help localize the residual fragments of stone in the kidney.

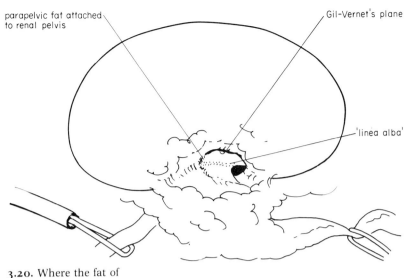

parapelvic fat attached to renal pelvis

Gil-Vernet's plane

'linea alba'

3.20. Where the fat of the renal sinus is densely attached to the renal pelvis, it may have to be dissected with a knife before Gil-Vernet's space is opened up.

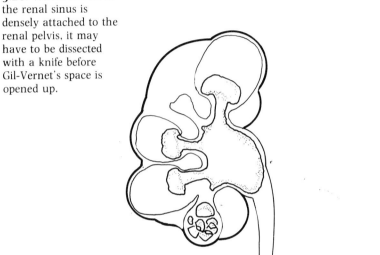

3.21. Difficult stag-horn stones.

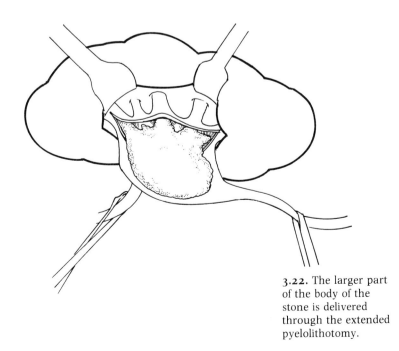

3.22. The larger part of the body of the stone is delivered through the extended pyelolithotomy.

The films are developed, and brought back to the operating room as soon as possible. It often helps if a small bit of stone is placed on the edge of the kidney so that one can differentiate an artifact and a stone. Do not close the incision in the renal pelvis until the films have been seen, and it is certain that their quality is such that a small stone left behind would have been detected.

The difficult staghorn stone

Begin with a generous incision. Be prepared for a prolonged dissection of the kidney, and start off by entering the peritoneum so that the colon or duodenum can be protected. When there has been a previous extended pyelolithotomy, Gil-Vernet's plane may be difficult to reopen, and the renal pelvis may be concealed in hard white fibrous tissue. The trick is to find the ureter a little way from the kidney, dissect the adventitia from its muscular wall, and follow the sub-adventitial plane up into the renal sinus. The sinus fat in such a patient is often very adherent especially at the border of the kidney—Gil-Vernet's 'linea alba' (3.20). One may have to dissect this from the pelvis with a fine knife. Sometimes the fat around the sinus is so stiff that it cannot be retracted easily, and must be divided in a radial direction: if this seems likely, make sure that the fatty tissue has been undermined, so that there is an edge into which a suture may be placed in case unexpected bleeding is encountered. There are often huge veins in this tissue. Now lift the fat and parenchyma from the renal pelvis with malleable copper strips, or with the special retractors designed for the purpose.

Continue the dissection in Gil-Vernet's plane up into the renal sinus as far as necessary, according to the size and shape of the calculus (3.21). If the staghorn has a long process reaching out into a calix, continue to develop the plane so that the neck of the calix can be opened up.

The incision in the renal pelvis is made more or less parallel with the long axis of the kidney. It is sometimes useful to make a T-extension to this incision in order to deliver a bulky staghorn, but one should avoid crossing the pelviureteric junction lest stenosis develops there later on.

When the main body of the stone has been eased out through the incision in the renal pelvis, hold it in a suitable forceps and try to wriggle it free (3.22). Occasionally the entire staghorn calculus can be extracted intact—a most gratifying achievement—but there is no prize for removing the specimen whole. Have no hesitation in breaking it into smaller bits. Most large calculi are friable and firm pressure with heavy scissors will crack them into smaller pieces that are more easy to remove (3.23). A uric acid stone, and some oxalate stones, are so hard that the lithotrite may be needed to break them. I have on occasion even made use of a hammer and osteotome. Thorough irrigation with a bulb syringe will wash away the little fragments which are detached when breaking up a larger calculus.

Now that the main body of the stone has been removed, adjust the retractors so that you can see the openings of the major calices. The broken-off neck of a stone is easily seen sitting in its calix (3.24). If a small outlying calculus is seen, extract it through the neck of the calix with suitable forceps. It may be necessary to stretch the caliceal neck, or even slit it up, but one must avoid tearing it by forcible removal of a bit of stone that is too large to go through the neck, for this will tear the vessels that run beneath the mucosa and cause bleeding that is difficult to control.

Rather than attempt such forcible removal of a large 'mushroom' extension of a calculus, it is better to break up the stone *in situ*, or make a nephrotomy and remove the stone through the renal parenchyma.

To break up the stone as it lies in the calix, one can use scissors and artery forceps, but a neater way to remove such a stone is by using the ultrasonic lithotriptor, which has the advantage that it aspirates the fragments of stone and does not injure the calix.

A useful adjunct to this stage of an extended pyelolithotomy is the flexible endoscope. With a little skill and practice one can direct a narrow flexible choledochoscope into each calix to identify small peripheral calculi and make sure that all the fragments have been removed.

Finally, if the hand-held ultrasound probe is available, it may be used to search the kidney for tiny outlying fragments of stone; when one is located, it may be identified with the assistance of the endoscope, and destroyed with the ultrasound probe.

These adjuncts will not be available to every surgeon who sets out to remove a branched calculus from the kidney, and in many cases he must perform a nephrotomy to remove large outlying fragments. Two principles should be borne in mind here: first, always have control of the renal artery before you start, so that if severe bleeding is encountered, it can be

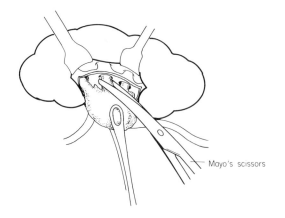

3.23. Extensions of the staghorn stone which are attached to large mushroom outcrops are broken off.

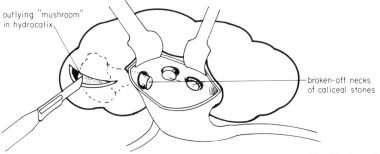

3.24. The big 'mushroom' is removed through a calicotomy.

stopped at once; second, make the incisions in the direction that will avoid the main segmental arteries. In most instances the parenchyma overlying the mushroom extensions of a staghorn is so thin that the stone is easily felt with the finger-tip. In such a case make a radial incision on to the stone, retract the edges of the parenchyma with narrow copper retractors and lift out the stone. Irrigate the calix thoroughly and inspect it carefully to make sure no little fragments are left behind (3.25).

By these two manoeuvres the entire kidney can be cleared in nearly every case. The main difficulty arises when a small peripheral fragment of stone cannot be located. An X-ray is taken *in situ*, but the little piece of stone cannot be seen with the flexible endoscope nor felt

3.25. Each hydrocalix is thoroughly irrigated and cleared of outlying bits of stone.

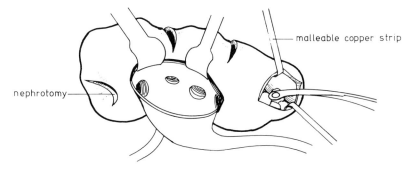

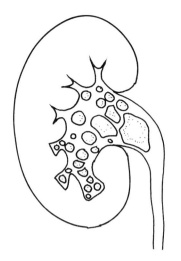

3.26. Multiple small calculi in kidney.

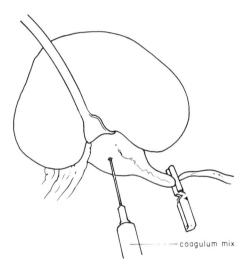

3.27. Coagulum mix is injected into pelvis.

— coagulum mix

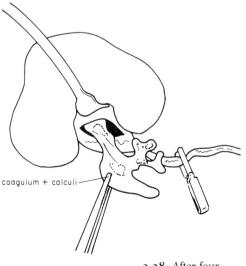

coagulum + calculi —

3.28. After four minutes the coagulum and the entrapped calculi are removed through an incision in the pelvis.

with the finger or a stone forceps. In such a case if an arterial clamp is placed on the renal artery for a minute or two, it will become flaccid and soft, as the blood drains out of it, and this simple trick often allows you to feel the calculus through the now soft and thin parenchyma. Do not rest until the radiograph shows that the kidney is completely cleared.

Coagulum pyelolithotomy

Some stones (3.26) pose a different problem: there may be one or two large calculi, but a large number of small peripheral ones, often smooth and round, and easily missed. There is a real danger that these little smooth 'pebbles' may be missed, and in the post-operative days may pass down the ureter to give rise to endless trouble and a persistent urinary fistula.

One useful manoeuvre in such cases is to fill the entire collecting system with a stiff co-agulum before incising it. There are several methods of doing this, but the technique I prefer is as follows.

Human dried fibrinogen solution, reconstituted with 50 ml sterile water gives a fixed concentration of 4.4 g fibrinogen per 100 ml. This is the least volume that will dissolve the fibrinogen. About 19 ml of this solution are mixed with 1 ml of a thrombin solution containing 5000 units of topical bovine thrombin in 100 ml sterile normal saline (concentration fifty units per millilitre).

A butterfly needle is inserted into the exposed renal pelvis after making the Gil-Vernet dissection. As much of the urine inside the pelvis is withdrawn as possible. In a 50 ml syringe, 19 ml of the fibrinogen and 1 ml of the thrombin solution are taken up as swiftly as possible, and then injected into the butterfly needle (3.27). This whole process must be completed within thirty seconds or it will clot. A drop of methylene blue added to the fibrinogen solution makes it easy to see the otherwise colourless coagulum. Then the pelvis is opened in the usual way, and the coagulum and the stones extracted after allowing about four minutes for the coagulum to reach its maximum strength (3.28) (Norris *et al.* 1981).

Peripheral calculi in a thick parenchyma

Large peripheral stones over which the parenchyma is not atrophied are encountered in children and young adults, especially those with metabolic disorders such as hyperoxaluria or hyperparathyroidism. The large peripheral stone will not pass through the neck of the calix without causing undue damage, and the parenchyma is so thick that it is difficult to feel the stone (3.29). Even when it has been found, to reach the stone it is necessary to cut through a considerable thickness of healthy parenchyma. To make a complete clearance of the kidney needs more than the fifteen or twenty minutes of safe ischaemia permitted at normal body temperature. But by cooling the kidney, the period of safe ischaemia is prolonged well beyond the time needed for the most dilatory procedure. Many methods for cooling the kidney have been described. One of the most simple and effective is to surround the kidney with sterile ice slush, which is easily prepared by putting three-litre bags of saline or glycine in the refrigerator forty-eight hours before they are likely to be needed. The ice-cold slush cools the kidney surface, and has been found to be a tried and trusty method of cooling the organ. However, there is a risk of over-cooling the surface parenchyma and causing frost-bite.

An equally simple method of cooling the kidney that needs only apparatus that is to be found in every operating room was devised by Politano and developed by Marshall (Marshall & Blandy 1974). Overnight have 2 or 3 three-litre bags of saline, water, or the glycine used for TUR, put into the refrigerator to cool it to about 4 °C. When you need to cool the kidney, occlude the renal artery with an arterial clamp, and allow the ice-cold liquid to trickle over the surface of the kidney through one blood-giving set, while through a second set in parallel, the same ice-cold solution is allowed to irrigate the interior of the kidney through the pyelotomy incision made to remove the body of the stone. It is easy to measure the temperature of the renal parenchyma with a thermocouple, and the irrigation can be stopped when the temperature falls to about 10 °C, a temperature which allows at least an hour of safe ischaemia (3.30).

Since nurses are only human, you may one day find that your scrub nurse has forgotten to put the requisite fluid into the refrigerator ahead of time. In such circumstances you merely run the fluid through disposable blood-warming coils (that are always available) which are immersed in a bucket of ice sprinkled with salt. In practice this simple system works well, and will cool the saline from room temperature to about 5 or 6 °C, quite cold enough to lower the temperature of the kidney to safe limits (3.31).

One precaution should be observed when

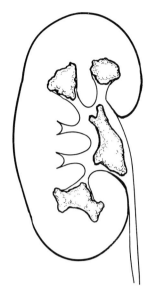

3.29. Peripheral stones with thick parenchyma.

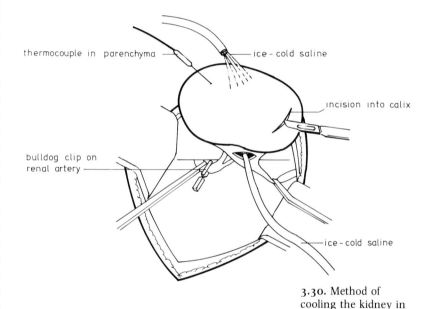

thermocouple in parenchyma

ice-cold saline

incision into calix

bulldog clip on renal artery

ice-cold saline

3.30. Method of cooling the kidney in the wound.

using any of these cooling methods: make sure the patient's body temperature is measured. Twice I have unwittingly caused a severe hypothermia: your anaesthetist should be aware of this risk and ready, when necessary, to take suitable measures to warm the patient up afterwards.

Nephrotomy

Usually when the kidney has been rendered bloodless and cold, it is easy to feel through the parenchyma for the outlying parts of the stone. One may cut down boldly upon the stone, making the incision in a radial direction parallel with the lines of the renal arterial segmental branches (3.32).

These incisions may be planned with even

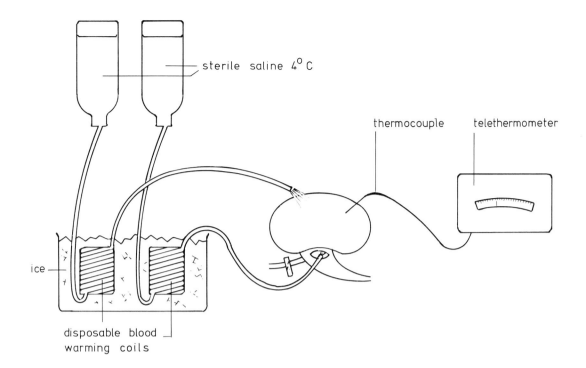

sterile saline 4° C

thermocouple   telethermometer

ice

disposable blood
warming coils

3.31. Simple system
of cooling the kidney
in situ.

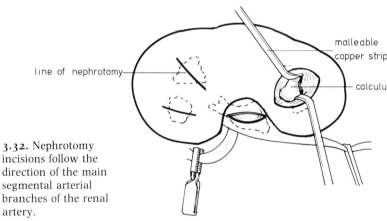
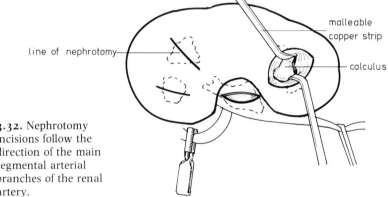

malleable
copper strip

line of nephrotomy

calculus

3.32. Nephrotomy
incisions follow the
direction of the main
segmental arterial
branches of the renal
artery.

more care and precision by mapping out the
segmental arteries. They are located with a
hand-held Doppler ultrasound probe (3.33). It
takes only a few minutes to track the various
segmental arteries, mark them on the surface
of the kidney with methylene blue, and then,
when the arterial clamp has been applied,
make the incision between the lines (3.34)
(Thuroff *et al.* 1982).

Bisection of the kidney

From time to time one is obliged to remove a
branched big calculus that occupies several
adjacent calices, and is so hard that it cannot
easily be broken into smaller manoeuvrable
fragments. Rather than make a number of
radial nephrotomies, it may be simpler to bisect
the kidney by joining two radial nephrotomies

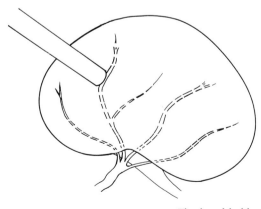

3.33. The hand-held
Doppler ultrasound
instrument detects the
four major segmental
arteries on the front
of the kidney.

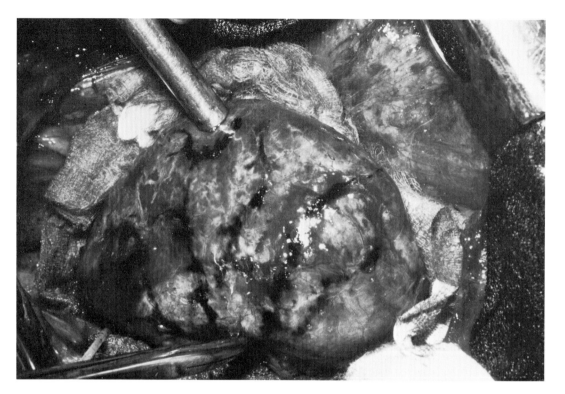

3.34. Operation photograph: the arteries have been mapped on the kidney with methylene blue, using Hohenfellner's method with the Doppler ultrasound instrument.

together (3.35). By doing this the kidney is taken apart into two halves, the stones are prized out from their hiding places and the kidney is thoroughly irrigated. Just as in an ordinary partial nephrectomy, care is now taken to catch up and suture-ligate every small vessel that has been transected (3.36). By making the nephrotomies between the 'tramlines' that have been mapped with the Doppler probe, no major arteries need be secured, but there will always be a number of veins to be sutured. Release the clamp intermittently to identify all the little veins; obtain

complete haemostasis and then, when the opposing surfaces of the kidney are quite dry, sew them together first with a layer of 4-0 catgut to the collecting system, and then with a layer of 4-0 catgut through the capsule (3.37).

Closure of a nephrotomy

Most nephrotomies do not bleed, and it is only necessary to approximate the capsule with a

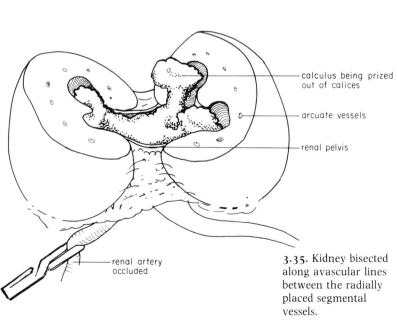

— calculus being prized out of calices

— arcuate vessels

— renal pelvis

— renal artery occluded

3.35. Kidney bisected along avascular lines between the radially placed segmental vessels.

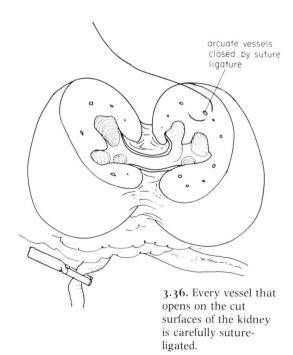

arcuate vessels closed by suture ligature

3.36. Every vessel that opens on the cut surfaces of the kidney is carefully suture-ligated.

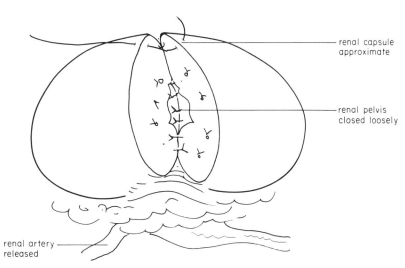

renal capsule
approximate

renal pelvis
closed loosely

renal artery
released

3.37. The renal pelvis is approximated, then the capsule, after complete haemostasis has been obtained.

few 4-0 chromic catgut sutures (3.38). Indeed, by the time the operation is drawing to its close, one often finds that the little parenchymal incisions have become sealed off with clot and need no sutures. If, however, a radial nephrotomy has cut across a larger vein or, by mischance, a segmental artery, the edges of the nephrotomy must be retracted and the vessels meticulously suture-ligated, before the nephrotomy is closed.

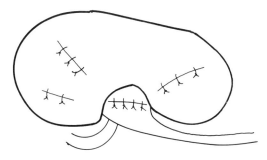

3.38. Closure of nephrotomies and pyelotomy.

Nephrostomy

Most cases require no nephrostomy, but when there is a solitary kidney, when renal function is precarious, or when clearance has been less than complete a nephrostomy tube should be left in. Bring it out through one of the lower calices, to emerge in a straight track to the skin. The tube should be about 24 Ch. It is secured to the skin before continuing with the operation. Later on a percutaneous tube may be passed along the nephrostomy track and residual fragments removed with a flexible nephroscope.

Omental wrapping

If there is good reason to anticipate that the kidney may have to be explored at some time in the future—and in all large series of staghorn calculi there is a 15–20% chance of recurrent stone formation—then it may be prudent to take a little extra trouble to wrap the kidney up in omentum. These are just the cases in which the operation will have started off by opening the peritoneum, so it only takes a moment to reach in, seize the omentum, detach it from the transverse colon, and fold it around the kidney. I have now had to re-explore several kidneys that were protected in this way and there is no doubt at all that the plane of omentum makes the second exploration incomparably more easy.

Closure of the wound

Use catgut throughout, never any non-absorbable material. Provide dependent drainage. If the pleura has been opened, lead the drain to an underwater seal, having expelled all the air in the pleura before closing it.

Hazards of the operation

During any operation for stone in the kidney, sudden, unexpected, and torrential haemorrhage may occur when dissecting in the renal sinus. Always make sure of the renal artery in all but the most accessible and easy stones in the renal pelvis. Knowing that you have an arterial sling around the renal artery means that unexpected bleeding is easily stopped, and can be dealt with safely, without haste or loss of blood. Emergency enforced nephrectomy, and even loss of life, were by no means uncommon in former times when operating for stones in the kidney.

Venous ooze may obscure the view during operations for renal calculi. This may be caused by angulation and obstruction of the renal vein when it is rotated forwards to display the interior of the pelvis. Roll the kidney back into its normal position and compress it for a minute or two, and the bleeding will stop.

Bits of stone left behind

To leave a bit of stone behind is a mistake, but not the unmitigated disaster that is sometimes described. Of course one must try as hard as possible to get out all fragments of stone, but intraparenchymal calcification, as seen in renal tubular acidosis and hyperoxaluria, lies outside the collecting system, and cannot be removed completely. Often too, the calcification that is revealed in the operative X-rays lies just under the epithelium of the renal papillae—Randall's plaques. Be ready to use a little surgical common sense, and know when to call a halt. Stones recur whether the kidney has been completely cleared or not. Tiny fragments often pass down the ureter spontaneously, and many a small fragment left behind remains unchanged year after year and causes no further trouble. Recurrence of stones is nearly always due to uncontrolled infection with *Proteus mirabilis* or failure to control some severe underlying metabolic disorder. Only two out of twenty patients, in my series of infective calculi that were incompletely cleared, grew new stones (Woodhouse *et al.* 1981). Of twenty kidneys with obviously metabolic causes for their stones, one regrew a staghorn, and one with cystinuria and one with hyperoxaluria formed recurrent small calculi. Of twenty-four patients with mixed infective and metabolic causes for their stones, seven developed recurrences.

Partial nephrectomy

When there is more than one stone in a lower pole (3.39) or when the lower pole is badly scarred, then it ought to be removed (Marshall

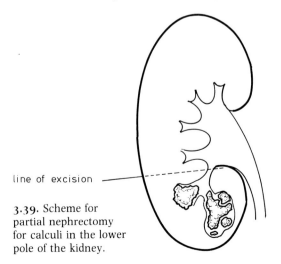

line of excision

3.39. Scheme for partial nephrectomy for calculi in the lower pole of the kidney.

et al. 1976). But partial nephrectomy is no longer indicated as a method of preventing recurrence of calculus according to the 'stone nest' theory of former times. Partial nephrectomy is equally rarely indicated today for tuberculosis, since chemotherapy will cure all but the most severely damaged kidneys, and nephrectomy is then required rather than any form of conservative operation.

For well-differentiated tumours of the renal pelvis and calices, partial nephrectomy has a useful but limited place (Petkovic 1978; Wallace *et al.* 1981). It is also indicated when there are small, strictly localized parenchymal carcinomas, especially if they affect both kidneys simultaneously (Puigvert 1976; Schiff *et al.* 1979).

Special precautions

If a partial nephrectomy is likely to be difficult, or when one anticipates requiring a frozen section in order to make sure that the limit of resection of a tumour is clear of growth, then arrange cooling in order to give ample time for the operation and avoid the need for any haste. (See page 50.)

Position

The patient is placed in the lateral position, as for a straightforward nephrectomy.

Incision

The 12th rib-bed incision gives excellent access.

Steps of the operation

Mobilize the kidney fully and secure the ureter and renal artery early on in the dissection. Make sure that suitable arterial clips are ready for the renal artery.

Lower pole resection

Where you are going to cut across the kidney will depend on the pathological process. The line of resection will not correspond with the territory supplied by the segmental arteries of the kidney, and there is no point in seeking to ligate the lower pole vessel in the renal hilum —it makes a pretty dissection but does not help at all. Look at the X-rays and measure where the parenchyma needs to be divided in relation to the position of the stone, the tumour, or the tuberculous lesion.

Dissect into the renal sinus, and separate the ureter and pelvis from the lower pole parenchyma. Occlude the renal artery. Take a large knife blade, and amputate the chosen part of the lower pole cleanly and carefully, so as to leave a smooth flat surface (3.40). The flat cut surface of the kidney now shows a number of small vessels cut across, some obliquely. Their

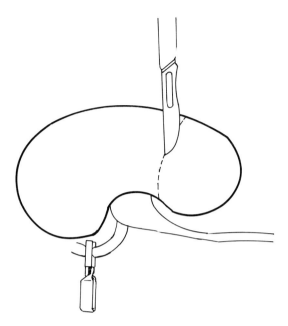

3.40. With the renal artery occluded, a clean guillotine amputation of the lower pole is performed.

mouths lie open, the arteries empty and the veins oozing a little. Every one of these open vessels is now meticulously closed with a suture ligature of 4-0 chromic catgut. Since the renal parenchyma is soft, like cheese, these sutures must be placed with great care and gentleness: a cross-stitch is placed across each vessel, and as the knot is tightened, make sure the catgut does not tear the parenchyma (3.41).

There are always several large vessels near the hilum and a number of arcuate arteries

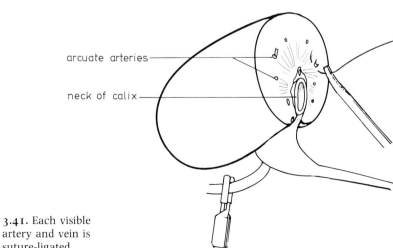

arcuate arteries

neck of calix

3.41. Each visible artery and vein is suture-ligated.

along the demarcation line between cortex and medulla. When every one of these little vessels has been closed, release the clip on the renal artery for a moment. This will show one or two vessels that escaped observation, and these too must be closed. In most cases this entire procedure takes about fifteen minutes, well within the time limit of warm ischaemia.

After the main vessels have all been secured, there is often a tiresome ooze from the cut surface. Let your assistant compress the kidney gently between finger and thumb, now compressing and now releasing it until all the remaining tiny vessels have been sutured. Apply a gauze swab to the raw surface for four minutes or so, and the bleeding will all have stopped. Close the calix with 4-0 catgut (3.42).

Note that there is no place in modern surgery for the classical 'kidney' sutures that compressed the kidney, and caused damage by

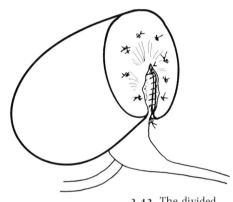

3.42. The divided caliceal neck is closed with fine catgut.

ischaemia. Nor is there any need to reflect the renal capsule and bring it over the raw surface: this invites infection under a haematoma, and risks secondary bleeding (Maddern 1967).

When performing a partial nephrectomy for a stone, it is a wise precaution to obtain a radiograph of the remaining portion of kidney before closing the wound; it is surprisingly easy to leave a fragment of stone behind.

Partial nephrectomy for tumour

Partial nephrectomy for a tumour in the renal parenchyma or renal pelvis requires more time, and one must provide some method of cooling the kidney with irrigation or slush. In a renal parenchymal tumour it is difficult to know just where the boundary of the tumour is situated, and one will need to verify naked eye appearances by a frozen section.

In planning partial nephrectomy for a localized tumour in a calix, however good the preliminary radiographs, it is wise to open the renal pelvis and examine all the lining of the collecting system before deciding just where the calix should be amputated. For this the flexible endoscope is (in my hands at least) of far more use than the rigid one, but if this instrument is not available, an excellent view of the calices may be obtained with a child's cystoscope using 0° and 70° telescopes. Occasionally this preliminary examination will reveal that the tumour is arising from a narrow pedicle and there is, in the event, no need to sacrifice any parenchyma.

Bench surgery for tumour

Challenging, exciting, and fashionable, the concept of cutting the kidney out, dealing with multifocal tumour with the assistance of an operating microscope, and then replacing it as an autotransplant, has caught the imagination of urologists all over the world. In fact the indications for such a performance are exceedingly few, for with an adequate incision everything that needs to be done to the kidney can be done on the kidney *in situ* and there is no need to cut the ureter or divide the renal vein. However, surgeons should bear in mind that this exotic procedure is an option to be thought of in the exceptional case (Wickham 1975).

Drainage after partial nephrectomy

One can only guess how many nephrons will continue to make urine from the amputated surface of the kidney and so it is essential to provide a means for this urine to get out. A drain is led from the region of the cut surface of the kidney and left in position for four days. It is then shortened and removed over the next forty-eight hours. The wound is always closed with catgut, never with non-absorbable material.

Variants of the operation

Injury to the renal artery or vein can be prevented by dissecting carefully into the renal sinus before removing either pole. Knowledge of the renal arterial anatomy and complete control over haemorrhage, thanks to early dissection of the renal artery, makes it possible to adapt the principles described above for lower pole partial nephrectomy to the removal of almost any part of the kidney. The removal

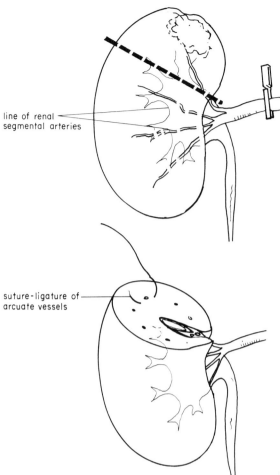

line of renal segmental arteries

suture-ligature of arcuate vessels

3.43. Upper pole partial nephrectomy.

of the upper pole, for example, is exactly the same as for the lower pole, except that particular care must be taken not to injure the main renal arterial branches in their rather oblique course (3.43). Similarly, one may remove the middle of the kidney (3.44) perfectly easily. Having chosen which bit to take out, make two guillotine incisions through the kidney, and then, after stopping all the bleeding by meticulous suture-ligature, join the two remaining portions together again (3.45).

Hazards of partial nephrectomy

In former times partial nephrectomy was notorious for giving rise to secondary haemorrhage. Maddern (1967) clearly showed that this was the result of ischaemic necrosis and haematoma that resulted from the then classic method of performing the partial nephrectomy, and the thick compression sutures employed to stop bleeding. A flat guillotine amputation and precise suture-ligature of every tiny vessel avoids this risk, and I have not had a single example of secondary haemorrhage since adopting Maddern's method more than sixteen years ago.

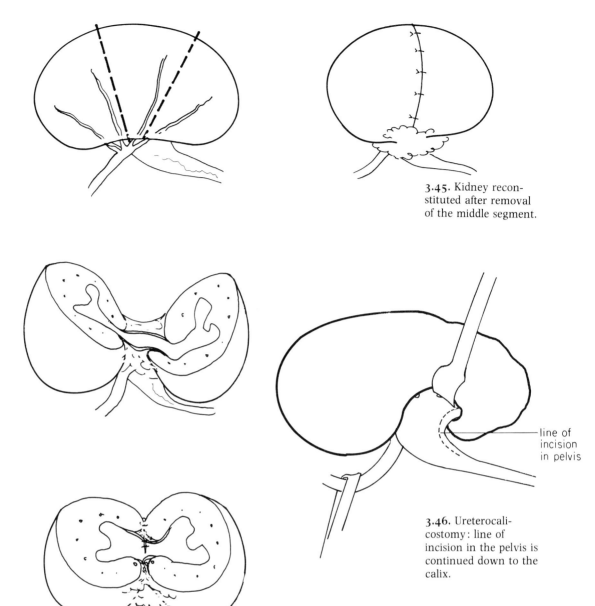

3.45. Kidney reconstituted after removal of the middle segment.

3.44. Removing the middle segment of the kidney by partial nephrectomy. Haemostasis is obtained on each cut surface before they are apposed and the renal pelvis sewn up.

line of incision in pelvis

3.46. Ureterocalicostomy: line of incision in the pelvis is continued down to the calix.

Urinary fistulae are today equally rare. If they persist longer than seven to ten days after removing the drainage tube, suspect obstruction downstream in the ureter and perform a retrograde ureterogram. If obstruction has been ruled out, then a ureteric catheter may be left *in situ* for a few days until the fistula has dried up soundly.

Ureterocalicostomy

Indications

A stone may form in a hydronephrosis as a result of narrowing at the pelviureteric junction but by the time the obstruction is present it may be difficult to know which came first,

the hydronephrosis or the stone. A formal pyeloplasty is seldom feasible because the tissues are too soggy and friable to allow a precise and accurate anastomosis. One answer to this difficulty is to anastomose the upper few centimetres of the ureter to the inferior calix. This is also very useful when an operation for hydronephrosis (done elsewhere of course) has gone wrong, and you are faced with a difficult gap between ureter and kidney, and no spare pelvis to bridge it with.

Steps of the operation

Expose and mobilize the kidney, place an arterial sling around the renal artery and ureter. Develop Gil-Vernet's plane towards the lower calix (3.46). Clear the upper few centimeters of the ureter, if necessary opening the peritoneum first. Secure the ureter down towards the pelvis and follow it up; the tissues are often very scarred and fibrous in the type of case for which ureterocalicostomy is going to be considered.

To make the incision along the lower edge of the pelvis and run it down into the ureter, first clip the renal artery to give yourself a few minutes ischaemia. Insert a right-angled forceps into the inferior calix, and cut along its groove (3.47). Now suture-ligature the cut inferior segmental artery, and pick up all the other little vessels that the incision has cut through, just as you would in a partial nephrectomy, until the incision is completely dry. The lower calix is now opened up like a book, from the renal pelvis down to the tip of the papilla (3.48). The slit-up ureter is anastomosed to the edge of the mucosa of the lining of the renal calix. Put the posterior layer of stitches in first (3.49). Try and keep the knots outside the lumen, using 3-0 or 4-0 chromic catgut. Interrupted sutures are easier to place neatly than a continuous row.

The mucosa of the lining of the calix is easy to stitch near the pelvis, but as you approach the periphery, it becomes thin and friable. Now insert a Cummings nephrostomy tube (3.50). It serves as a splint, and its long tail goes down the ureter. The anterior layer of sutures are then placed between calix and ureter (3.51). Again, it is easy to stitch the caliceal neck to the ureter, but the stitches do not hold as they approach the most peripheral part of the calix and papilla (3.52). This does not matter because the Cummings tube serves as a splint, urothelium quickly grows across any raw gap, and the scarred renal parenchyma so commonly met with in these cases holds sutures very effectively. The wound is closed in the usual way with drainage down to the anastomosis. The Cummings tube is left in position for ten to fourteen days, and the drain comes out on the fifth day.

Hazards of the operation

The main danger of ureterocalicostomy is bleeding from the incision in the lower pole of the kidney. This can be very confusing and it is therefore essential to get control of the main renal artery before making this incision.

Goodwin's operation—ileal substitution for the ureter

Indications

In a small proportion of patients nothing stops the stones from coming back when there is a

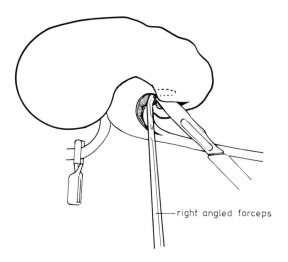

right angled forceps

3.47. With the renal artery occluded, the calix is slit down.

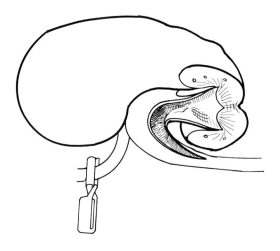

3.48. The calix is opened out; divided vessels are suture-ligated at this stage.

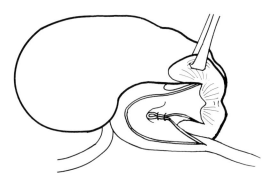

3.49. Anastomosis of the back layer of ureter to the mucosa of the calix.

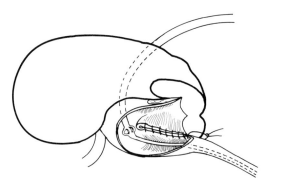

3.50. A Cummings tube is passed before the anastomosis is completed.

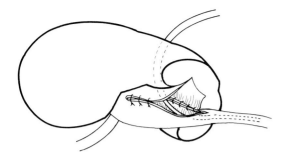

3.51. Completion of the ureterocalicostomy.

3.52. The ureter attached to the inferior pole parenchyma.

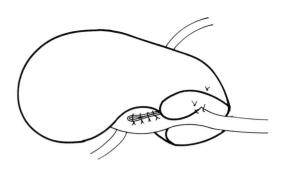

3.53. Incision for Goodwin's operation to replace ureter with ileum.

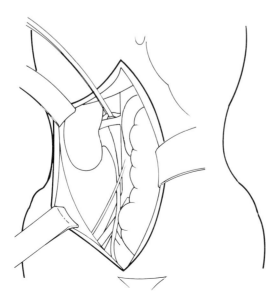

persistent and ineradicable infection with *Proteus mirabilis*. First a thick matrix of sludge appears, throwing a soft-tissue shadow in the urogram. Inexorably within the next few months the matrix calcifies and a new stag-horn stone begins to form. Sometimes the underlying problem seems to be an inability of the ureter to carry off the sludge matrix. Goodwin proposed to replace the ureter by a length of ileum so that ileal peristalsis could convey the sludge away. Goodwin's consider-able experience with this operation and our more limited series makes me recommend it, but only for exceptional cases, since it is always a big and difficult procedure, not to be lightly undertaken (Skinner & Goodwin 1975).

Special preparations

In addition to the usual preparations for a major abdominal operation, prepare four units of blood, have the bowel cleansed and pre-pared for a bowel resection and provide the usual antibiotic cover.

Position

The patient lies supine with a sandbag under the affected side.

Incision

Use a long paramedian incision from xiphi-sternum to pubis (3.53).

Steps of the operation

Entering the peritoneal cavity mobilize the colon and duodenum to expose the kidney which, in these cases, is always surrounded by very dense adhesions from previous operations. Dissect out the kidney and pass a sling around the renal artery (3.54). Make a wide incision in the renal pelvis, carrying it into the inferior calix if needs be, and make certain that there is perfect haemostasis along the incision into

3.54. Exposure of the right kidney and ureter ready for ileal replacement of the ureter. Secure the renal artery early in the dissection.

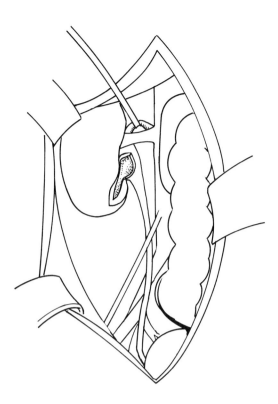

3.55. With control of the renal artery, an opening is made into the renal pelvis, and continued down into the inferior calix.

the calix as described above for ureterocalicostomy (3.55). Remove as much calculous and matrix material as possible, if necessary searching for outlying bits of sludge and stone with the flexible endoscope. In my experience it has been impossible to mobilize the whole kidney in some of these cases, and removal of the stone has had to be less than complete. Nevertheless the result has still been good.

There is no need to meddle with the ureter. It may be left *in situ*. Mobilize the colon down to the bladder. The round ligament in a female needs to be divided. The bladder is opened between stay sutures, any small bleeding vessels in its edges being secured by suture ligature. Ileum is used to bridge the gap on the right side, but on the left the descending colon is conveniently situated and easier to use.

On the right side, a loop of ileum is made in the usual way (see page 144) measuring the distance between renal pelvis and bladder, and marking this off along the bowel. Err on the generous side because it is easier to resect a little extra bowel than to try to elongate too short a segment.

Try to preserve two major branches of the superior mesenteric artery in the mesentery of the isolated ileal loop. The small bowel is made to lie without tension against the renal pelvis, and is brought behind the caecum and ascending colon (3.56).

On the left side the descending colon is mobilized, and the splenic flexure divided between ligatures, until the whole transverse

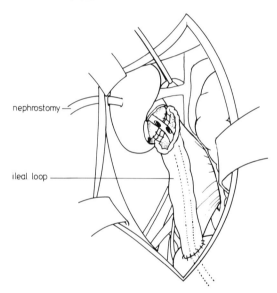

3.56. The proximal end of the ileal loop is anastomosed over a splinting nephrostomy tube, to the pelvis and inferior calix. The distal end of the loop is anastomosed to the bladder.

and descending colon is loose. A suitable length of colon is chosen, isolated on its mesentery, taking care to preserve the inferior mesenteric vessels. The transverse colon is then anastomosed to the sigmoid end-to-end with an all-coats layer to the mucosa and interrupted thread or silk to the serosa.

Each end of the chosen length of bowel is anastomosed with catgut over a suitable splint which should be brought out as a nephrostomy through the loin. Omentum is usefully added as an extra layer outside each of the anastomoses. The wound is closed in the usual way with drainage and a vesical catheter. These patients often develop rather prolonged ileus afterwards and the closure should be reinforced with tension sutures.

Hazards of the operation

The chief difficulty is in dissecting the renal pelvis for there are always dense adhesions from preceding operations and the kidney is always scarred and stiff. An anterior approach makes it possible to ensure the colon and duodenum are safe. The catheter may become blocked afterwards, with lumps of inspissated mucus, and stones may form in the bladder and need to be crushed and evacuated. Absorption of urine from the long length of bowel may give rise also to hyperchloraemic acidosis especially in the very patient most in need of this sort of operation, who starts off with less than perfect renal function. Nevertheless it stops reformation of stones and may be worthwhile when the only alternative must be dialysis and transplantation.

In the future one hopes that the Dornier extracorporeal method of dissolving calculi will make this, and other difficult and unpleasant stone operations, unnecessary.

References

Alken P., Hutschenreiter G., Gunter R. & Marberger M. (1981) Percutaneous stone manipulation. *J. Urol.* **125**, 463.

Blandy J.P. & Tresidder G.C. (1967) Extended pyelolithotomy for renal calculi. *Brit. J. Urol.* **39**, 121.

Chaussy C., Brendel W. & Schmiedt E. (1980) Extracorporeally induced destruction of kidney stones by shock waves. *Lancet*, ii, 1265.

Chaussy C., Schmiedt E. & Jocham D. (1982) First clinical experience with extracorporeally induced destruction of kidney stones by shock waves. *J. Urol.* **127**, 417.

Cook J.H. III & Lytton B. (1977) Intraoperative localization of renal calculi during nephrolithotomy by ultrasound scanning. *J. Urol.* **117**, 543.

Gil-Vernet J.M. (1964) Nuevas diectrices en la cirugia del rinon litiasico. *Annal. Med. Cirurg.* (Barcelona) **40**, 391.

Maddern J.P. (1967) Surgery of the staghorn calculus. *Brit. J. Urol.* **39**, 237.

Marshall V.R. & Blandy J.P. (1974) Simple renal hypothermia. *Brit. J. Urol.* **46**, 253.

Marshall V.R., Singh M., Tresidder G.C. & Blandy J.P. (1976) The place of partial nephrectomy in the management of renal calyceal calculi. *Brit. J. Urol.* **47**, 759.

Norris R.W., Colvin B.T., Kenwright M.G., Flynn J.T. & Blandy J.P. (1981) In vitro studies on optimum preparation of coagulum for surgery of renal calculi. *Brit. J. Urol.* **53**, 516

Petkovic S.D. (1978) Treatment of bilateral renal pelvic and ureteral tumours. A review of 45 cases. *European Urology*, **4**, 397.

Puigvert A. (1976) Partial nephrectomy for renal tumor: 21 cases. *European Urology*, **2**, 70.

Schiff M., Bagley D.H. & Lytton B. (1979) Treatment of solitary and bilateral renal carcinoma. *J. Urol.* **121**, 581.

Skinner D.G. & Goodwin W.E. (1975) Indications for the use of intestinal segments in management of nephrocalcinosis. *J. Urol.* **113**, 436.

Thuroff J.W., Frohneberg D., Riedmiller R., Alken P., Hutschenreiter G., Thuroff S. & Hohenfellner R. (1982) Localization of segmental arteries in renal surgery by Doppler sonography. *J. Urol.* **127**, 863.

Wallace D.M.A., Wallace D.M., Whitfield H.N., Hendry W.F. & Wickham J.E.A. (1981) The late results of conservative surgery for upper tract urothelial carcinomas. *Brit. J. Urol.* **53**, 537.

Wickham J.E.A. (1975) Conservative renal surgery for adenocarcinoma: the place of bench surgery. *Brit. J. Urol.* **47**, 25.

Wickham J.E.A. & Kellett M.J. (1981) Percutaneous nephrolithotomy. *Brit. med. J.* **283**, 1571.

Woodhouse C.R.J., Farrell C.R., Paris A.M.I. & Blandy J.P. (1981) The place of extended pyelolithotomy (Gil-Vernet operation) in the management of renal staghorn calculi. *Brit. J. Urol.* **53**, 520.

Chapter 4
Operations for hydronephrosis

Pyeloplasty aims to make a wide elliptical anastomosis between the ureter and the renal pelvis in such a way that the ureter drains the lowest part of the pelvis, avoids the polar vessels, and does not sacrifice parenchyma. With any anastomosis in the urinary tract the scar shortens to about one-third of its original circumference. End-to-end anastomosis is invariably followed by a pinhole stenosis and only a long ellipse will leave an adequate lumen (4.1).

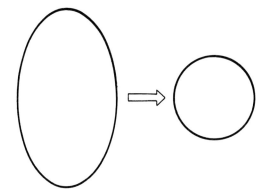

4.1. A suture line exposed to urine must be expected to contract to about one-third of its original length. To keep the lumen the same calibre, the anastomosis must begin by being made in the form of a long ellipse.

Indications and selection of method of operation

It is futile to take up a dogmatic stance and declare that any one particular operation is best for all kinds of hydronephrosis. The principles that make the Anderson–Hynes operation so successful are no different from those of Culp's operation: a wide gusset is made of surplus renal pelvis and inserted into the slit-up ureter (4.2). The Culp procedure can deal with a long stenosis in the ureter, but needs a capacious renal pelvis to provide a long flap (Culp & deWeerd 1951). When faced with a difficult case, operated on two or three times before, an anastomosis between the spatulated ureter and the inferior calix of the kidney may bridge the gap (page 57). One should feel free to select the procedure that seems most suited to the case in hand. There is no point in being dogmatic about the use of a splint or nephrostomy and much hot air has been wasted by argument over them. If the case seems to merit a splint, use one. If it does not, then do without. My own practice is to use a splint in nearly every anastomosis because, since adopting a uniform technique that involves a Cummings nephrostomy-splint, I have never lost a kidney or had to revise the anastomosis, but I am well aware that many other surgeons get excellent results without either.

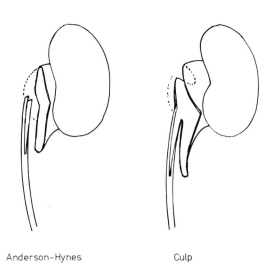

Anderson–Hynes   Culp   modified Culp

4.2. The three standard pyeloplasty methods all have in common the insertion of a long dependent ∩-shaped flap into the spatulated upper end of the ureter.

Choice of incision

Use the approach to the kidney that seems most appropriate to the case in hand. In children and slim patients with a big hydronephrosis, when the enlarged pelvis has rotated the kidney forward and down, the anterior transverse incision favoured by Anderson & Hynes (1949) avoids the need to mobilize the upper pole of the kidney, allows the suturing to be done almost at the level of the skin, and gives splendid access (4.3). On the contrary, in a thick, tough, muscular young male whose kidney is tucked up under the 12th rib, the anterior approach is difficult and the 12th rib-tip incision much easier.

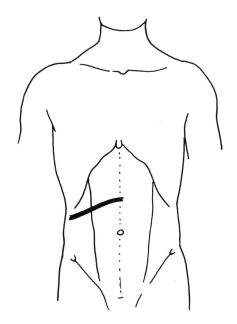

4.3. Anderson's anterior approach for pyeloplasty.

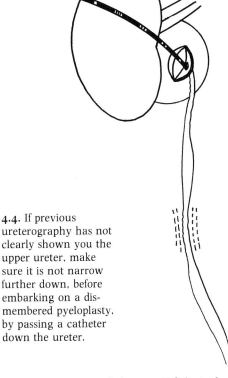

4.4. If previous ureterography has not clearly shown you the upper ureter, make sure it is not narrow further down, before embarking on a dismembered pyeloplasty, by passing a catheter down the ureter.

Steps of the operation

There has been endless debate on the advantages of the Anderson–Hynes dismembered pyeloplasty versus techniques that keep the tissues in continuity. This is entirely irrelevant. The essential feature of a pyeloplasty is a generous flap of pelvis that hangs down without tension and is long enough to enlarge the complete length of the narrow part of the ureter. Whether the ureter is cut off at the pelviureteric junction or not is of no consequence, but one must know exactly the extent of the narrow part of the ureter. This may be obvious from the pre-operative X-rays, but if the upper end of the ureter is not clearly depicted (and it seldom is in an idiopathic hydronephrosis) then a ureterogram should be made before proceeding. It is my practice to do this immediately before the operation. Even so, one may be in doubt, in which case the wise thing to do is to open the renal pelvis, and pass a small catheter down the ureter to make sure that there is no long narrow segment present near to the pelviureteric junction, or even, as is sometimes the case, lower down the ureter (4.4).

When there are large lower pole vessels you must divide the ureter at the pelviureteric junction so that the anastomosis lies in front of them. When no large lower pole vessels cross the pelviureteric junction you may choose, according to the appearances of the tissues, whether to divide the pelviureteric junction or not. The important thing is to design the flap right. In the usual Anderson–Hynes operation the apex of the flap is close to the pelviureteric junction, but this may not give a flap long enough to fill a very long

narrow segment of ureter. Culp's technique allows a much longer flap to be formed from the redundant pelvis, and there is no reason at all why one should not combine the advantages of a dismembered pyeloplasty with a long Culp flap when it seems indicated.

When there are lower pole vessels the dissection begins by separating the ureter and polar vessels, often stuck together by firm connective tissue (4.5). Narrow silicone rubber

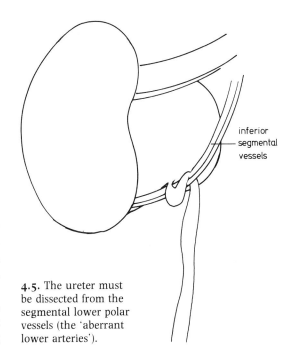

inferior segmental vessels

4.5. The ureter must be dissected from the segmental lower polar vessels (the 'aberrant lower arteries').

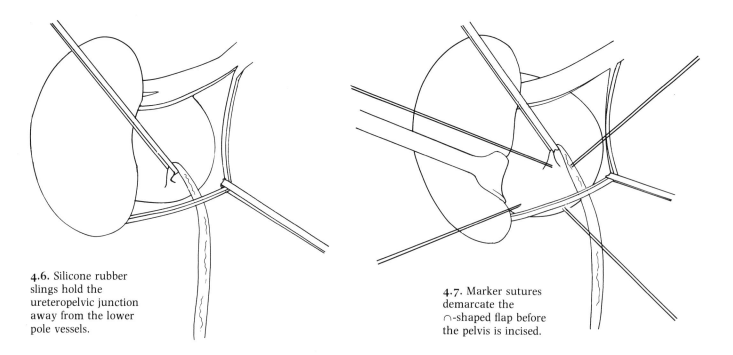

4.6. Silicone rubber slings hold the ureteropelvic junction away from the lower pole vessels.

4.7. Marker sutures demarcate the ∩-shaped flap before the pelvis is incised.

slings are useful for this dissection (4.6). Having defined the anatomy, place marker sutures before cutting off the ureter or defining the intended flap. It is a great help at this stage to fill the renal pelvis with saline using a syringe and needle. Place three marker sutures at the corners of the intended flap, and a fourth at the medial aspect of the ureter (4.7). Cut off the ureter at the pelviureteric junction and thread it in front of the lower polar vessels. Carefully dissect the pelvis clear of the thick

connective tissue adventitia which is always present. Following under this tissue leads you to Gil-Vernet's plane in the renal sinus, and it is very useful to put a Gil-Vernet retractor into this plane to bring the kidney into the wound during the subsequent anastomosis.

The flap should form a ∩-shape with a broad base and curving apex (4.8). Take care not to encroach on a calix—an easy mistake in a distended hydronephrosis. When the flap is made, the surplus renal pelvis (4.9) is left

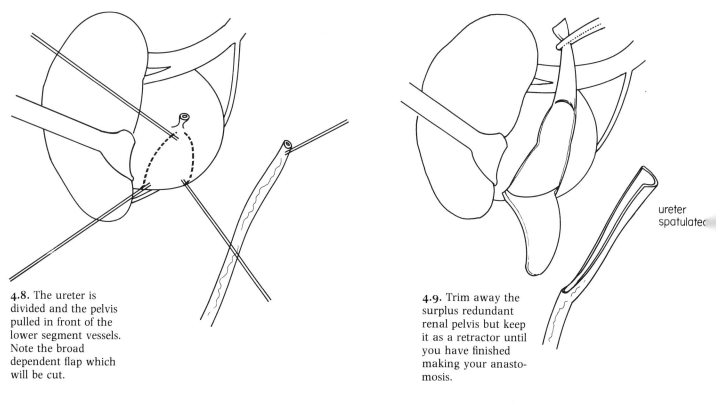

4.8. The ureter is divided and the pelvis pulled in front of the lower segment vessels. Note the broad dependent flap which will be cut.

4.9. Trim away the surplus redundant renal pelvis but keep it as a retractor until you have finished making your anastomosis.

ureter spatulated

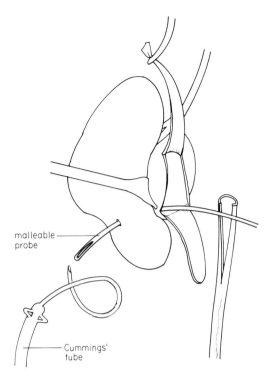

4.10. Introducing the Cummings tube through the inferior calix.

attached at its upper end to the pelvis, to serve as another useful retractor to keep the kidney up and into the wound while the anastomosis is completed.

The ureter is slit along its lateral aspect, the distance being judged according to the length of the narrow segment and the length of the flap of pelvis: ureter and pelvic flap should lie against each other without any tension at all.

Nowadays I always use a Cummings splint-cum-nephrostomy. It is introduced through the parenchyma by first passing the eye of a malleable probe from within out through the parenchyma (4.10). The tail of the Cummings tube is stitched to the eye and drawn through the parenchyma of the kidney into the renal pelvis. The wings of the Malecot part of the Cummings tube are now pulled straight and it is brought into the pelvis. The tail is passed down the ureter.

The anastomosis is made in a single layer of continuous 4-0 chromic catgut. Following the advice of Anderson & Hynes, the suture is started a little way from the apex of the flap, and the slit in the ureter, so that this, the most important part of the anastomosis, does not lie adjacent to a knot. The knot is put on the outside of the anastomosis. The ureteric tail of the Cummings tube prevents inadvertent catching-up of the opposite side of the ureter (4.11). The suture line is not drawn up too tightly, and from time to time it should be locked so that the anastomosis cannot bunch up. Once round the apex of the flap a second catgut suture is started (4.12). The defect in

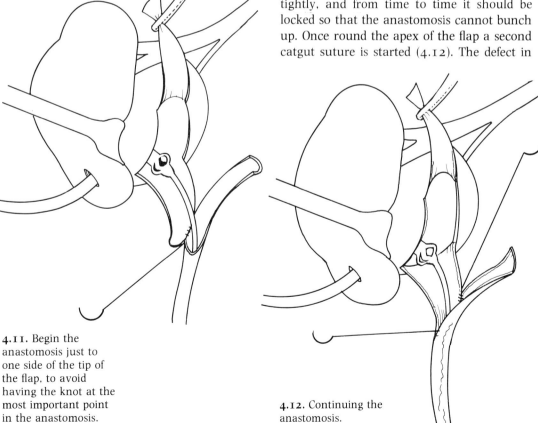

4.11. Begin the anastomosis just to one side of the tip of the flap, to avoid having the knot at the most important point in the anastomosis.

4.12. Continuing the anastomosis.

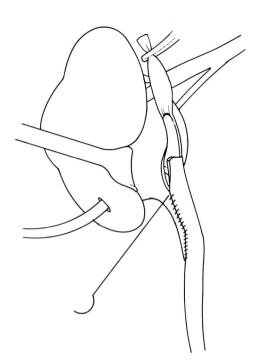

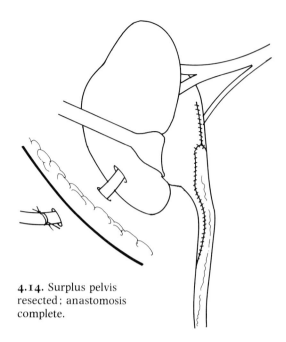

4.13. Completing the front row of the anastomosis.

4.14. Surplus pelvis resected; anastomosis complete.

the pelvis is closed only after thoroughly washing all clots out with a bulb syringe (4.13). Check that the Cummings tube is patent with a syringe, bring it out through a separate stab, and stitch it securely to the skin before doing anything else (4.14). Close the wound in layers with catgut, leaving a drain to the vicinity of the anastomosis.

Culp pyeloplasty

In the Culp pyeloplasty a long dependent flap is fashioned from the redundant pelvis by taking the incision obliquely across the pelvis, if necessary going round the corner on to its posterior wall. This is particularly suited to patients with a long narrow segment in the upper end of the ureter (4.15, 4.16). It can be perfectly well combined with dismemberment of the pelviureteric junction; the principle is the shape and plan of the flap, not the dismemberment! The important decision that must be made is whether or not you need to take the flap up on to the upper part of the pelvis, for a flap cut in the Anderson–Hynes shape cannot be extended. The diagrams show

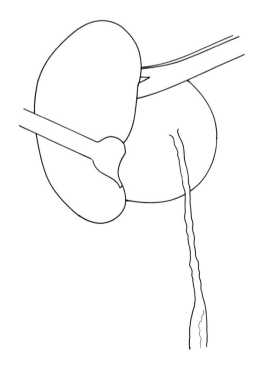

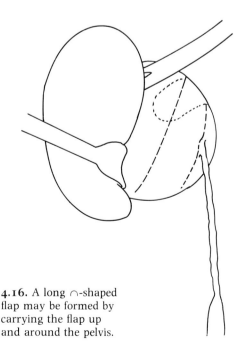

4.15. Culp anastomosis for a longer narrow segment at the upper end of the ureter.

4.16. A long ∩-shaped flap may be formed by carrying the flap up and around the pelvis.

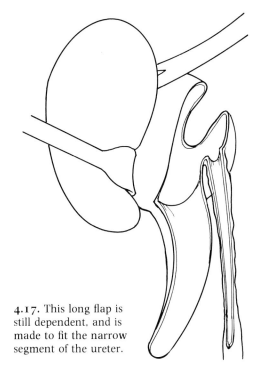

4.17. This long flap is still dependent, and is made to fit the narrow segment of the ureter.

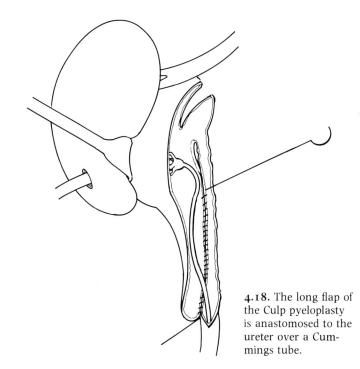

4.18. The long flap of the Culp pyeloplasty is anastomosed to the ureter over a Cummings tube.

better than words why one must decide early on in the dissection how the flap is to be designed before you start to cut it out (4.17, 4.18).

Once the flap has been formed, the rest of the anastomosis is exactly as described above for the usual Anderson–Hynes operation (4.19, 4.20).

Hazards of the operation

A small tear in the peritoneum may be made when the kidney is approached from the an-

terior incision. It is of little consequence, and indeed in children many paediatric surgeons routinely approach the hydronephrosis across the peritoneal cavity.

When the lower pole vessels are damaged the pole will be infarcted, with the risk of a urinary fistula early in the post-operative period and of hypertension as a late sequel. These lower pole vessels do not cause pelvi-ureteric obstruction though they may sometimes make it worse. Dividing the vessels together with ureterolysis used to be a method of dealing with hydronephrosis and was some-

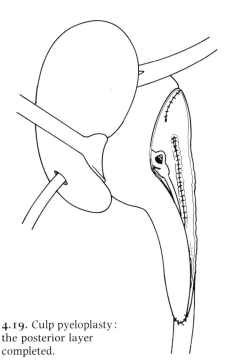

4.19. Culp pyeloplasty: the posterior layer completed.

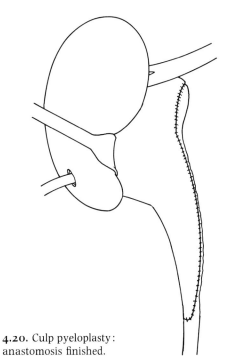

4.20. Culp pyeloplasty: anastomosis finished.

times successful, but carried an unacceptable risk of hypertension and fistula (Notley 1976).

Clots left behind in the pelvis may pass down the ureter and give rise to colic, but this is of no importance as long as there is a nephrostomy in position.

It is our practice to leave the nephrostomy tube in position for ten days and then clamp it. If the patient has no pain or fever, the nephrostomy is removed. If there is a persistent leak of urine or pain or fever, a 'nephrostogram' may be obtained to make sure there is no leakage from the anastomosis, but it really is not necessary in every case.

Ureterocalicostomy

In a revision pyeloplasty dense adhesions in the vicinity of the lower pole of the kidney may rule out any attempt at a new flap pyeloplasty. Direct anastomosis of the upper end of the ureter to the lower calix (page 57) may save a kidney. The secret of this operation is to secure the renal artery as the first step in the dissection.

Davis' intubated ureterotomy

Davis (1943) demonstrated that a long narrow segment of ureter could be slit up, splinted, and allowed to regenerate around the splint in such a way that a new ureter of adequate calibre would be formed. Two points about this operation are crucial to success. First, the material used for the splint must be inert. Red rubber will provoke an intense fibrosis followed by stricture, and many plastics contain plasticizers and anti-oxidants that are no less toxic. Second, the tube must be left in long enough not only for connective tissue to grow around the tube, but for it to mature and finish contracting. Otherwise the sheath that is formed around the splint will shrink and stenosis will return. The splint should therefore be made of silicone rubber, and should be kept in position for at least six weeks. Today the double-J tube type of indwelling splint offers an ideal solution to the problem: it is placed in position at operation, and protected by a nephrostomy for two weeks. After the nephrostomy is removed, the patient is allowed to go home, to be readmitted eight weeks later for the double-J tube to be removed (4.21, 4.22).

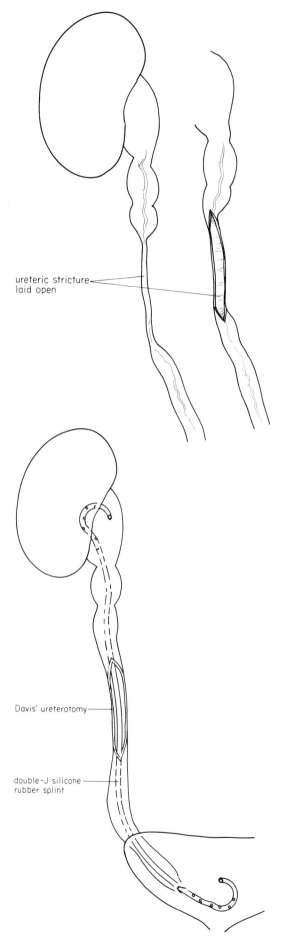

ureteric stricture laid open

4.21. Davis' intubated ureterotomy. The ureteric stenosis is incised for its complete length.

Davis' ureterotomy

double-J silicone rubber splint

4.22. Davis' intubated ureterotomy. Nowadays a double-J silicone splint is passed up and down the entire length of the ureter, and left *in situ* for a minimum of six weeks.

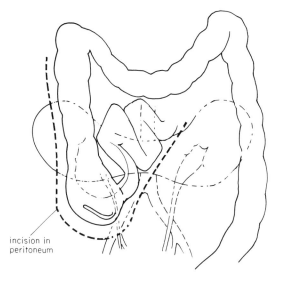

4.23. Exposure of a horseshoe kidney. The peritoneum is incised along the lateral border of the right colon, and along the line of the mesentery.

incision in peritoneum

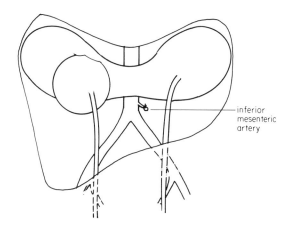

4.24. Retracting the bowel upwards displays the entire extent of the horseshoe kidney. Note that it may be necessary to divide the inferior mesenteric artery between ligatures.

inferior mesenteric artery

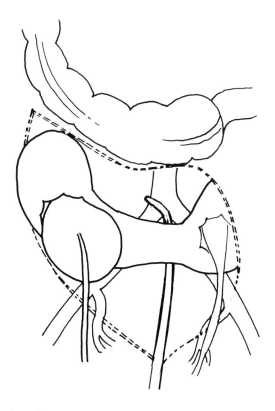

4.25. The isthmus lies in front of the aorta and cava and is easily separated if it must be divided to get at the aorta. The isthmus is quite irrelevant to hydro-nephrosis associated with horseshoe kidney.

Hydronephrosis in a horseshoe kidney

Although horseshoe kidneys are fairly common, and cause no trouble unless access is needed to the aorta for an aneurysm, they tend to be associated with other congenital anomalies in the urinary tract, especially pelviureteric junction obstruction. The obstruction to the pelviureteric junction is situated well away from the isthmus, and the isthmus has nothing whatever to do with the obstruction.

Exposure of the horseshoe kidney

One must make a generous incision to expose a horseshoe kidney in its entirety. When, as is often the case, both sides need to be dealt with, the entire kidneys must be exposed. To do this make a very long transverse or midline incision (4.23). Mobilize the intestines by dividing the reflexion of the peritoneum along the ascending colon, and continue this incision along the left side of the mesentery until the small and large bowel can be lifted out of the abdomen and laid in a protective moist pack on the chest (4.24).

The arrangement of arteries of a horseshoe kidney is often strange and puzzling to the surgeon. Graves (1971) has pointed out that they are in fact the standard five segmental arteries of the normal kidney, but that they come off unexpected great vessels including the aorta and common iliacs. Not uncommonly one or more of these arteries may seem to be closely related to the pelviureteric junctions (Castro & Green 1975).

The dissection of the pelviureteric junctions and the formation of a suitably shaped Anderson–Hynes or Culp type of flap is no different in a horseshoe kidney than a normal one. The anastomoses are made over Cummings tubes in the usual way, and the site of anastomosis is protected by a drain (4.25). After completion of the anastomoses the bowel is carefully replaced and secured in its correct anatomical position with a few 3-0 catgut sutures. There is no need to repair the peritomeal incisions exactly. Merely make sure the bowel is correctly positioned and the peritoneum will look after itself.

Retrocaval ureter

By a curious irony this, the rarest of all causes of hydronephrosis, was what made Anderson & Hynes devise their procedure.

There is an excess of renal pelvis, and no difficulty in finding tissue to bridge the gap.

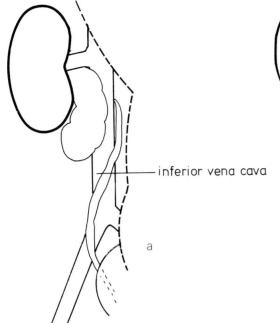

inferior vena cava

a

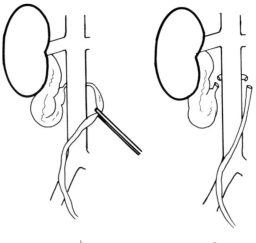

b c

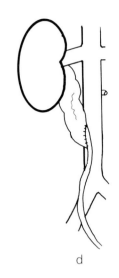

d

The segment of ureter behind the vena cava is quite useless, and no time should be wasted in trying to fish it out from behind the vena cava (Feldman *et al.* 1982).

Through an appropriate long transverse or paramedian incision mobilize the right colon medially. Find the lower part of the ureter and pass a sling around it. Dissect the upper bulging pelvis until it disappears down behind the inferior vena cava (4.26). Cut it off there. You now have a normal distal ureter and a huge excess of proximal renal pelvis. Fashion a long elliptical flap from the excess pelvis and anastomose it over a Cummings tube to the spatulated lower part of the ureter.

4.26. (a) Retrocaval ureter. Disregard the atretic segment behind the cava but (b) dissect each end of the ureter where it goes behind the cava and (c) cut it off there, leaving the atretic segment *in situ*; (d) a long elliptical anastomosis is made to join the ureter together again.

Nephrectomy for hydronephrosis

In a bulky hydronephrosis the renal parenchyma may be reduced to a mere shell of useless tissue, in which perhaps infection has destroyed the remaining vestige of function. In setting out to remove such a kidney do not try to get it out intact and entire. First, make the smallest incision that will allow safe access to the kidney shell (4.27). Aspirate the contents with trochar and sucker to reduce its bulk to a shrivelled-up crumpled bag, a fraction of its former size. Deliver the empty bag

4.27. Nephrectomy for hydronephrosis. (a) Empty the sac first with trochar and aspirating cannula which will reduce its bulk (b) and make it easy to remove through a relatively small incision (c).

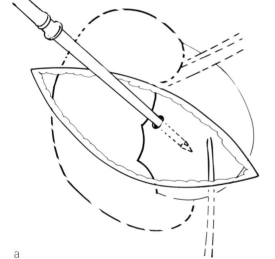

a

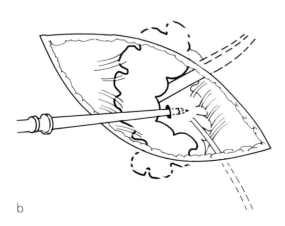

b

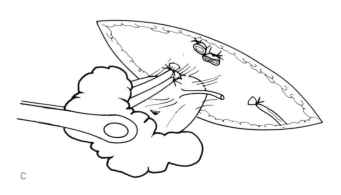

c

into the wound, secure the blood supply with double catgut ligatures, and close the incision with an appropriate drain.

If the kidney is infected, that is a pyonephrosis, the procedure is more safely performed in stages. First, the pyonephrosis is drained with a percutaneous nephrostomy tube and then, after a suitable interval, the nephrectomy is performed. On one occasion I aspirated more than four litres of pus from a giant hydronephrosis, left in a tube for a month, and was then able to remove the useless remnants of kidney through a small and inconspicuous incision.

Nephrostomy

Indications

Today there are very few indications for a formal open nephrostomy, thanks to the introduction of percutaneous methods (4.28). Every urologist should make himself master of

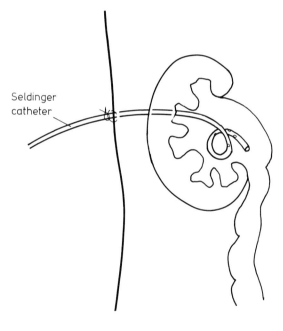

Seldinger catheter

4.28. Percutaneous nephrostomy.

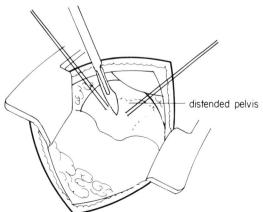

distended pelvis

4.29. Nephrostomy: open the renal pelvis between stay sutures.

this simple technique. Under radiological control, a fine needle is introduced into the kidney under local anaesthetic. Through the needle a Seldinger wire is passed, the needle withdrawn, and a suitable catheter slid over the Seldinger wire to lodge in the kidney. Even if very thick pus is present, repeated aspiration and irrigation will usually allow effective drainage to take place, and avoid the need for an open operation.

Open nephrostomy

Through a short 12th rib-tip approach to the kidney, open Gerota's fascia, retract the peritoneum forward, and feel the distended tense kidney under your finger. Very occasionally the renal cortex is paper thin, and all that is needed is to introduce a trochar and cannula directly into the distended bag of pus, insert a catheter, and close the wound.

Unfortunately, in most cases where a formal nephrostomy is needed, this cannot be done, and blind attempts to force a catheter into the lumen of the renal pelvis from outside may well enter the plane between calices and parenchyma rather than the collecting system itself.

Hence in most cases it is better to spend a little time deliberately identifying the renal pelvis: roll the kidney towards you; clear the pelvis of its surrounding often very stiff and oedematous tissue; insert two stay sutures and open the pelvis between them (4.29). Now pass a right-angled forceps (or a probe with an eye) through the renal parenchyma from within outwards, seize a Malecot catheter, and bring it into the pelvis of the kidney (4.30).

Ring nephrostomy

For a permanent nephrostomy, Tresidder's loop technique has the advantage that it allows the tube to be changed easily (4.31) but it does call for a greater dissection of the kidney. Pass a forceps through the upper calix and draw a polyethylene tube into the pelvis. Pass the forceps through the inferior calix and draw in a second tube. Sew the two tubes together, and use one to draw the other out through the inferior calix. A side hole in the middle of the polyethylene tube is adjusted to lie in the middle of the renal pelvis, which is now closed. Each end of the polyethylene tube is brought out, in an even half-circle, through a separate stab incision in the skin and secured there with a suture. The ends of the polyethylene tube are attached to a Y-connection

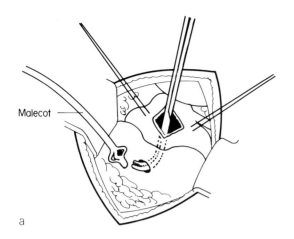

Malecot

a

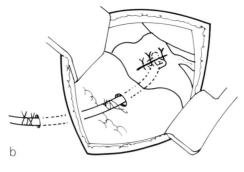

b

4.30. The right-angled forceps grasps the nephrostomy tube and draws it into the renal pelvis (a), where it is sutured (b).

leading to a sterile collecting bag.

When the time comes to change the tube, a second tube of identical length is prepared. Measure off the length of protruding tubing, attach the new tube to the old, and use the old one to draw in the new until it occupies exactly the position of its predecessor.

References

Anderson J.C. & Hynes W. (1949) Retrocaval ureter; case diagnosed preoperatively and treated successfully by plastic operation. *Brit. J. Urol.* **21**, 209.

Castro J.E. & Green N.A. (1975) Complications of horseshoe kidney. *Urology*, **6**, 344.

Culp O.S. & DeWeerd J.H. (1951) A pelvic flap operation for certain types of ureteropelvic obstruction: preliminary report. *Mayo Clinic Proceedings*, **26**, 483.

Davis D.M. (1943) Intubated ureterotomy; a new operation for ureteral and ureteropelvic stricture. *Surgery Gynecology Obstetrics*, **76**, 513.

Feldman S.L., DiMarco E.R., Tencer T. & Ross L.S. (1982) Retrocaval ureter; radiographic techniques directing surgical management. *Brit J. Urol.* **54**, 212.

Graves F.T. (1971) *The arterial anatomy of the kidney.* Wright, Bristol.

Notley R.G. (1976) Anatomy and physiology of the ureter. In *Urology* (ed. by Blandy J.P.), p. 568. Blackwell Scientific Publications, Oxford.

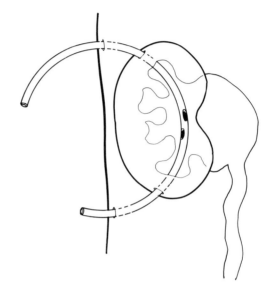

4.31. Tresidder's ring nephrostomy.

Chapter 5
Operations on the renal artery and vein

Indications

Few topics in contemporary urology are more controversial than the right indications to operate on the renal artery for *renal artery stenosis*. Just as the introduction of digital subtraction imaging techniques has made it possible to detect renal artery stenosis with minimum disturbance to the patient, the advent of the technique of forcibly dilating narrowed renal arteries with a balloon passed under radiographic control challenges the traditional position of open reconstructive techniques for treating stenosis of the renal artery (Castaneda-Zuniga *et al.* 1980; Tegtmeyer *et al.* 1980).

Renal artery aneurysm poses similar problems. Instead of the strongly held opinion that all these aneurysms should be operated on in case they burst (Charron *et al.* 1975), more recent reports suggest that only those greater

than 2.0 cm in diameter need be treated (Hubert *et al.* 1980). Often when the other kidney is healthy, a nephrectomy is the best procedure.

Exposure of the renal vessels

Special preparations

Anticipate loss of blood and have at least four units cross matched. Most patients are already on anti-hypertensive medication and the anaesthetist will need to take due notice of the ganglion-blocking agents that are being used, and if necessary, discontinue them for a few days before operation. Facilities for measuring the fall in pressure across the stenosis will be needed, as well as flow-meters that can be applied outside the vessels. Means of cooling the kidney are required, and if a prolonged dissection of the renal artery is anticipated, ice-cold perfusion fluid should be made available with which to preserve the kidney as for transplantation.

Position on the table

The patient is supine, with a sandbag under the affected side. Prepare the skin over each thigh in case the saphenous veins need to be used for grafting.

Incision

Either a high transverse or a long paramedian approach can be used according to the build of the patient.

Mobilization of the bowel

As already described (page 25) for carcinoma, the bowel is reflected by dividing the peritoneum along the lateral border of the colon. Divide the splenocolic and hepatocolic ligaments. On the right side, continue the incision along the left side of the mesentery to allow the small bowel to be swung out of the abdomen (5.1).

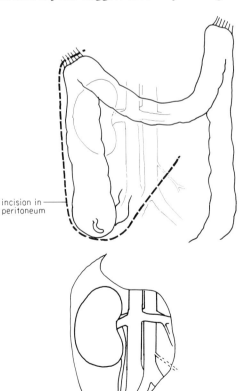

incision in peritoneum

5.1. Exposure of the right renal artery. The peritoneum along the right side of the colon and mesentery is incised, and the bowel displaced medially to expose the right renal artery.

Dissection of the renal vessels

On the *right* side, the origin of the renal artery is found by lifting up the left renal vein, and searching between the vena cava and the aorta (5.2). The distal part of the right renal artery is found under the right renal vein which must be mobilized and retracted out of the way.

On the *left* side, the left renal vein is dissected off the front of the aorta and held up in a sling (5.3). If the adrenal and gonadal veins are divided between ligatures the dissection is made more safe and easy. The left renal vein is retracted down to display the left renal artery where it springs off the side of the aorta, under a stiff sheath of fibrofatty tissue that must be carefully dissected away. Each small vessel must be carefully sealed to avoid an ooze that may obscure the rest of the operation.

Renal artery stenosis

What can be done depends upon the state of the other kidney, the general condition of the patient, and the exact anatomy of the stenosis (Davies & Kapila 1983). Sometimes nephrectomy may be best for the particular patient on the table. Sometimes it will be better to enlarge the stenosed segment by a patch, or to bypass the obstruction. A patch will not suit a long series of stenoses extending to the branches of the artery, and a bypass operation needs a healthy distal lumen to the artery if there is to be a good run-off. It may be impossible to come to a decision without measuring the renal arterial blood flow, and it will certainly be necessary to measure it after reconstruction to ensure that the flow has been improved.

Bypass operations

Splenic artery

The splenic artery is usually supple and free from atheroma. For a short stenosis at the origin of the left renal artery with a healthy distal artery, the splenic artery can be anastomosed end-to-end to the renal artery. Mobilize the spleen just sufficiently to gain access to the splenic artery (5.4). Ligate the distal branches of the splenic artery, and place a DeBakey clamp across its proximal end. The artery is now gently mobilized until it can be apposed without tension to the renal artery. There is no need to remove the spleen. Ligate the renal artery near its origin, and trim away the offending atheromatous tissue until healthy

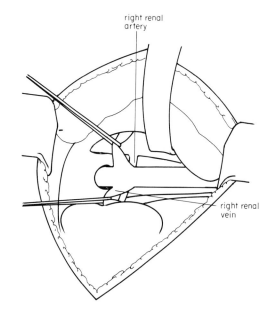

5.2. Exposure of the right renal vessels.

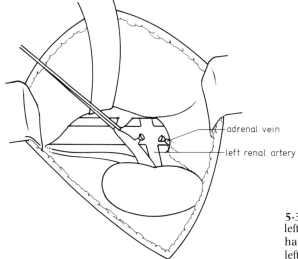

5.3. Exposure of the left renal vessels, having retracted the left renal vein.

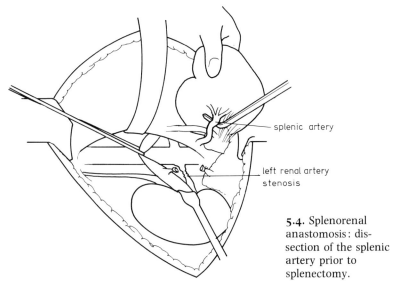

5.4. Splenorenal anastomosis: dissection of the splenic artery prior to splenectomy.

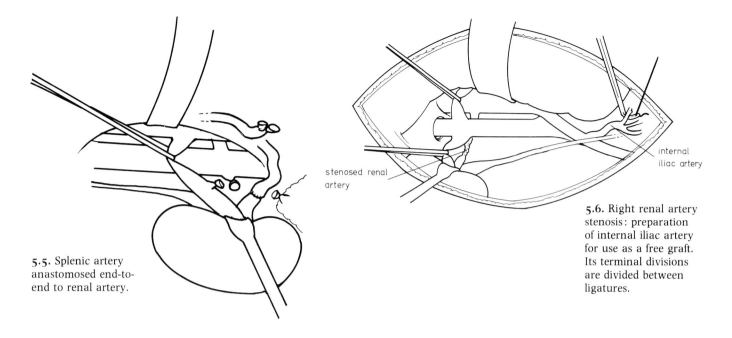

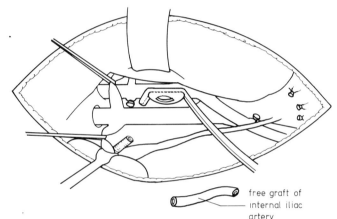

5.5. Splenic artery anastomosed end-to-end to renal artery.

5.6. Right renal artery stenosis: preparation of internal iliac artery for use as a free graft. Its terminal divisions are divided between ligatures.

5.7. The renal artery prepared to receive the free graft of internal iliac artery, which will be anastomosed to a hole cut in the side of the aorta, held in a Satinsky clamp.

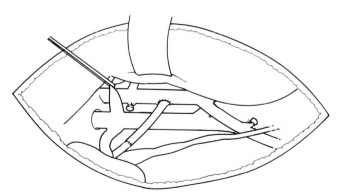

5.8. Completion of internal iliac artery by-pass graft, between side of aorta and end of renal artery.

renal arterial lumen is found. After irrigating both ends with heparinized saline, anastomose the splenic to the renal artery with 5-0 Tevdek or silk (5.5).

Internal iliac artery

A segment of internal iliac artery makes a useful by-pass for the renal artery (5.6). Divide the internal iliac artery close to its origin from the common iliac artery. Trim the terminal branches from the segment of internal iliac artery and irrigate it with heparinized saline. Then sew one end to the side of the aorta, which is held in a Satinsky or DeBakey clamp (5.7) while the other end is anastomosed to the renal artery end-to-end or end-to-side (5.8).

Saphenous vein

The saphenous vein may also be used to bridge the gap between aorta and renal artery. It is exposed through a vertical incision in the thigh, its tributaries all carefully individually ligated. The vein is distended with heparinized saline, and all the adventitia trimmed away. Being certain that the vein is reversed, to prevent the venous valves acting as an obstruction, the upper end of the vein is anastomosed to the side of the aorta and the lower end to the renal artery.

Dacron or Gortex

A Dacron or Gortex prosthesis may be used to bridge the gap between aorta and renal artery.

Patch grafts

Stenosis of the renal artery in its course, or at its origin from the aorta can be dealt with by means of a patch. Multiple narrow zones, seen in fibromuscular stenosis, which extend right out into the kidney, are unsuited to this type of reconstruction. A patch is conveniently taken from the saphenous vein, trimmed to size, and sutured into the opened-out renal artery (5.9, 5.10).

Autotransplantation

There have been numerous accounts of lesions of the renal artery which have been dealt with by dividing the renal artery distal to the obstructed part, and joining it on to the internal iliac artery as in an ordinary transplant. In such operations the renal vein is reunited to the external iliac vein, but there is no need to divide or reimplant the ureter. Care is of course taken to make sure that the new course of the ureter does not become kinked (see page 99).

Renal artery aneurysms

Nephrectomy may be the best way to deal with a large and complex aneurysm in the middle of the kidney. From time to time an aneurysm is found in the line of a segmental artery for which partial nephrectomy is easily performed, as described on page 54. Partial nephrectomy is also suited to an aneurysm on one of the segmental arteries supplying the middle of the kidney. First, a dissection is made into the renal sinus, having secured the main renal artery in a sling. The segmental branches are dissected out, and the artery supplying the aneurysm ligated. When the blanched segment of the kidney has become clearly demarcated and shows exactly which part of the kidney should be removed, a partial nephrectomy is performed removing the ischaemic part of the parenchyma along with the aneurysm, and the remainder of the kidney is reconstructed. Extra time is afforded by cooling the kidney.

Sometimes an aneurysm forms a saccular dilatation on the main renal artery, extending along one or more of its segmental branches. In such patients the renal vascular system can be reconstructed, but will need time. There is no need to remove the entire kidney to a bench. The main renal artery can be divided, reconstructed and remodelled. Excess aneurysmal tissue may be trimmed away and the branches modelled over a suitable catheter. The kidney can be perfused (if the vein is

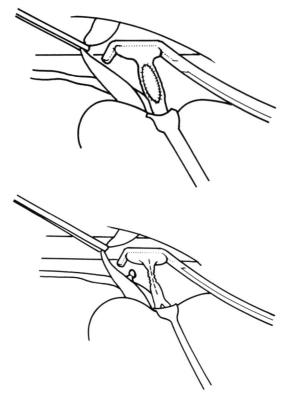

5.9. Left renal artery stenosis: line of incision for patchplasty.

5.10. Vein graft used as patch for renal artery.

divided) as for a transplant; it can be cooled by Marshall's method or by the use of iceslush (page 50). Only very exceptionally is there any need to perform 'bench surgery'.

Hazards of renovascular operations

In addition to the complications of any operation involving displacement of bowel and prolonged retraction, one must anticipate deterioration in renal function, leading to acute tubular necrosis, unless care is taken to protect the kidney by hypothermia. Unless facilities are available for post-operative dialysis, reconstruction of the renal vessels should probably be referred to centres that are so equipped.

References

Castaneda-Zuniga, Formanek A., Tadavarthy M., Vlodaver Z., Zollikofer C. & Amplatz K. (1980) Mechanism of balloon angioplasty. *Radiology*, **135**, 565.

Charron J., Belanger R., Vauclair R., Leger C. & Razavi A. (1975) Renal artery aneurysm. *Urology*, **5**, 1.

Davies R. & Kapila H. (1983) Investigation of hypertension. *Brit. J. Hosp. Med.* **29**, 428.

Hubert J.P., Pairolevero P.C. & Kazmier F.J. (1980) Solitary renal artery aneurysm. *Surgery*, **88**, 557.

Tegtmeyer C.J., Dyer R., Teates C.D., Ayers C.R., Carey R.M., Wellons H.A. & Stanton L.W. (1980) Percutaneous transluminal dilatation of the renal arteries: techniques and results. *Radiology*, **135**, 589.

Chapter 6
Renal transplantation

Transplantation should be thought of by every doctor concerned with the management of patients who are likely to die without cancer, infection, or severe hypertension. In practice today patients who die after multiple road accidents, severely injured, with severe hypotension, are unsuitable donors. Nowadays the main source of kidneys for transplantation are the medical teams taking care of young people with isolated head injuries or subarachnoid haemorrhage. The dangers of transplantation are multiplied if kidneys do not function soon after transplantation because then it is difficult to distinguish rejection from vascular obstruction or tubular necrosis. One tends to treat patients for rejection with increasing doses of immunosuppressive agents, thus increasing the hazards of haemorrhage and peptic ulceration. Many transplant teams consider it unethical to graft kidneys *not* obtained from patients with a beating heart. Legislation to make it possible to remove kidneys from patients with cerebral death, subject to certain wise and sensible safeguards, are now in general use, for Great Britain at least, where they are set out in an admirable pamphlet 'Cadaveric Organs for Transplantation, 1983'.

Since cadaveric kidneys are now virtually all obtained from 'brain dead' cadaver donors, the rules for the diagnosis of brain death must be carefully followed. The rules are now clearly codified: two senior doctors unconnected with the transplant team must satisfy themselves that certain criteria for brain death have been met. These include the following: checking for reaction of pupils to light, corneal reflexes, movements of the eyes on caloric testing, motor responses in cranial nerve distribution in response to stimulation of face, limbs or trunk, and gag and cough reflexes. There are stringent precautions to rule out reversible causes of coma that include allowing sufficient time to elapse before considering the diagnosis of brain death. Carefully drawn-up check lists are now available, and should be followed scrupulously by those concerned with removing cadaver kidneys. In particular, the surgeon on the transplant team must know that his responsibility includes making sure by personal examination of the body that the patient is dead, and that the coroner has given consent where his consent is necessary.

Many transplant surgical teams offer to speak to the relatives when they have been told by the doctors in charge of the patient's treatment that their loved one is dead, as they sometimes find it easier to undertake this harrowing but necessary task. Today it is rare to meet refusal on the part of the relatives, and when it is encountered it is essential not to bring any pressure to bear upon people already overwrought and distressed. The transplant surgeon must use the utmost tact when discussing the matter with his clinical colleagues, who are themselves often emotionally concerned with the dead patient, frequently reproaching themselves, consciously or unconsciously, for having failed to save a life. It is never easy: many a kidney has been forfeited by a reluctance on the part of the distressed doctors to contemplate the possibility of transplantation.

Special precautions

Prolonged hypotension, anuria, cancer, infection, and evidence of renal disease may make kidneys unusable. Be specially careful of the potential donor who has died of a subarachnoid haemorrhage: the kidneys may be polycystic. Make gentle enquiry as to whether the kidneys were palpable prior to death. Pretreatment of the donor in times past gave rise to misgivings on the part of those involved in renal transplantation. The very sensible rules laid down by the Working Party in 'Cadaveric Organs for Transplantation' have cleared some of the worries and confusions on this score. They point out that:

'The maintenance of normal homeostasis, by ensuring adequate fluid intake, normal blood pressure and the monitoring of urine output by catheter collection, is part of the standard medical care of the patient where brain death has not been conclusively established. It is also important to maintain the function of organs for transplantation.

After a patient is dead there is no legal objection to administering any drugs necessary to maintain the condition of the organs or to conducting the necessary diagnostic tests.

Sometimes a patient thought to have irreversible brain damage, and who would be a suitable donor, stops breathing before it has been possible to make the necessary enquiries. In most cases of this kind brain death will not yet have been diagnosed and it will not be possible to say with certainty that it will inevitably occur. In such cases initiation of artificial ventilation as part of resuscitation is justified because it is of potential benefit for the patient.'

Different transplant units have different views about the best way to prepare the cadaver before the kidneys are removed. All agree that the cadaver should be well-hydrated and many would advise administration of an alpha-blocker, for example phenoxybenzamine.

Equally, all agree that as blood is being taken anyway for various tests relevant to the treatment of the patient, it is not unethical to ask that blood should be sent for tissue typing and hepatitis antigen determination at the earliest possible moment.

For HLA antigen determination 10 ml of blood are taken into a plain glass bottle which is defibrinated by being gently twirled for ten minutes. This is better than having it taken into a heparinized tube. The blood is sent as rapidly as possible to the nearest HLA laboratory for determination of the HLA and blood group antigens.

Removal of the cadaver kidney is performed in a sterile operating room by a fully scrubbed transplant surgical team who need a full set of instruments and as much light and assistance as for any major operation.

Cadaver donor nephrectomy *en bloc*

A long midline incision from xiphisternum to pubis may be extended by a transverse incision if necessary to get extra exposure (6.1). Haemostasis is obtained step by step with artery forceps and diathermy. The entire bowel is now carefully mobilized: there is no need for haste today in removing cadaver kidneys. Circulation and respiration are maintained throughout the procedure.

Mobilize the right colon fully, and continue

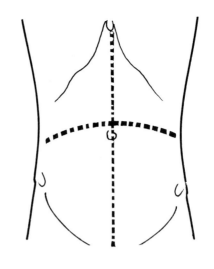

6.1. *En-bloc* removal of the kidneys: the cruciform incision.

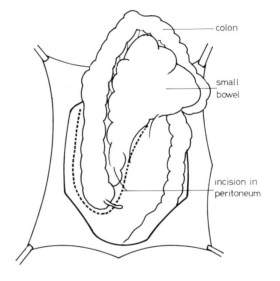

6.2. Mobilization of the bowel by dividing the peritoneum over the colon and medial to the mesentery of the small bowel. The inferior mesenteric artery is divided between ligatures.

the incision along the left side of the mesentery. Divide the inferior mesenteric artery between ligatures, to allow the entire small bowel and the right and transverse colon to be brought out of the abdomen and placed on the chest and covered with a large pack (6.2).

The superior mesenteric vessels are now doubly clamped and divided. Both ends are ligated with strong thread (6.3). The aorta above the origin of the superior mesenteric artery is now followed up and the coeliac axis similarly clamped and divided (6.4). Now a large curved aortic clamp is gently passed around the aorta, as high as possible, and left open. A second aortic clamp is placed across the aorta well below the renal vessels but above its bifurcation and closed. The first aortic clamp is closed. Ice-cold Marshall's solution, which has been prepared and attached to a giving set, is now brought near. The lower end of the aorta is cut through, the cannula containing the perfusate inserted into the aorta, and a clamp applied. Now the kidneys are perfused *in situ* (6.5).

6.3. Retracting the bowel upwards displays the superior mesenteric artery which is divided between ligatures.

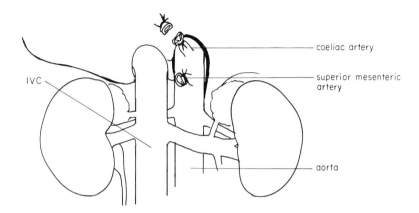

superior mesenteric artery

crura

6.4. Cadaveric transplant nephrectomy. The superior mesenteric artery and coeliac artery are divided between ligatures.

coeliac artery

superior mesenteric artery

IVC

aorta

6.5. Cadaveric transplant nephrectomy. After cross-clamping the aorta, ice-cold Marshall's solution is run in through a Foley catheter tied into the aorta.

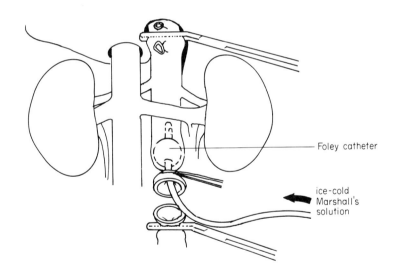

Foley catheter

ice-cold Marshall's solution

A pair of clamps are similarly placed on the vena cava above and below the renal veins. The entire block of tissue, containing kidneys, ureters, cava and aorta, is removed from the cadaver by dividing the lumbar arteries and veins to which they remain attached (6.6).

The pair of kidneys are now perfused until the effluent from the cava is blood free. The kidneys are separated by dividing the aorta in the sagittal plane and the cava similarly. Large lumps of adherent fat are removed. The renal arteries and veins are carefully in-

spected, and note made of the presence of more than one on each side for the future transplant.

A lymph node and a 3 cm cube of spleen are also removed for purposes of tissue typing. Each kidney, carefully labelled, is inserted in a pair of sterile nylon bags, closed, and placed in the polystyrene transport containers containing ice chips.

The wound is closed carefully with a continuous suture.

Live donor nephrectomy

Indications

Undoubtedly the short- and long-term results of using kidneys from living related donors are better than those from cadaver kidneys. Today more and more relatives, aware of these facts, and aware of the long waiting time that so many people have to endure before a suitable cadaver kidney becomes available, come forward asking to give a kidney. Every would-be donor needs a most careful investigation: it is obvious that one must check that their ABO and HLA antigens are suitable (and one must be tactful when one finds that, from time to time, they are not). The renal function and general health of the would-be donor are carefully investigated and from time to time some serious disorder may call for treatment on its own account. Underlying disease in one kidney may not be an absolute bar to transplantation but it certainly calls for very careful discussion with the patient. The courage and generosity of the would-be living donor not only elicit the utmost respect from the surgeon but also place upon him a heavy additional responsibility, and there is universal agreement that there are few operations so stressful to the transplant team than a living donor transplant.

All things being equal, it is easier to use the left kidney because its renal vein is longer, but before deciding which one to remove, a careful pre-operative angiogram is performed to detect multiple renal arteries. Few transplant surgeons would consider it justifiable to remove a patch from the aorta, so that, whenever possible, one should take the kidney with the single artery.

Position on the table

The lateral position is used.

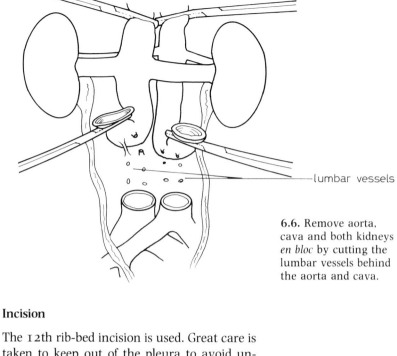

6.6. Remove aorta, cava and both kidneys *en bloc* by cutting the lumbar vessels behind the aorta and cava.

Incision

The 12th rib-bed incision is used. Great care is taken to keep out of the pleura to avoid unnecessary morbidity.

Steps of the operation

The kidney is gently but completely mobilized. Great care is taken to preserve the precious triangle of fat in which run the branches of the inferior segmental artery to the ureter, upon which its viability depends. Every small efferent vessel is carefully sealed.

On the left side the adrenal and gonadal veins are divided between ligatures, and the left renal vein followed across the front of the aorta to its entry into the vena cava. From time to time one will meet the unpleasant surprise of a circumcaval renal vein, one division passing behind the aorta, the other in front. It is not difficult to deal with this anomaly as long as one recognizes it (6.7). The vein

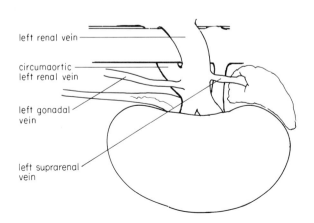

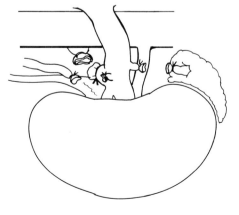

6.7. Living donor transplant nephrectomy. Circumaortic renal veins may cause difficulty. The vein that runs behind the aorta is divided between ligatures.

running behind the aorta is carefully doubly ligated and divided, and the one in front used to join on to the external iliac vein at the time of transplantation.

The renal artery is slowly and carefully dissected free from its stiff investment of fibrous tissue, until its origin from the aorta can be plainly seen. The lateral aspect of the aorta is now cleaned, to make sure that there are no small additional renal arteries that have escaped detection in the angiogram.

At this stage, we let the putting-in team know the anatomical arrangements. They, in turn, operating in another room, tell us when they have exposed the recipient vessels. When all is ready, the ureter is transected about 15 cm down from the kidney, care being taken not to be rough, or to injure the delicate artery and vein of the ureter. Then the renal artery is doubly ligated and cut across as close to the side wall of the aorta as is compatible with safety. Two ligatures of o linen thread are used on the aorta and the kidney side of the artery is not tied. The renal vein is similarly doubly ligated and cut across.

The kidney is now plunged into a basin of ice-cold saline, which itself is immersed in a second bowl full of ice slush (6.8). Sterile, ice-cold Marshall's solution is now irrigated into the open end of the renal artery until the kidney is completely perfused and the effluent from the renal vein is clear. The kidney in its bowl of ice-cold sterile saline is taken to the second operating room where the other team is waiting to put it into the recipient.

With careful attention to haemostasis, the wound is closed in the usual way. No drain is needed.

Post-operative care

The main post-operative complications concern the chest. As usual, it is painful to cough, and there is a tendency for sputum to be retained in the basal segments of the lower lobe of the lung on the affected side. Physiotherapy, encouragement to cough, and above all, relief of pain, soon clears the lung. Ileus may last for forty-eight hours, but seldom longer.

It is usual for the donor to have a slight rise in the plasma creatinine following transplant nephrectomy. It is of no consequence, and remains slightly higher than the pre-operative level.

The donor needs much reassurance, and often needs special encouragement and sympathy during rejection episodes affecting the function of the kidney in the recipient who is

a child or sibling. Later, when everything is going well, it is necessary to emphasize again that expectation of life for a transplant donor is normal, and that life assurance companies should not attempt to load a premium later on.

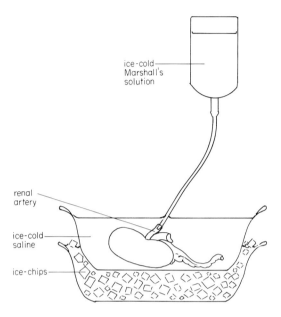

6.8. Once the kidney is removed from the donor it is plunged into ice-cold saline, which is kept cold by being surrounded with ice in a second bowl. Ice-cold Marshall's solution is run into the lumen of the renal artery through an intravenous giving set, until no more blood can be seen issuing from the renal vein.

Renal transplantation

Indications

This is not the place to recount the indications for renal transplantation in general or the care needed to get a recipient ready for it. The management of end-stage renal failure today is a skill of its own. Successful transplantation calls for the utmost collaboration between nephrologists and surgeons (Hamburger *et al.* 1983). To decide when a patient will be better off with a transplant than on dialysis calls for the measured evaluation of many factors, not all of them medical. Most surgeons are glad to acknowledge that the brunt of the work falls upon those with the day-to-day responsibility for dialysis. Not every urological surgeon will find himself obliged to transplant kidneys from live or dead donors, but the technique of renal transplantation is one with which he should have a working knowledge since it allows him to share more fully that fruitful partnership with nephrology which makes urology today such a rewarding field of medicine. Furthermore, circumstances may arise in ordinary urological practice that call for moving the kidney from loin to groin, and he ought to know how it is done.

Special preparations

The recipient will have been selected after a long process of which tissue typing is an essential part. There will have been a full evaluation of the urological system, and any source of sepsis within the urinary tract will have been removed. Bladder outflow obstruction, reflux, calculi, diverticula, and urethral strictures may all call for preliminary attention before the patient is got ready for a transplant. The recipient should have been recently dialysed; he or she should be well hydrated; at least three units of blood should be ready; and the correct dose of immunosuppressive agents should be calculated according to the patient's body weight. At the time of writing the standard is still 5 mg/g azathioprine together with 400 mg hydrocortisone intravenously immediately before the clamp on the renal artery is removed (Calne 1976).

Position on the table

Supine. Shaving and preparation of the skin is deferred until the patient is asleep. A small 16 Ch catheter is placed in the bladder and connected to a giving set and half-litre bottle of sterile saline, clipped off until the moment comes to distend the bladder prior to implantation of the ureter.

Incision

The Alexandre incision is generally used nowadays since it cuts no muscle and is followed by almost no haematoma (6.9). The vertical limb of the incision exposes the junction of external oblique aponeurosis and rectus. The lower limb of the incision is carried across medially through the rectus aponeurosis, and the rectus muscle fibres are retracted. The inferior epigastric vessels are doubly ligated and divided.

Steps of the operation

The external iliac vein and artery are displayed by sweeping back the peritoneum, dividing its attachment at the internal ring and the round ligament in a female. In a male the vas deferens and testicular vessels are pre-

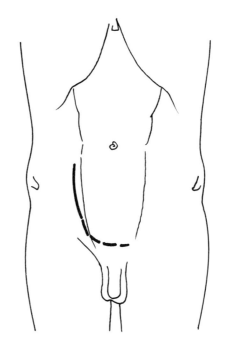

6.9. Alexandre incision for renal transplantation.

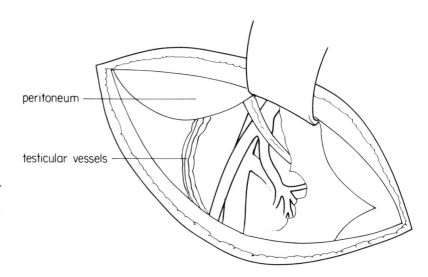

peritoneum

testicular vessels

6.10. Retract the peritoneum to display the common, external and internal iliac vessels.

served (6.10). The fascial sheath over the external iliac artery is opened so as to display the junction of the common and internal iliac arteries. This dissection is continued proximally to mobilize the last 2 cm of the common iliac artery round which a silicone rubber vascular sling is placed. The internal iliac artery is carefully palpated to see if it is sufficiently free from atheroma to be used.

If the internal iliac artery is soft and healthy (and often it is not, in a would-be recipient of a transplant), then it is mobilized down to its terminal divisions (6.11). These are each ligated with o-thread, and a DeBakey clamp placed gently across the internal iliac artery at its origin. The main trunk of the artery is cut across just proximal to its division into branches. Wash it out with heparinized saline.

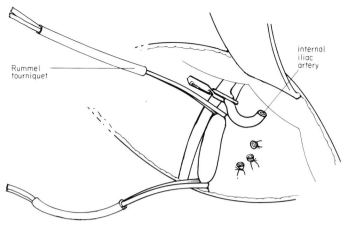

6.11. The internal iliac artery is mobilized by dividing its terminal branches.

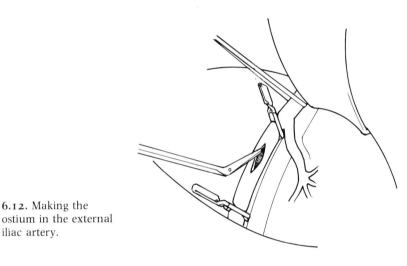

6.12. Making the ostium in the external iliac artery.

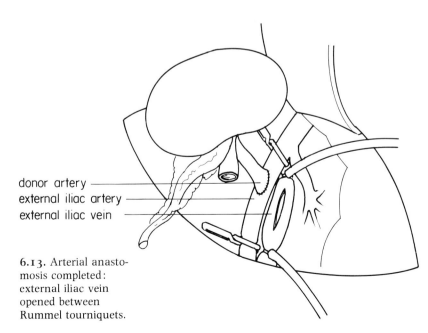

donor artery
external iliac artery
external iliac vein

6.13. Arterial anastomosis completed: external iliac vein opened between Rummel tourniquets.

If the donor arteries are multiple, and arrive on a Carrel patch of aorta, or if the recipient has a very atheromatous internal iliac artery, the external iliac artery should be used for the transplant. Mobilize it gently. Tape it above and below the site chosen for the transplant. Make the opening in the artery between two DeBakey clamps, twice as long as the width of the donor artery (6.12). Irrigate it well with heparinized saline.

Mobilize the external iliac vein up to its junction with the internal iliac vein and down to the inguinal ligament, taking care to divide between ligatures all tiny tributaries, including a not-so-tiny one that enters it from behind. Mobilize the vein completely. To occlude the vein gently and safely, with least damage to the intima, we prefer to use a pair of Rummel tourniquets made with silastic slings and rubber tubing.

The cadaver kidney is now removed from the sterile container in which it has been transported and carefully examined in a sterile bowl of ice-cold saline. Make sure all the tributaries of the renal vein have been ligated. Check that no small polar vessel has been severed. Trim off excess fat without trespassing on the precious triangle of tissue between the lower end of the kidney and the ureter in which runs the ureteric blood supply. Trim away excessive aortic and caval wall.

Hold the kidney in a large pack soaked in ice-cold saline to stop it warming up during the anastomosis.

The arterial anastomosis is made with 5-0 Tevdek or similar arterial suture material. Two mattress sutures are placed to appose the endothelium of donor and recipient vessel, and the suture line is completed with running or interrupted sutures (6.13). Care is taken to include in each suture the intima and any atheroma present. Pull up the sutures firmly, and make sure that they are regularly and neatly placed. Before the anastomosis is completed, irrigate the lumen of the vessels to get rid of clot and air.

The venous anastomosis is made in the same way, placing mattress sutures to appose the endothelial surfaces, and using a running unlocked suture. Because the far side of the anastomosis is tethered, it may be easier to sew it from within rather than turn the kidney over in the wound (6.14).

Remove the clamps in logical order, those with the lower pressure preceding those with the greater. The Rummel tourniquet is released first from the distal vein, then the proximal one. The arterial clamp is taken off first the

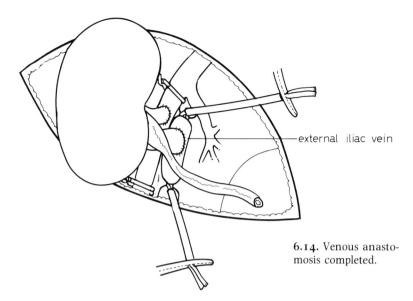

—external iliac vein

6.14. Venous anastomosis completed.

distal artery, then the proximal one. Place a swab over the anastomosis to control the inevitable small pin-hole leaks that seal themselves within a few minutes.

As soon as the arterial clamp is removed, the kidney becomes suffused with blood and turns a healthy pink. Pulsation returns to the parenchyma. Small, hitherto unnoticed veins in the hilum may bleed and should be picked up and tied. After three minutes, remove the swab and look at the anastomosis: occasionally a tiny leak will call for a recovery suture or two. There should be good pulsation in the recipient artery and its branches: if there is none, then something is wrong. There may be an unnoticed dissection of the intima of the donor artery, perhaps caused by traction when removing it from the cadaver. At once replace the clamps, cut through the suture line, trim back the injured artery, and do the anastomosis over again taking great care to include the intima in the sutures, and if necessary performing a limited end-arterectomy.

A poor but regular flow through the recipient artery is often seen in kidneys kept for a prolonged time on ice, especially if the donor has had prolonged ante-mortem ischaemia. This may presage a week or two of anuria from tubular necrosis, but is not incompatible with an excellent long-term result.

If the arterial inflow is good, but the vein is obstructed, the kidney becomes engorged. One may have made too small an opening in the recipient vein. The remedy is to reapply the clamps, irrigate well with heparinized saline, and revise the anastomosis after making the venous opening larger.

Ureterovesical anastomosis

Many methods have been described for joining the ureter to the bladder, but the most convenient and reliable is that described by Calne (1976) which is the same as the classic Leadbetter ureterosigmoidostomy so familiar to an older generation of urologists.

First, find the bladder. In an anuric patient whose bladder has been empty for several years, it helps to have a catheter in the bladder. Allow 200 ml or so of sterile saline to run into the bladder. This makes it easy and safe to incise the muscle and find the plane between muscle and mucosa with which to make the valvular anastomosis.

Place a tissue forceps on the bladder to hold it in the line of the ureter, and divide the muscle fibres slowly until the vesical mucosa pouts out (6.15). Snip off a tiny circle of mucosa at the distal end of the tunnel. Slit the lower end of the ureter to make a long oval which will lie comfortably without any tension in the tunnel.

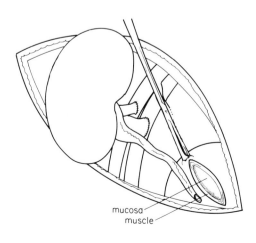

mucosa
muscle

6.15. Tunnel prepared for ureter in the vault of the bladder.

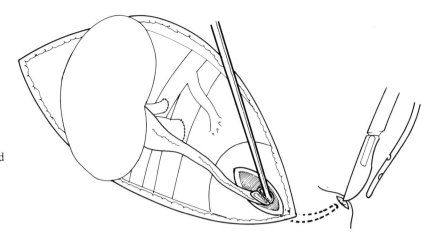

6.16. Ureter spatulated and anastomosed to mucosa of bladder: Gibbon catheter introduced as splint.

In my department these anastomoses are always protected by a splint, although many transplanters prefer to do without this protection, fearing the risk of infection. To introduce the splint, pass a right-angled forceps into the bladder: make it emerge through the abdominal wall to seize the tip of a 6 Ch Gibbon catheter which is passed up the ureter (6.16) and secured to the lining of the bladder with a 4-0 catgut suture to prevent subsequent angulation. The wings of the Gibbon catheter are trimmed and used to secure it to the skin.

Sew the spatulated ureter to the mucosa of the bladder with 4-0 chromic catgut. The ureter is buried in the tunnel with a series of 4-0 chromic catgut sutures tied over a small rubber tube to ensure that the tunnel is not closed too tightly (6.17), after which the tube is slipped out.

Before closing the wound in layers with catgut, make sure that all bleeding has been controlled. Check the vascular anastomoses but do not fiddle with them if they are dry, for this may lead to further bleeding. The kidney lies in its extraperitoneal pocket, and the ureter should run unkinked from pelvis to bladder. A drain alongside the kidney is brought out through a separate stab lateral to the main incision and connected to a sterile closed drainage system.

Today when most donor kidneys come from 'beating heart' cadaver donors, one must expect a diuresis. Leave the Foley catheter in the bladder, connected to a closed drainage system.

Hazards of the operation

There are many hazards to transplantation but some of the homely and practical ones need to be described in this chapter. Polar arteries cause trouble if they are not noticed when removing the cadaver kidney. If there is an ischaemic pole persisting at the end of the operation when the arterial clamp is removed, one may be able to find the polar artery and anastomose it to the main renal artery or to a branch of the internal iliac. These branches are sometimes very small, and an operating loupe or microscope may help with the interruped sutures needed for the anastomosis.

A tear is easily made in the main renal vein in the hilum of the kidney at the time of nephrectomy which may bleed furiously when the clamps are removed. Replace the vascular clamps, suture the laceration in the vein, and proceed as before.

If the blood supply to the lower end of the ureter has been injured there will be necrosis

6.17. The muscle of the bladder is sewn over the ureter to form a tunnel: a small Jaques catheter prevents you from making this tunnel too tight.

Gibbon catheter as ureteric splint

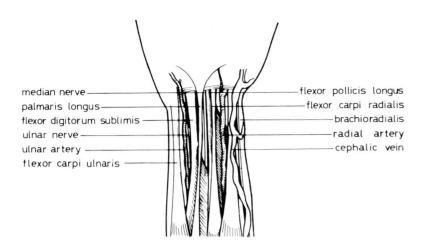

median nerve
palmaris longus
flexor digitorum sublimis
ulnar nerve
ulnar artery
flexor carpi ulnaris

flexor pollicis longus
flexor carpi radialis
brachioradialis
radial artery
cephalic vein

and leakage of urine. Ureteric complications occurred in 4% of a series of two hundred consecutive transplants in our department, although many of these were related to late rejection involving the ureteric tissue. These results would suggest that the use of a splint may diminish the risk of urinary leak. If a leak takes place, the wound should be re-explored without delay. It may be easy to resect the ischaemic segment of ureter and reimplant it into the bladder, with a small Boari flap (page 106). It may be better to join the donor ureter to the patient's own one left behind, protecting the anastomosis with a Cummings tube that serves as splint and nephrostomy in one. When exploration has been delayed, or when there is infection, one may still save a transplant kidney by packing the wound loosely, after inserting a nephrostomy, and closing it by secondary suture some days later.

A rare difficulty arises when one has unknowingly transplanted a kidney that has an unsuspected pelviureteric junction obstruction. In one patient in the London Hospital series this led to necrosis of the renal pelvis and a urine leak. But by trimming away the necrotic tissue, and anastomosing what was left of the pelvis to the recipient ureter over a Cummings tube the kidney was saved with an excellent long term result.

Access for dialysis

Haemodialysis

There have been many developments in the craft of providing vascular access for haemodialysis since the introduction of the Quinton–Scribner shunt (Quinton *et al.* 1960) and the description of the Cimino shunt (Breschia *et al.* 1966). Today each haemodialysis centre has its own preferences (see Farrell *et al.* 1983).

The Scribner shunt

Anaesthesia

General, local, or regional block anaesthesia may be used.

Incision

A leg or arm vessel may be used for the insertion of the shunt, which is today rarely used except for short-term dialysis, pending the maturation of a Cimino or similar fistula. The incision is made well up the forearm so that the loop of the shunt is clear of the patient's wrist (6.18). The radial artery is dissected with great care, making sure that all its minute branches are individually ligated rather than torn, and that its intima is not injured by clumsy handling. The cephalic vein is similarly dissected, its tributaries individually ligated and divided and its distal end ligated. The Teflon cannulae (6.19) are now chosen and attached to the Silastic loop pieces. It takes some skill and judgement to make sure

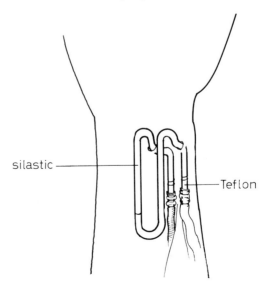

silastic

Teflon

6.19. Insertion of the Quinton–Scribner shunt.

6.20. Formation of the Cimino–Brescia fistula.

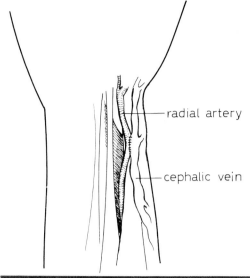

radial artery

cephalic vein

6.21. Tenckhoff Silicone-rubber-Dacron-velour cannula.

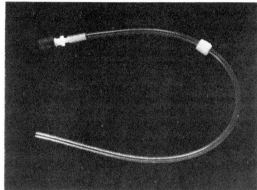

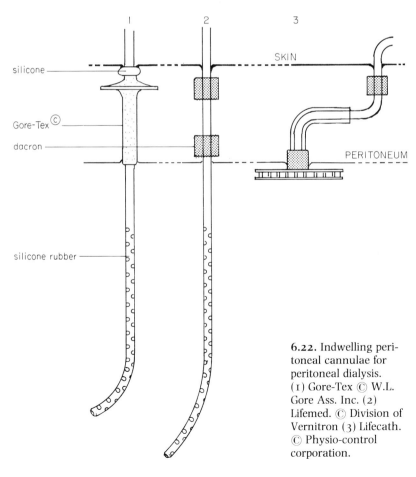

silicone

Gore-Tex ©

dacron

silicone rubber

1   2   3

SKIN

PERITONEUM

6.22. Indwelling peritoneal cannulae for peritoneal dialysis. (1) Gore-Tex © W.L. Gore Ass. Inc. (2) Lifemed. © Division of Vernitron (3) Lifecath. © Physio-control corporation.

that the loop runs easily through the incisions in the skin and that the cannulae are not kinked as they enter the vein or the artery. Very scrupulous care is taken in the early post-operative days to unclog a clotted shunt. Later on stenosis or thrombosis at the end of the venous cannula may call for revision. For these reasons, few departments now use the Scribner shunt except as a temporary form of vascular access, but it is a technique that every urologist should master and be able to offer his nephrological colleague when the need arises.

The Cimino fistula

Anaesthesia and access to the vessels are as in the Scribner shunt. The vessels selected are according to local circumstances, but in general one should start as far down the arm as possible, so that if the fistula closes up, another one may be made further up the arm. Similarly it is wise to use the patient's left arm, if he is right handed, and *vice versa*. Having dissected out the radial artery and cephalic vein with the greatest care an anastomosis is made from side-to-side between radial artery and cephalic vein (6.20), a manoeuvre which is much facilitated by the use of a binocular loupe. Many surgeons feel that it is better to ligate the distal limb of the radial artery after making the anastomosis to prevent the sore thumb phenomenon which sometimes arises from vascular 'steal'.

According to the calibre of the artery and vein, one must usually wait three to four weeks before the forearm veins have enlarged to a size that permits them to be repeatedly needled for haemodialysis.

Peritoneal dialysis

As with vascular access for haemodialysis, so with peritoneal dialysis, there have been many developments in the technology of the cannula used to run the dialysis fluid in and out of the peritoneal cavity (6.21, 6.22). In most cases a modified Tenckhoff silicone rubber cannula is used, which is attached to the rectus sheath by means of one or two Dacron-velour collars.

Having emptied the bladder first (if necessary) the abdominal wall is prepared with all aseptic care. A site is selected below the umbilicus and infiltrated with lignocaine. A short 3 cm incision is made in the skin crease which just exposes the rectus sheath. This is nicked, allowing the Tenckhoff trochar and cannula to be introduced into the peritoneal cavity. The catheter is made to lie in the pelvis and is irrigated to make sure that it is not kinked. The cannula is made to run through a short subcutaneous tunnel to diminish the risk of infection. The Dacron collar is fixed to the rectus fascia with one or two 2-0 chromic catgut sutures (6.23).

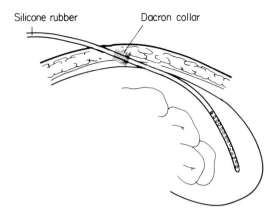

Silicone rubber   Dacron collar

6.23. Insertion of the Tenckhoff cannula: note that the skin hole is some distance away from the velour cuff.

References

Breschia M.J., Cimino J.E., Appel K. & Harwich B.J. (1966) Chronic hemodialysis using venupuncture and a surgically created arteriovenous fistula. *New Eng. J. Med.* **275**, 1089.

Calne R.C. (1976) Renal Transplantation. In *Urology* (ed. by Blandy J.P.), p. 433. Blackwell Scientific Publications, Oxford.

Farrell E.M., Rubio P.A., Flynn C.T., Harmon W.E., Hussey J.L., Kramer M.S. Kwaan J.H.M., Longnecker R.E., Twardowski Z.J. & Van der Werf B. (1983) What form/forms of vascular access do you favor? Why? *Dialysis & Transplantation*, **12**, 330.

Hamburger J., Crosnier J., Bach J.-F. & Kreis H. (1983) *Renal Transplantation Theory and Practice*, 2nd edn. Williams & Wilkins, Baltimore.

Quinton W., Dillard D. & Scribner B.H. (1960) Cannulation of blood vessels for prolonged hemodialysis. *Trans. Amer. Soc. Artific. Int. Organs*, **6**, 104.

Tenckhoff H. & Schechter H. (1968) A bacteriologically safe peritoneal access device. ibid. **14**, 181.

Chapter 7
The ureter

The first deliberate operation on the ureter was that of Sir John Simon, in 1852, who made a fistula between ureters and rectum in a neglected extrophy of the bladder. Ureteric surgery had to wait for radiography and the development of non-irritating materials for ureteric splintage. For a long time the surgery of the ureter held a peculiar dread for surgeons and the usual remedy for injury or neoplasm of the ureter was nephrectomy, few surgeons being bold enough to attempt to reanastomose the ureter or join it to the bladder. The next generation of urologists became obsessed with the minutiae of anastomosis of ureter to bowel, as this for a time became the method of choice not only for urinary diversion, but also for dealing with a ureteric injury. Only when the long term biochemical aftermath of uretero-sigmoidostomy was appreciated did the operation fall into disrepute. During the Second World War the great French urologists Couvelaire, Kuss and their colleagues showed the rest of the world how to make use of segments of large and small bowel in reconstruction of the urinary tract—discoveries that were quickly imitated by others (Bricker 1950; Wells 1956). To these new operations were added the use of the pedicled bladder flap, first suggested by Boari (1894) and developed by Ockerblad (1936). Today the urologist is confident to operate on any part of the ureter, and is armed with a wide range of procedures that may be adapted to almost any anatomical problem that confronts the surgeon after almost any pathological process.

The ureter can be trusted to heal without leak or stricture as long as certain basic principles are followed. Its blood supply is tenuous, depending mainly on the longitudinal vessel that comes down from the inferior segmental branch of the renal artery. In mobilizing the ureter meticulous care must be taken to preserve the connective tissue sheath containing these vessels.

Tension on the ureter will lead to narrowing of this artery, and in making any ureteric anastomosis, there must be absolutely no tension at all. This is particularly important to remember when operating in a previously scarred field, when the ureter is thickened and fibrous. After it has been dissected clear of its surroundings it will often shorten considerably, and the gap to be closed is longer than it appeared to be when the operation began.

In making any anastomosis involving the ureter a long ellipse must be formed by spatulating the ureter, or a stricture will result as the scar shrinks.

Reflux should be prevented where possible by always forming a submucosal tunnel at the site of anastomosis of ureter to bowel or bladder. There are some situations when this is unnecessary or impossible, notably in uretero-ileal anastomosis.

Splinting the ureter is a good precaution against urinary leak, but if a splint is used, it must be made of non-irritating material: ideally silicone rubber should be used, but whatever material is chosen, the splinting tube must not be too large. In my practice every anastomosis involving the ureter is splinted, since I feel that the advantages far outweigh the theoretical disadvantages of infection.

Operations for stone in the ureter

Indications

Calculi in the ureter more than 0.5 cm diameter seldom pass spontaneously. Whatever its size, a stone must be removed if there is obstruction upstream of it as well as infection, since this combination invites septicaemia and scarring in the renal parenchyma.

On the other hand, stones under 0.5 cm diameter which are making progress down the ureter need not be interfered with surgically unless there is evidence of progressive dilatation of the upper urinary tract, repeated and incapacitating attacks of pain, or some other particular complication. There is seldom any difficulty in deciding when a stone is too large to go down the ureter but there are many calculi whose management calls for the wisest judgement and the most masterly restraint. One thing is *never* an indication for surgery—

the impatience of the patient. Nobody who has been obliged to deal with the dreadful complications of operations for stones in the ureter will ever permit himself to be bullied by a patient into operating just so that the patient can go on holiday. Remember these complications whenever you are tempted to use a stone basket. Long faces at a urological congress mean that your colleagues are exchanging anecdotes about Dormia basket disasters. Make sure you do not qualify to join them.

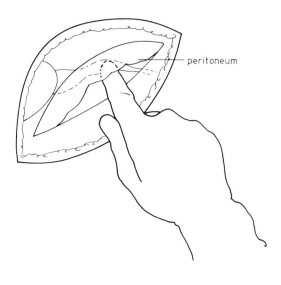

7.1. Exposure of a stone in the upper third of the ureter. Find the stone with your finger-tip.

Stone in the upper third of the ureter

Special precautions

Confirm the diagnosis even if it requires a ureterogram, or passage of a catheter alongside the stone with X-rays in two planes. Always insist that a plain radiograph is taken *en route* to the operating room. Stones have a way of passing back to the kidney when least expected.

Position on the table

Lateral, as for nephrectomy.

Incision

Use a short 12th rib-tip incision (page 14).

Steps of the operation

Take a shrewd look at the X-ray and note the position of the stone in relation to the tip of the 12th rib and the upper edge of the iliac crest.

After incising skin and muscles, open Gerota's fascia, push the peritoneum forward and feel for the stone, where the X-rays make you think it ought to be. Feel carefully, lest you dislodge the stone back up to the kidney. Feel forwards, for the ureter is always carried forwards stuck to the back of the peritoneum (7.1).

As soon as the unmistakable hard thing which is the stone has been felt, keep a finger on it. Get an assistant to insert a narrow Deaver's retractor to retract the peritoneum medially, revealing the tip of the finger on the stone (7.2).

Incise the sheath of the ureter to expose its wall. With a right-angled forceps, pass a silicone rubber sling around the ureter upstream of the stone (7.3), and have the assistant pull gently on it to kink the ureter and prevent the stone slipping upwards. Dissect the ureter over the stone until its wall can be clearly seen.

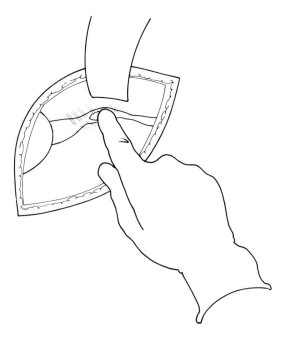

7.2. Slide a Deaver retractor over your finger and retract the peritoneum; keep your finger-tip on the stone.

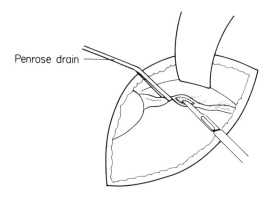

7.3. A thin Penrose drain is slung around the ureter above the stone to prevent it being dislodged upwards. Cut down directly on to the calculus.

Make sure that three implements are ready: a long-handled small-bladed knife, a Watson-Cheyne dissector, and a ureteric catheter.

Cut directly down on to the stone through the full thickness of ureteric wall. Do not attempt to 'milk' the stone up or down. Let the knife grate on the calculus. Use the flat blade of the dissector to prise the stone out of its nest of oedematous epithelium in the wall of the ureter (7.4). The stone can now be lifted out. A gush of urine often follows which must be cultured in case it is infected.

Keep the retractor still, and run a ureteric catheter up to the kidney and down to the bladder to make sure other particles of stone are not present (7.5).

If only a tiny incision has been made in the ureter, there is no need to close it. If the ureter is thick and dilated, its wall should be closed with two or three 5-0 catgut sutures placed just through the muscle, not the mucosa.

Close the wound with interrupted catgut and a drain to the hole in the ureter.

The drain is left in position for four days, after which it is removed for half its length, and taken out entirely on the sixth day. By this time a solid track has formed around the drain and there is no risk of a urinoma forming. If a ureteric drain is left longer than this, it invites a tiresome persistent fistula. (Draining a ureter is not like draining pus from an abscess which, as every novice surgeon knows, must be left in position until it stops draining.)

Hazards of the operation

With a stone in the upper ureter the main hazard is that it may slip back into the kidney. If this is detected before the patient is anaesthetized no harm is done and the operation is postponed until the stone once more lodges in a favourable position, or it is planned with the object of exposing the renal pelvis for pyelolithotomy (page 41).

The real difficulty arises when the incision has been made and the exploring finger fails to find the stone because it has slipped back up into the kidney in the interval between taking the precautionary X-ray and positioning the patient on the table.

Sometimes you only need to get the sling round the ureter, draw it towards you, and feel upstream along the course of the ureter, and the stone will be found somewhat higher up than expected. Alas, much more often, the stone has slipped right back into the kidney. Such a patient usually has rather a distended upper ureter and kidney, and on reaching the

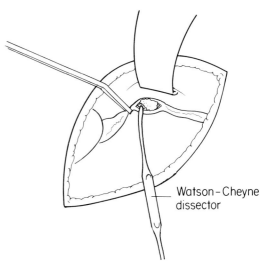

Watson–Cheyne dissector

7.4. Liberate the jagged calculus from the ureteric mucosa with a Watson–Cheyne dissector.

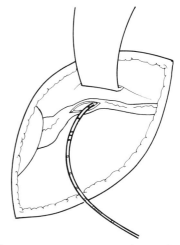

7.5. Make sure no other bits of stone have gone down the ureter by passing a catheter down its lumen.

lower part of the pelvis, when it is incised between stay sutures, out gushes urine, bringing the stone with it. If this does not occur, gently search the pelvis with stone forceps: it can often be found without further trouble.

If still hidden, at this stage the flexible endoscope can be of great assistance. It allows the interior of the kidney to be examined in a stream of water at leisure; the stone will be located, and a forceps guided down on to it.

If all these manoeuvres fail to reveal the stone, it is necessary to give some thought to the whole situation of the patient before proceeding further. When the tissues are very inflamed and the patient has been operated on because of pyonephrosis, it may be best not to enlarge the wound and make a formal dissection of the entire kidney as for a pyelo-lithotomy, since this might be dangerous in the presence of active inflammation. It may be wiser to pass a nephrostomy through the renal substance and close the wound, planning perhaps a percutaneous lithotripsy (page 40) on a later occasion. In other patients there is nothing to prevent extending the wound and carrying out a formal pyelolithotomy.

Stone in the middle third of the ureter

Special precautions

A radiograph is taken *en route* to the operating room. If there is any doubt as to the diagnosis, a ureterogram should be performed before proceeding.

Position

The patient is supine with a cushion or sand-bag under the loin on the side of the stone.

Incision

Study the radiograph to see where the stone lies in relation to the 12th rib and the iliac crest. Make a short muscle-splitting incision in the skin crease (7.6).

Steps of the operation

Carry the incision through skin and fat. Split the oblique muscles as you would for appendicectomy. When splitting the transversus begin well posteriorly, deepening the incision until the finger enters the retroperitoneal fat without opening the peritoneum. Wipe the peritoneum from the back of the transversus to which it is always firmly attached. Then complete the division of the transversus muscle along the length of the incision.

Having decided where the stone is likely to lie from the radiograph and the bony landmarks, feel along the back of the peritoneum until you meet the hard thing which is the stone (7.7). Have the peritoneum retracted up and medially with a Deaver's retractor until finger tip and stone are displayed. Slip a silicone rubber sling around the ureter upstream of the stone. Incise directly on to the stone. Prize it out with a Watson-Cheyne dissector and slip a ureteric catheter up and down to make sure the ureter is clear in both directions. Close the wound with catgut and a drain down to the ureterotomy.

The only difficulty one meets with in this

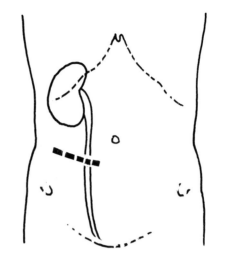

7.6. Choose your incision for a stone in the middle third of the ureter according to its position in the X-ray in relation to the bony landmarks.

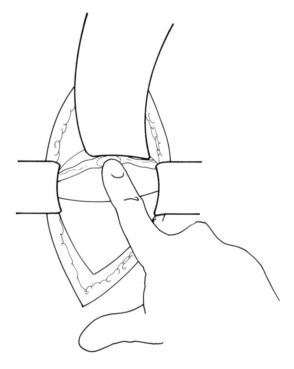

7.7. Feel for the stone with your index finger.

operation is inadvertent tearing of the gonadal vein which may have to be carefully dissected off the ureter before it can be clearly seen and cleanly incised (7.8).

Stone in the lower third of the ureter

Position

Supine.

Incision

The Pfannenstiel incision gives excellent access to the lower end of the ureter and an excellent cosmetic scar (7.9). Satisfactory access may also be obtained with a lower paramedian or

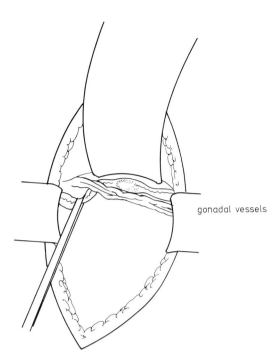

gonadal vessels

7.8. Dissect the ureter away from the gonadal vessels and place a Penrose drain sling proximal to the calculus to prevent it from being dislodged.

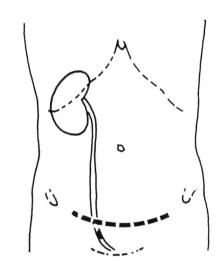

7.9. Stone in the lower ureter: a Pfannenstiel incision gives the best exposure.

midline incision, and when the patient is badly scarred from previous surgery the Alexandre incision described for transplantation (page 82) gives excellent access.

Special precautions

Always have an X-ray *en route* to the operating room. It is easy for a stone to slip into the bladder when least expected. It can be removed in seconds with an Ellik's evacuator and the patient excused any open operation. Stones, even in the lower end of the ureter, may also slip back to the kidney.

Steps of the operation

Having made the incision (page 115), retract the peritoneum, dividing the round ligament in a female or the processus vaginalis in a male. Dissect along the external iliac artery to the bifurcation of the common iliac artery, retracting bladder and peritoneum medially. The ureter is found where it crosses the bifurcation of the common iliac artery, lightly tethered to the underside of the peritoneum. A stone in this situation is easily felt and removed as described above.

More often it is impacted in the ureter further down towards the bladder and not so easily found. The secret of making this operation easy is to divide the superior vesical vessels. Retract the bladder medially, putting the obliterated hypogastric artery on the stretch. Follow it down to the superior vesical pedicle (7.10), which should be doubly ligated and divided. The ureter is now released and can be easily followed down to the bladder (7.11). Two or three smaller vessels may need to be divided as the ureter is traced distally. Eventually the stone is found, always much

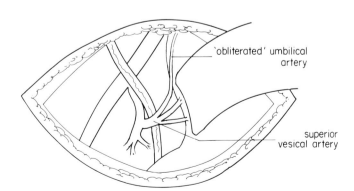

'obliterated' umbilical artery

superior vesical artery

7.10. The superior vesical vessels must be divided before you can dissect the lower 5 cm of the ureter.

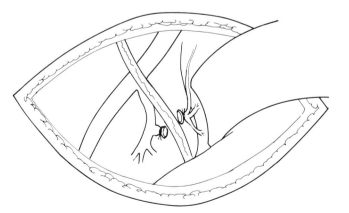

7.11. Once the superior vesical vessels are divided between ligatures the ureter can be easily mobilized.

further down than expected.

When the stone is in the extreme lower portion of the ureter some of the bladder muscle fibres must be cut before the stone is exposed, and it is often necessary to coagulate a small artery (7.12). When the calculus is exposed, cut down on it, free it with a dissector in the usual way and take it out. Do not suture the ureter, but close the wound with drainage in the usual way.

Hazards of the operation

The key to this operation is early division of the superior vesical pedicle. Until this is done one cannot mobilize the lower 5 cm of the ureter and it may be unbelievably difficult to feel the stone, let alone remove it. If the superior vesical vein or artery are torn, there can be confusing and frightening bleeding. There is no need to open the bladder or slit up the ureteric orifice, though this procedure was formerly advocated. Nor is it wise to open the ureter proximal to the stone in the hope that it can be milked back or retrieved with stone forceps. If the simple step of first dividing the superior vesical pedicle is followed, neither of these manoeuvres are necessary.

Endoscopy of the ureter and the Dormia basket

Although urologists have been using various snares and baskets to remove stones from the ureter for more than 50 years, they have earned themselves an evil reputation because it was so easy to catch the wall of the ureter along with the stone, and lacerate or even avulse it. The most recent addition to the armamentarium is the ureteroscope (7.13). This is essentially a very long thin Hopkins rod lens telescope with an irrigating channel and a channel for a instruments such as a basket, forceps, electro-hydraulic electrode, ultrasound probe etc.

Under general or spinal anaesthesia the ureteric orifice is dilated using a Fogarty or angioplasty catheter to about 16 Ch. The rigid ureteroscope is then introduced along the urethra: the ureteric orifice is located and the instrument gently passed up the ureter under direct vision, following the lumen all the way, until the stone is seen.

In most instances the stone is engaged in a Dormia stone basket, and when the wires are seen to have surrounded the stone, the basket is withdrawn, bringing the stone with it. Using the ureteroscope provides an extra margin of safety because one can see at once if the ureter

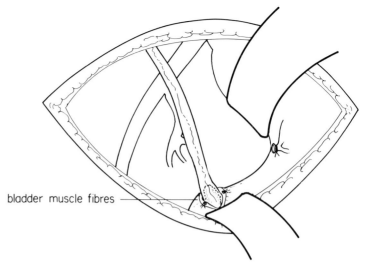

bladder muscle fibres

7.12. Follow the ureter right down to its entry into the wall of the bladder, dividing some vesical muscle fibres if you need to. In this way the whole length of the intra-mural ureter can be seen.

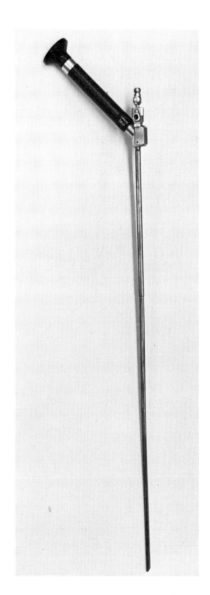

7.13. Direct viewing ureteroscope, by Karl Storz.

has been caught. Stones may now be extracted safely even when they are situated right up near the kidney. It is now possible to break up larger stones with the electrohydraulic lithotriptor or the ultrasound probe, so that today stones once regarded as far too large for endoscopic removal may be extracted safely.

At present many departments will not have been able to buy the ureteroscope, and must continue to use the Dormia basket in the standard way. Under general anaesthesia, using an operating cystoscope, the basket is introduced into the ureteric orifice, and gently passed above the stone (7.14). Once past the stone the basket is opened and moved up and down carefully, to free the stone from the wall of the ureter to which it is often attached rather firmly. Eventually the X-ray screen shows that the stone has been freed and is caught in the basket: it is then slowly withdrawn.

Frequently the stone is held up in the last centimetre of the intramural ureter. To set it free the ureteric orifice is incised with the blade of the optical urethrotome (7.16, 7.17). Hold onto the wire of the basket, withdraw the operating cystoscope over it, and then pass the optical urethrotome alongside the wire up the urethra and into the bladder. Sometimes the stone is too big to be washed out of the bladder and has to be crushed with a strong forceps or Mauermayer's punch.

Before using the Dormia basket or the ureteroscope always think very carefully whether they are really indicated. Remember that 98% of stones in the ureter under 5 mm in diameter will pass spontaneously given time and patience. Remember how often the ureter has been avulsed, and how the common iliac artery, peritoneum and bowel have all been damaged. Used with intelligence and care, in well-selected cases, these devices are invaluable, but they are never indicated merely for the private patient in a hurry (Dormia 1982).

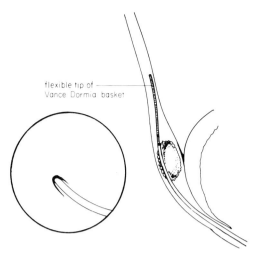

7.14. The stone basket is advanced into the ureteric orifice with the basket closed.

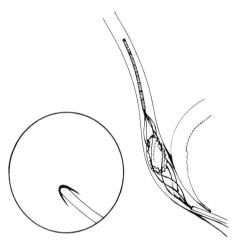

7.15. Once safely past the calculus the basket is opened and moved gently up and down until the stone is seen on the TV screen to be engaged.

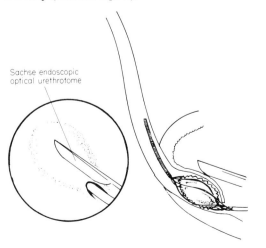

7.16. Stone jammed in ureteric orifice. Cut down on the stone with the Sachse optical urethrotome.

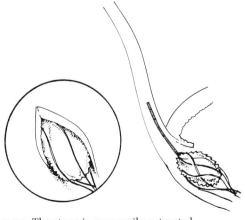

7.17. The stone is now easily extracted.

Operations for vesicoureteric reflux

Indications

When and when not to operate for reflux in a child demands more prolonged and careful consideration than would be appropriate to a book about general urological operations (Wallace *et al.* 1978). Reflux and urinary infection give rise to intractable scarring in a child, but if infection can be controlled, the scarring is seldom progressive, and indeed, in most cases, by the time the diagnosis has been made, the damage has been done, and will not get worse. In many children with well-documented reflux, when urine does not enter the renal parenchyma, no scarring follows so long as infection is controlled with appropriate antimicrobials (Edwards *et al.* 1977). The special importance of intrarenal reflux and the crucial significance of the anatomy of the renal papillae has made sense out of what was formerly an area charged with anomalies and paradoxes (Ransley 1978).

In adults reflux by itself is less harmful, and I have observed several patients for periods of up to fifteen years with continuing reflux, but no worsening of renal scarring. On the other hand, I have performed anti-reflux operations many times in the hope of mitigating the effects upon the kidney in patients whose childhood reflux has persisted into adult life: scarring has inexorably continued, and parenchymal damage has continued to get worse despite prevention of infection and correction of reflux. Only one symptom seems to have been helped—pain in the loin when voiding.

In children with a narrow ureter, the simplest reimplantation can be performed with a good result. When the ureter is very dilated, something must be done to make it more narrow and variations on the tapering operation of Hendren (1975) are employed. In adults these are notoriously apt to be followed by ischaemic necrosis of the lower end of the ureter.

Reflux prevention in a child with a narrow ureter

Position

Supine.

Incision

Pfannenstiel (7.18).

Steps of the operation

The bladder is opened between stay sutures in the midline and a self-retaining ring-retractor inserted (7.19). A ureteric or soft rubber catheter is passed up the ureter. A 4-0 catgut stay suture is placed in the lower edge of the ureteric orifice (7.20), which is now circumcised until the ureter can be drawn into the

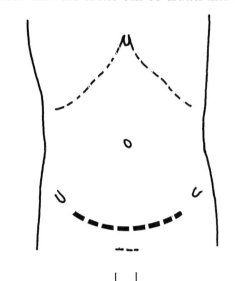

7.18. Pfannenstiel incision for anti-reflux operations.

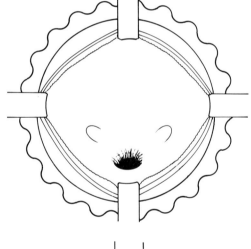

7.19. Bladder opened: ring-retractor inserted.

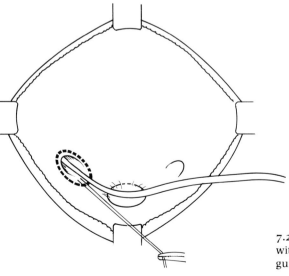

7.20. Ureter mobilized with catheter as a guide.

bladder with gentle traction on the suture (7.21), aided by a few snips of the dissecting scissors to free the intramural ureter completely. When it is quite loose, a right-angled forceps is passed up alongside the ureter, outside the bladder, and made to tent up the wall of the bladder 6 or 7 cm up and lateral to the original ureteric orifice. Cut down upon the tip of the forceps (7.22) so that it merges into the bladder and can grasp a stout catgut suture, which is tied to the stay suture on the ureter.

A submucosal tunnel (7.23) is made between the new entry of the ureter and the normal ureteric orifice, using curved dissecting scissors, and through this tunnel the ureter is drawn on its stay suture. The hole in the mucosa is closed, and the ureter sutured to its old place (7.24) (Politano & Leadbetter 1958).

This operation is the classical one, but a simpler variant (one of many) is that of Cohen (1969). In Cohen's method the intramural ureter is freed, just as in the Politano–Leadbetter method, but instead of being drawn in through a new extravesical route, the tunnel is made across the bladder to the opposite side (7.25). The principle is the same, but Cohen's method avoids the hazard of making the extravesical tunnel in the wrong place, or kinking the ureter over a fibrous band or blood vessel.

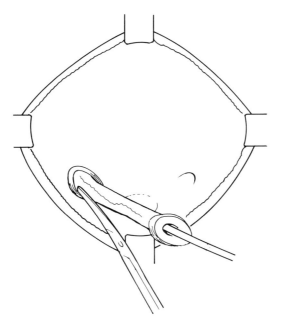

7.21. Ureter drawn into bladder until it is completely free.

7.23. A submucosal tunnel is created between the site of the old ureteric orifice and the new entry of the ureter.

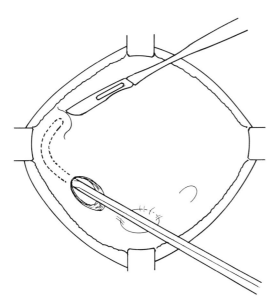

7.22. A new opening is made for the ureter with a right-angled forceps.

7.24. The ureter is sutured to the bladder mucosa turning back a short cuff. The small hole made for its re-entry is closed.

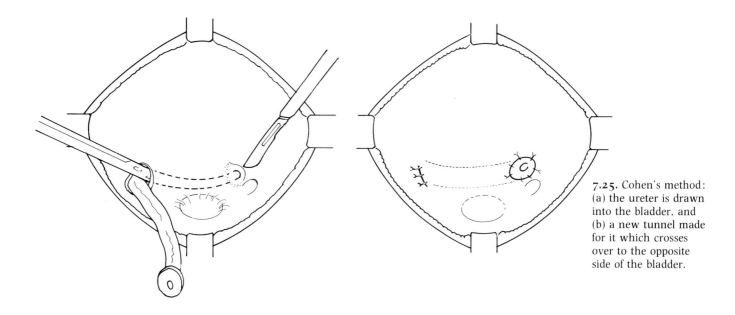

7.25. Cohen's method: (a) the ureter is drawn into the bladder, and (b) a new tunnel made for it which crosses over to the opposite side of the bladder.

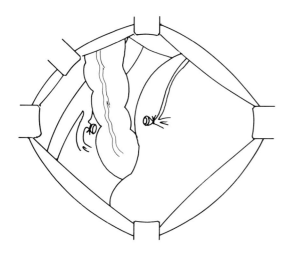

7.26. A wide ureter is mobilized outside the bladder by dividing the superior vesical vessels first.

Reflux prevention in a child with a wide ureter

Begin with an extravesical dissection, finding the ureter where it crosses the common iliac vessels. Liberate it by dividing the superior vesical vessels between ligatures, and dissect it with the utmost gentleness down to the bladder (7.26). The lower end of the ureter must be divided and the muscle layer closed carefully to avoid subsequent diverticulum formation.

Tapering the ureter needs patience and care (Hendren 1969). It must be tapered for at least the length of the tunnel, and in doing so, care is taken to preserve its longitudinal blood vessels (7.27). The ureter must be handled

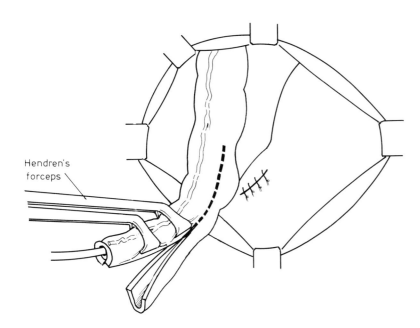

Hendren's forceps

7.27. The ureter is divided and the lower end carefully closed in two layers to prevent later formation of diverticulum.

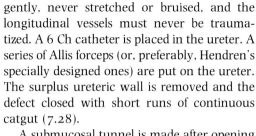

7.28. The ureter is narrowed by resecting the surplus on the side opposite its longitudinal vessels. The ureter is closed in short runs of 5-0 catgut.

gently, never stretched or bruised, and the longitudinal vessels must never be traumatized. A 6 Ch catheter is placed in the ureter. A series of Allis forceps (or, preferably, Hendren's specially designed ones) are put on the ureter. The surplus ureteric wall is removed and the defect closed with short runs of continuous catgut (7.28).

A submucosal tunnel is made after opening the bladder, beginning well away from the old ureteric orifice on the posterolateral wall of the bladder (7.29). It helps to put the bladder on the stretch as the scissors are worked into the plane between submucosa and muscle, but when the bladder is tented up, one must allow extra length in designing the tunnel or it is easy to make it too short to prevent reflux (7.30, 7.31).

Reflux prevention in an adult

Position

Supine.

Incision

As a general rule the Pfannenstiel incision is the best, but occasions may require the use of a paramedian, midline, or oblique incision.

Steps of the operation

First find the ureter at the bifurcation of the common iliac vessels and follow it down, dividing and ligating the superior vesical vessels to free the ureter. Divide the ureter and close the

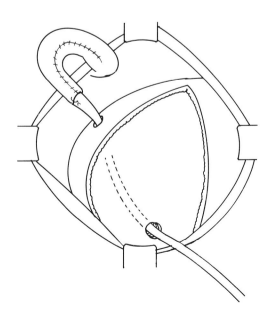

7.29. A long submucosal tunnel is made for the narrowed ureter along the lateral posterior wall of the bladder. A thin rubber tube is slipped over the ends of the scissors.

7.30. The narrowed ureter is drawn into the tunnel by the rubber tube.

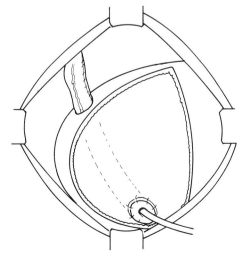

7.31. The narrowed ureter is everted and anastomosed to the vesical mucosa.

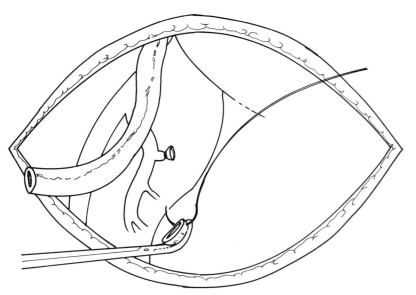

7.32. Reimplantation of a ureter in an adult: the ureter is mobilized extravesically and the old orifice carefully closed off.

defect in the bladder with catgut (7.32).

Open the bladder between stay sutures, and make a submucosal tunnel with dissecting scissors, beginning about 8 or 9 cm lateral to the old ureteric orifice on the outer and posterior aspect of the bladder. Dissect with scissors in the plane between mucosa and muscle, aiming for a point just medial to and distal to the old ureteric orifice (7.33). The length of the tunnel should be at least five times longer than the width of the ureter, so that it is necessary to allow for stretching of the wall of the bladder as the tunnel is made.

Push the end of an 8 Ch rubber Jaques catheter over the scissors, and withdraw both along the tunnel (7.34). Stitch the ureter to the tube, which now draws the ureter down the tunnel until it emerges at the chosen

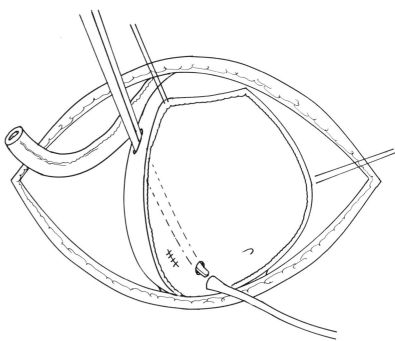

7.33. A new tunnel is formed for the ureter along the side and back of the bladder.

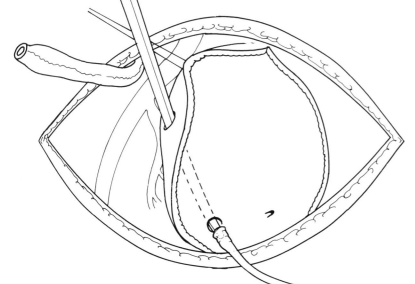

7.34. A thin rubber tube is slipped over the scissors.

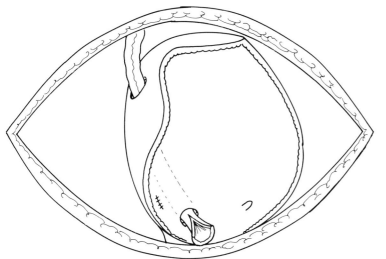

7.35. The ureter is spatulated before being everted.

position in the bladder. Remove any surplus ureter and slit it up to spatulate it (7.35). Turn back a cuff, and sew the ureter to the vesical mucosa with interrupted 4-0 chromic catgut sutures forming an everted nipple (7.36). It is a wise precaution to leave a 6 Ch or 8 Ch splinting catheter in the ureter. For this, the Gibbon urethral catheter is ideal. It is introduced retrogradely across the bladder on a right-angled forceps, and its plastic wings are sutured to the skin. The bladder is closed in catgut in one or two layers and drained with a urethral catheter. The wound is closed with a tube drain.

In children a Malecot suprapubic catheter is less likely to injure the urethra than a urethral one.

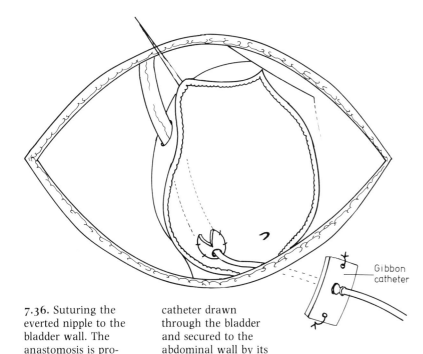

7.36. Suturing the everted nipple to the bladder wall. The anastomosis is protected by a Gibbon catheter drawn through the bladder and secured to the abdominal wall by its flanges.

Gibbon catheter

Retroperitoneal fibrosis

Indications

In retroperitoneal fibrosis one or both ureters are caught up in a hard white plaque of fibrous tissue which binds them on to the aorta and inferior vena cava, draws them towards the midline, and encases them in a rigid corset which prevents upwards or lateral movement. An identical radiological appearance is caused by retroperitoneal spread of carcinoma of the stomach, uterus, colon, or prostate. Often it is not known whether the obstruction is benign or malignant before the patient is explored: frozen sections on the table may mislead the pathologist, since the cancer cells may be widely dispersed in masses of fibrous tissue.

Preliminary investigations will have shown unilateral or bilateral ureteric obstruction in an ill patient with backache and a raised sedimentation rate. Retrograde catheterization is always surprisingly easy: the catheter and contrast medium readily pass up the ureter even though it is severely obstructed, a paradox which gives the diagnosis away. Hypertension is often present, uraemia may be so severe as to demand a percutaneous nephrostomy before any kind of operative intervention is begun.

In certain cases strong contra-indications to a major operation may call for the use of steroids when it seems highly likely, though perhaps not certain, that the diagnosis is idiopathic retroperitoneal fibrosis rather than malignant retroperitoneal obstruction by cancer (Tiptaft *et al.* 1982).

Special preparations

Successful management of retroperitoneal fibrosis calls for close collaboration with nephrologists. Anaemia and hypertension are often severe and salt-losing nephropathy may call for intensive treatment once the upper tract obstruction has been relieved. In former times, on occasion, dialysis was required to get the patient out of a critical state of renal failure but a percutaneous nephrostomy nowadays usually avoids the need for this.

Since it may be quite difficult to know whether the ureter has been entirely freed from its fibrous investment, a simple version of Whitaker's test may be useful, and a saline infusion and manometer should be made ready (Whitaker 1973).

At least four units of blood should be prepared: the dissection behind the bowel can be bloody, and one must be prepared to deal with an accidental hole in the aorta or vena cava, since neither of them can be identified under the stiff carapace of fibrous tissue. For equally sound reasons, make sure the bowel has been prepared before embarking on the operation.

Position on the table

Supine.

Incision

Make a long midline incision from xiphisternum to pubis.

Steps of the operation

In most of my cases both ureters have been obstructed, and it is usually necessary to plan the operation so as to deal with both (7.37).

Mobilize the colon medially, first on one side and then the other, right up to and across the hepatocolic and splenocolic ligaments, which must be divided carefully. The ascending and descending colons are fully mobilized and retracted medially.

The great omentum is detached from the transverse colon along its bloodless line of adhesion. A few tiny vessels may need to be sealed, and great care must be taken not to injure the middle colic artery and its branches.

The omentum is now divided in the midline into two halves, by carefully ligating each small vessel between ligatures, and dividing a few short gastric vessels.

First one ureter is liberated from its fibrous tissue encasement, then the other. Each must be freed from the kidney to the bladder. Find the normal part of the ureter, which is usually unscathed at the bifurcation of the common iliac artery, and pass a silastic sling around it at this point. To liberate the ureter from its constricting fibrous tissue can be very difficult or very easy: in some cases it is only necessary to ease a right-angled forceps between ureter and fibrous tissue, and the ureter strips out on the finger. In others, one must carve the ureter out of its fibrous casing with forceps and knife (7.38). Sooner or later the gonadal vessels are encountered, seldom before they are cut across, for the fibrous tissue is often most dense just at this point. On the right side, it is difficult to know where the inferior vena cava is, for the characteristic feel of that vein is absent, concealed by the fibrous

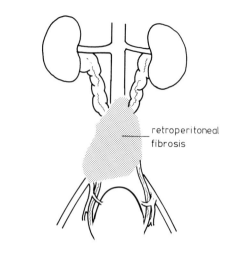

7.37. Idiopathic retroperitoneal fibrosis usually involves the middle third of the ureters.

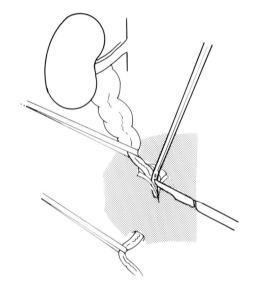

7.38. There is usually a plane of cleavage between the wall of the ureter and the fibrous tissue which can be found with right-angled forceps.

tissue. Be prepared to close a hole with a vascular suture.

On the left side the aorta presents a similar risk, for it is remarkably difficult to feel its pulsations through the fibrous casing.

When the ureter has been set free, hard lumps of fibrous tissue may still be attached, which must be peeled away until the ureter no longer feels like a hard cord, but is soft and pliable. If in doubt, make sure that it is liberated, by instilling saline through a needle upstream of the obstruction, connected to a manometer, and note whether the pressure rises as the saline is run in. Ideally the saline should be run in with a constant-rate syringe (7.39) (Whitaker 1973). If this test is carried out, then at the end of the operation a nephrostomy must be left *in situ* to protect against leakage of urine.

The ureterolysis must be taken from the renal sinus right down to the bifurcation of the common iliac artery. Once each ureter is completely free, the omental flaps are care-

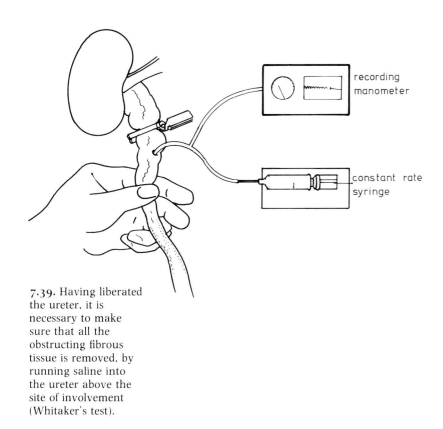

7.39. Having liberated the ureter, it is necessary to make sure that all the obstructing fibrous tissue is removed, by running saline into the ureter above the site of involvement (Whitaker's test).

fully wrapped round each one. Often it is necessary to divide several of the short gastric vessels between the greater curve of the stomach and the gastro-epiploic arch to give more mobility, (7.40, 7.41) but if this is done each flap of omentum can be brought without any tension to the kidney, folded round the ureter, and secured with a few 3-0 catgut sutures (7.42, 7.43). The abdomen is closed with a layer of interrupted nylon sutures to the anterior layer of the rectus sheath to prevent dehiscence.

Hazards of the operation

Difficulty may be encountered in dissecting the ureters from the fibrous tissue, but wrapping them in omentum is not difficult, though time consuming. If a hole has been made in the ureter, a nephrostomy should be placed on the appropriate side, and left *in situ* for eight days.

Follow-up

In our series (Tiptaft *et al.* 1982) of thirty-six ureters in twenty-one patients, we found late recurrence in 6% of renal units wrapped in omentum, 50% when they were simply placed

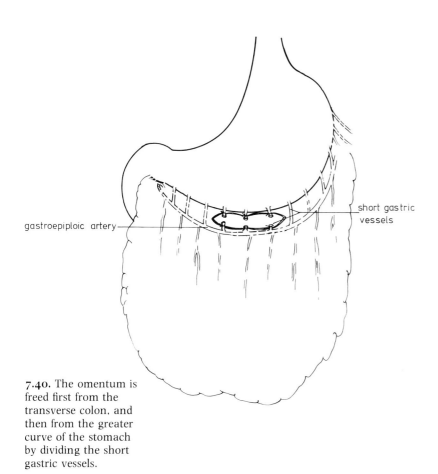

7.40. The omentum is freed first from the transverse colon, and then from the greater curve of the stomach by dividing the short gastric vessels.

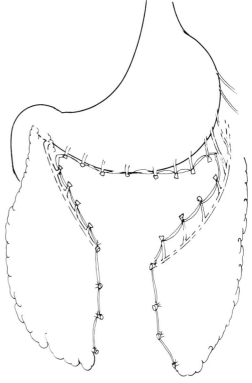

7.41. The gastro-epiploic arcade is divided between liga-tures, allowing the omentum to fall into two long flaps.

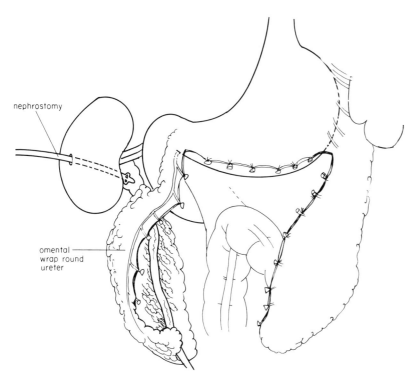

nephrostomy

omental
wrap round
ureter

7.42. Having divided the hepatocolic and splenocolic ligaments, each omental flap is brought out lateral to the colon, and used to wrap up the ureter from top to bottom. A nephrostomy is usually necessary when the ureter looks unhealthy.

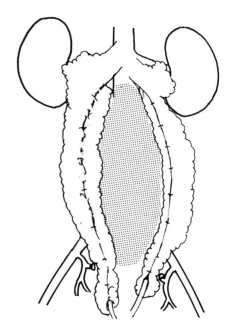

7.43. Each ureter is completely invested with a jacket of omentum. There must be no bare places. The omental covering extends from the renal sinus to the superior vesical vessels in the pelvis.

in the peritoneum, and 25% when the condition was treated only by steroids. These figures support the principle of wrapping the ureters in omentum, and also emphasize the necessity of a prolonged follow up. This seems to be a systemic disease, and late complications from hypertension and cardiovascular conditions are the rule.

Ureteric injury

Injury noticed at the time of operation

The ureter is injured from time to time in the course of surgical operations especially those in the pelvis. If the ureter has been cut during hysterectomy, and the two cleanly divided ends are seen in the wound, then it is perfectly feasible to sew them together (7.44). Nowadays one should use 4-0 chromic catgut interrupted sutures: spatulate the ends of the ureters, and provide an indwelling double-J silicone splint (7.45). If this type of splint is not available, an indwelling Gibbon catheter may be passed via the bladder as described for transplantation (page 85) or a nephrostomy may be performed (Bright 1982).

If the ureter is injured anywhere from the

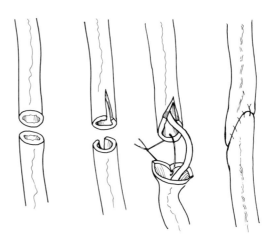

7.44. If the ureter is accidentally cut, and noticed at the time, it should be spatulated and anastomosed without tension over a suitable splint which can be withdrawn from the bladder later.

7.45. A double-J in-dwelling ureteric splint is left across the anastomosis, to be removed after a few weeks.

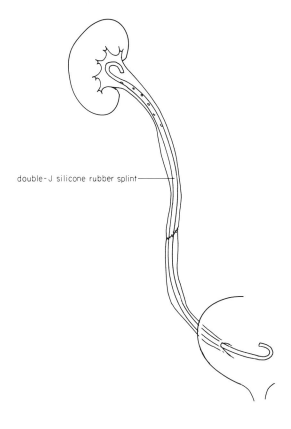

double-J silicone rubber splint

condition is recognized on the table, it is permissible merely to splint the ureter and hope that stricture will not result (7.46).

Nowadays ligature of the injured ureter is seldom indicated. It may give rise to pain, bacteraemia, and shock if the urine upstream of the ligature is infected, and it is often followed by enforced nephrectomy or a urinary fistula.

Delayed diagnosis of ureteric injury

Much more frequently the injury to the ureter is not noticed at the time of operation, when the ureter has been crushed, ligated, or caught up in the suture used to close the peritoneum. The injury is either near the uterine vessels or at the pelvic brim. Whatever injures the ureter also obstructs it. If the operation is on a patient with a single ureter, or if the injury is bilateral, the patient presents with post-operative anuria, and one may not be sure whether this is a result of loss of blood and shock or obstruction to both ureters.

In acute tubular necrosis from operative shock the anuria is usually of gradual onset, and *some* urine will be passed for the first few hours. In obstruction from ureteric injury a high-dose urogram will show *some* excretion, and delayed tomograms will show contrast medium in the renal pelvis and dilated ureter even six to twelve hours later.

Far more commonly the urologist is asked to see a patient several days after the operation at which the ureter has been injured. Characteristically the patient has been going

crossing of the common iliac artery to the bladder—common sites for injury during pelvic surgery—it is safer to reimplant it into the bladder rather than rely upon the rather precarious blood supply of the longitudinal artery of the ureter. My preference is for the Boari flap reimplantation (see page 106).

If the ureter has not been cut across, but merely crushed or ligated in error, and the

7.46. (a) When the ureter has been tied, it is sometimes possible merely to untie the ligature, and (b) leave a catheter indwelling up the ureter for ten or fourteen days.

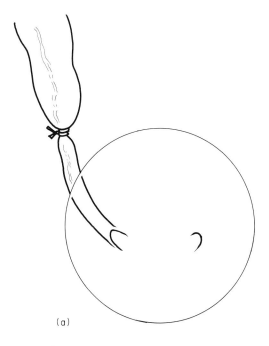

(a)

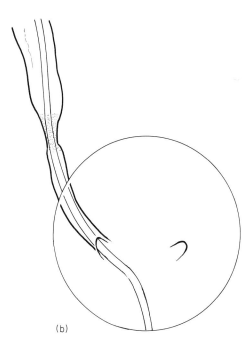

(b)

on quite well for five to six days when a vaginal discharge is noticed. Often there is confusion as to whether this discharge is urine, or merely serous or lymphatic loss from the upper end of the vagina after the hysterectomy. Many and confusing tests have been advocated to help make the diagnosis, involving insertion of several vaginal packs in tandem and of giving methylene blue intravenously or into the bladder. None of them are really helpful. The first and urgent test is to confirm that the fluid is indeed urine. Lose no time, have a small sample collected, if necessary by squeezing out a swab, and have a 'blood urea' measured on it by the clinical laboratory. If the fluid is urine it will have a higher 'blood urea' than the patient's plasma and the diagnosis is settled—there is a urine leak.

The next test is to have an IVU performed. If one ureter is dilated it will probably be the injured one. (Do not expect to see an actual escape of contrast medium into the vagina.)

Percutaneous nephrostomy

If there is some special cause for delay (see below) then a percutaneous nephrostomy should be performed on the obstructed side. This will gain time for the patient's general condition to improve, if it is not satisfactory, and will also gain time for the patient if necessary to be referred to a urological centre.

Early or late operation

It is my experience that the sooner these injured ureters are repaired the better. Not only are the tissues easier to dissect, but healing is rapid, and the patient does not have the prolonged misery of waiting at home with a urinary fistula, a time which is apt to generate bitterness and thoughts of medico-legal action. One should delay the repair only if there is massive local sepsis or if the patient has not recovered from the trauma of the original operation.

Preliminary investigations

In every case with a post-operative leak of urine one should suspect not only that a single ureter has been injured, but that both could have been, and that in addition there may be a vesicovaginal fistula. Before beginning the operative repair, therefore, always confirm the diagnosis exactly by means of cystoscopy and bilateral ureterography. At this cystoscopy, which is conveniently done at the same session planned for the repair operation, a careful search is made for a vesicovaginal fistula (see page 180). Then a bulb-ended Chevassu catheter is jammed in first one ureter and then the other, while contrast is injected and observed on the TV monitor of the image intensifier (7.47).

Low injuries of the ureter

The Boari–Ockerblad flap

This is the procedure of choice in our unit and therefore will be described first (Flynn *et al.* 1979; Bowsher *et al.* 1982).

Position on the table

The patient remains in the cystoscopy position with the legs almost straight.

Incision

Reopen whatever incision was used at the original operation. If the ureter has been injured during a vaginal hysterectomy then a Pfannenstiel incision will be found to give adequate access.

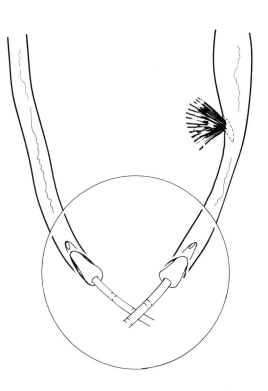

7.47. Before embarking on the repair of an injury to the ureter a ureterogram on both sides is a wise precaution and will show stenosis or extravasation.

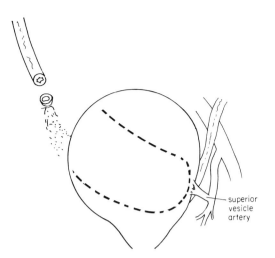

7.48. Boari flap. First, the superior vesical artery on the opposite side is divided between ligatures.

superior vesicle artery

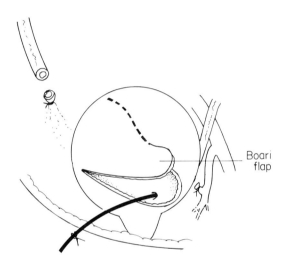

7.49. As the Boari flap is outlined, a precautionary measure is to pass a ureteric catheter up the good ureter.

Boari flap

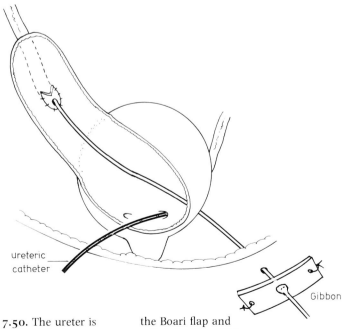

ureteric catheter

Gibbon

7.50. The ureter is implanted via an oblique tunnel into the Boari flap and splinted with a Gibbon catheter.

Steps of the operation

Open the peritoneum and pack away the intestines, taking care to divide previous adhesions in the pelvis. Find the offending ureter where it crosses the common iliac artery and trace it down, dividing the superior vessels to make this easier (7.10). The ureter will be found to vanish into dense fibrous tissue, and it is seldom possible to identify the offending ligature or site of injury. The ureter is marked with a stay suture and cut off at this point (7.48).

Now the Boari flap is marked out on the bladder. To make this easy, fill the bladder with 200 ml of saline and place three stay sutures at the corners of the ∩-shaped flap. It is essential that the flap should be long enough to bridge the gap without any tension, and this is why it is best to dissect and divide the damaged ureter, since it often shrinks back a little way, and there is a possibility that the flap may be designed too short (7.49).

As the incision is made through the wall of the bladder a number of small arteries are divided: these are suture-ligated rather than coagulated with diathermy.

The good ureter is now catheterized to protect it from inadvertent injury.

A submucosal tunnel is made with curved scissors beginning near the tip of the Boari flap, and emerging about 5 cm down the flap, with the object of preventing reflux subsequently. A rubber tube is slipped over the scissors, drawn through the tunnel, sutured to the tip of the ureter, and made to draw the ureter down the tunnel where its end is spatulated and sewn to the mucosa of the bladder with interrupted 4-0 chromic catgut. A Gibbon catheter is led through the abdominal wall to serve as a splint for the ureter. The Gibbon splint is secured to the wall of the bladder with one or two fine 4-0 catgut sutures to make sure it cannot kink (7.50, 7.51).

The bladder is closed with two layers of 4-0 and 3-0 catgut and drained with the urethral catheter. The wound is closed with catgut with a drain down to the suture line in the bladder.

Hazards of the operation

Complications are mercifully few with the Boari operation (Bowsher et al. 1982). In our series of sixty-two ureters in fifty-four patients we had one death from pulmonary embolism

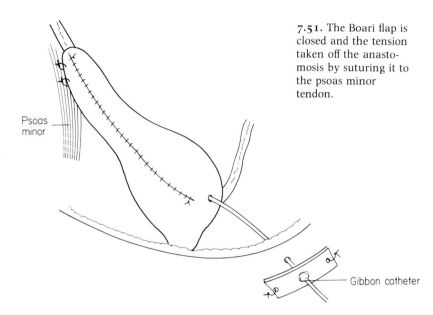

7.51. The Boari flap is closed and the tension taken off the anastomosis by suturing it to the psoas minor tendon.

Psoas minor

Gibbon catheter

7.52. The psoas hitch procedure: (a) the bladder is incised in the transverse axis and hitched to the tendon of psoas minor (b), taking the tension off the ureterovesical anastomosis.

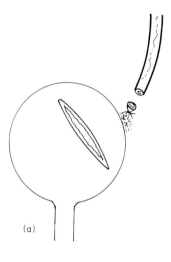

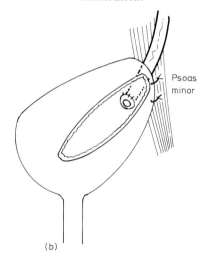

Psoas minor

(a)

(b)

in a man already grossly ill, and one failure to cure a persistent fistula when the operation was done in the presence of carcinoma. Infection in the urine and wound is, of course, common but seldom serious.

The major hazard of the Boari operation is the risk of injuring the opposite good ureter in the course of forming the flap, or of closing the bladder. It is for this reason that it is prudent to mark the position of the other ureter early in the operation.

Cukier (1966) and Bowsher *et al.* (1982) have reviewed the Boari procedure, and conclude that it is the operation of first choice for dealing with damage to the lower end of the ureter, but there are alternatives which should be kept in mind.

Reimplantation with the psoas hitch

Having dissected the ureter down to the site of injury in the way described above, instead of forming a ∩-shaped flap, the bladder is opened obliquely (7.52). It is pulled up to the site of injury, if necessary, having first divided the superior vesical pedicle on the opposite good side to mobilize the bladder. Tension is taken off the anastomosis, which is a short tunnel-and-cuff reimplantation (see page 100), by stitching the wall of the bladder to the tendon of psoas minor. There is very little difference between this and the Boari operation, and in experienced hands the results are equally good (Ehrlich & Skinner 1975).

Uretero–ureteric anastomosis

This operation has had distinguished advocates (Smith & Smith 1975) but it risks damage to the good ureter. It is easy and quick to do, and should always be in the urological repertoire for the exceptional case where it is relevant (Hodges *et al.* 1980).

Having mobilized the injured ureter, bring it medially behind the colon (7.53) and anastomose it to the side of the good ureter. It is very important that the anastomosis is wide, made neatly with very fine catgut, and that neither the good nor the damaged ureter are kinked.

Bilateral injuries to the ureter

Here it is essential that the double injury is recognized; hence the wisdom of *always* performing a ureterogram on both sides before setting out to repair a damaged ureter. According to the site of the injury, and the state of the patient's bladder, one may choose between making two Boari flaps (7.53a) or performing uretero-ureteric anastomosis above the bladder, and bringing the good ureter through the Boari flap (7.53b).

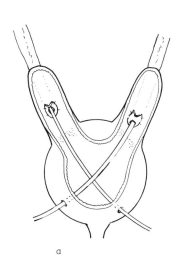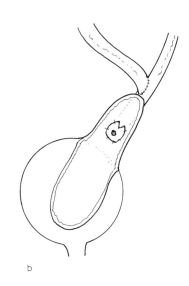

7.53. Bilateral ureteric lesions can be dealt with (a) by bilateral Boari flaps or (b) by trans-ureteroureterostomy followed by implantation of the longer ureter into one Boari flap.

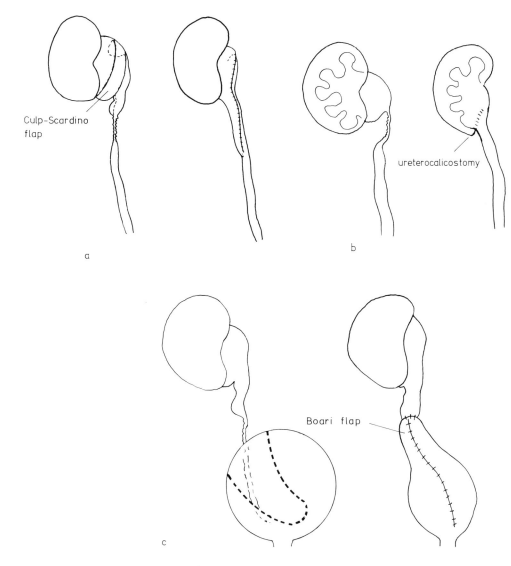

7.54. Alternative methods of coping with a high injury of the ureter: (a) by means of a long Culp–Scardino flap; (b) by ureterocalicostomy; (c) by a long Boari flap taken from a capacious bladder.

Ureteric stricture

A stricture in the upper end of the ureter is dealt with as for a hydronephrosis, with one or other variation of the Anderson–Hynes or Culp pyeloplasty (page 66). A stricture in the lower end of the ureter is treated with a Boari or psoas hitch reimplantation (see above). Very rarely does one come across a stricture that cannot be dealt with by either of these manoeuvres. Such a stricture may be seen following localized bilharziasis, or after previous operation for stone in the ureter. These conditions are rare, and it is impossible to set out hard-and-fast rules. One may, for example, create an exceptionally long Boari flap, and I have succeeded on one occasion in taking the bladder flap right up to the renal pelvis (7.54). On the other hand, when the renal pelvis is grossly dilated, a very long Culp flap may be formed that will extend down into the pelvis. To these manoeuvres one may always add the possibility of replacing the entire ureter with a loop of ileum or colon (page 58).

However, two smaller manoeuvres may be described which can be added to the armamentarium: each is easy and quick to do.

Appendix to bridge a ureteric gap

On the right side one sometimes finds a short bilharzial stricture just adjacent to the appendix. The caecum is rolled medially, and the damaged part of the ureter resected. The appendix is divided at its base, and the caecum is closed (7.55). The mesentery of the appendix is carefully preserved, and the appendix anastomosed to the ureter over a suitable double-J silicone splint (Weinberg 1976).

Pedicled patch of peritoneum for the ureter

It is not difficult to shape a piece of peritoneum to suit a narrowing in the ureter, and it may be kept viable by providing it with a pedicle made of adjacent fat. In the type of situation where such a patch is likely to be relevant—for example after several previous interventions—the adjacent peritoneum is usually thick and its supporting fat vascular and sturdy (7.56).

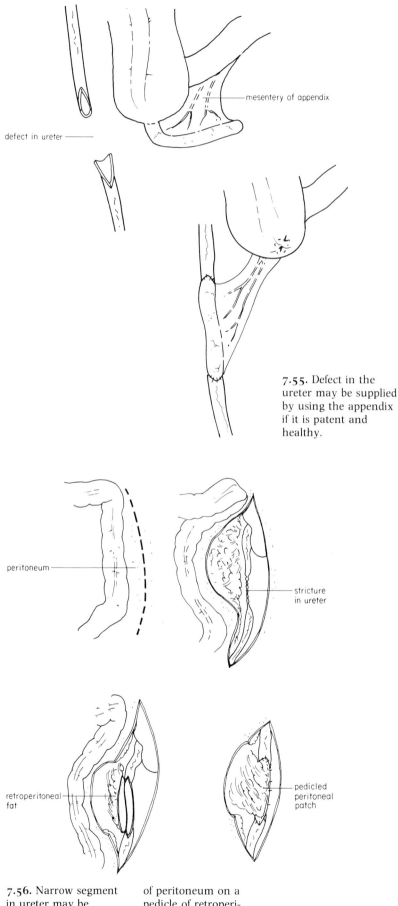

7.55. Defect in the ureter may be supplied by using the appendix if it is patent and healthy.

7.56. Narrow segment in ureter may be enlarged with a patch of peritoneum on a pedicle of retroperitoneal fat.

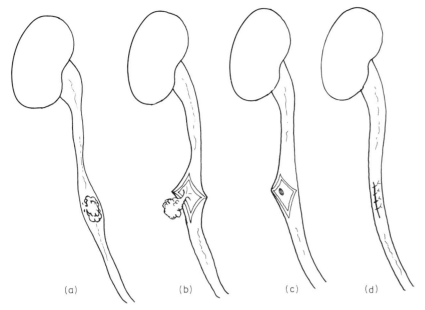

7.57. Conservative management of a pedunculated carcinoma of the ureter (a) is occasionally feasible. The ureter may be opened (b), the pedicle divided (c) and the ureter closed with drainage (d).

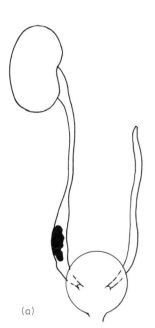
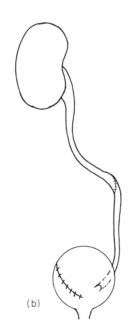

7.58. After ureterectomy for carcinoma in the lower third of the ureter (a), if there is a spare ureter it may be used to save the remaining kidney by transuretero-ureterostomy (b).

Conservative operations for carcinoma of the ureter

Indications

Until recently the notion of performing anything less than nephro-ureterectomy for carcinoma of the ureter was regarded as quite wrong, but today it is recognized that ureteric tumours fall into two distinct groups: those with a very anaplastic tumour and those with a well-differentiated tumour. The former must be treated as radically as possible, preceding surgery by radical radiotherapy, whilst the latter, the well-differentiated tumours, may be treated conservatively. It is for these, the well-differentiated G1 tumours of the ureter, that local resection may be contemplated.

Pedicled tumours in the mid-ureter

One of the striking features about a pedicled tumour in the mid-ureter is that there is always considerable dilatation of the ureter both above and below the growth (7.57). This makes it all the more easy to open the ureter between stay sutures, excise the tumour with, if necessary, its pedicle, and close it without significant loss of ureteric width.

Tumours in the lower ureter

Having removed a tumour from the lower ureter with a suitable cuff of healthy bladder (page 37) one should reimplant it into the bladder using a Boari flap, or into the opposite good ureter. Occasionally I have found myself with a stump of unused ureter on the good side, and have been able to solve the problem by uretero-ureterostomy (7.58).

Hazards of the operation

In all these conservative operations for carcinoma of the ureter it is necessary to start by getting histological material from the tumour with which to grade it, for it is pointless to embark on conservative surgery for a G3 tumour that demands more radical treatment. Cytology of the urine on the affected side, or a brush biopsy should always be obtained.

The problems of post-operative leakage and infection are common to all operations on the ureter. In carcinoma there is a particular need for adequate follow-up: during the follow-up of a tumour first detected in the kidney or ureter, there is almost certain to be recurrence in the bladder, so that in addition to regular urography, these patients need regular follow-up cystoscopy.

Ureterostomy

Ureterostomy has almost been replaced by percutaneous nephrostomy (page 71) for those indications that required temporary drainage of urine. As a permanent form of drainage, ureterostomy has almost no place, except as a method of last resort.

Ureterostomy *in situ*

Through an appropriate incision, the ureter is exposed, and taped above the obstruction. A short incision is made into it between stay sutures, and then a long oblique tunnel is made for a Gibbon catheter (7.59) which is inserted into the ureter and sewn to the skin. It is important that this ureterostomy-*in-situ* is allowed to become solid and well healed before an attempt is made to change the tube (Walsh 1969). It is equally important that the tube is replaced at once should it become dislodged, or the track will be lost. The tube must follow an easy curve from skin to ureter.

Loop ureterostomy in children

The indications for loop ureterostomy in children are decreasing with the advent of more bold reconstruction of the upper tract in children and better and earlier treatment of lower tract obstruction. However in the presence of intractable infection and persistent dilatation, a loop ureterostomy may still be occasionally needed.

Steps of the operation

Through a small incision in the loin, the ureter, which is always grossly varicose and dilated, is drawn into the wound. A side-to-side anastomosis is made between two adjacent loops, and the salient part is opened and sewn to the skin (7.60).

Later on, when the time comes, all that is needed is to circumcise the ureterostomy, close it, and drop it back into the wound.

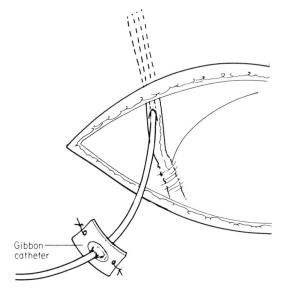

7.59. Ureterostomy *in situ*. A Gibbon catheter makes a good first ureterostomy tube, since it can be well anchored to the skin by its flanges. The line of the tube must fall along a gentle and even curve, without any sharp bends or kinks so that it can be replaced later on if need be.

Gibbon catheter

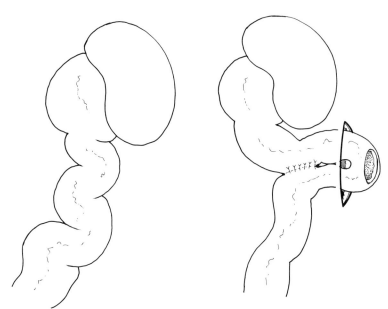

7.60. Temporary urinary diversion in infants with mega-ureters may be performed by a loop ureterostomy. Note that the two limbs of the loop should be anastomosed together.

Permanent end-ureterostomy

Of all forms of diversion of urine permanent ureterostomy must be among the worst, but that does not mean that it should never be performed. For example, after cystectomy, if it is impossible to form an ileal conduit, the patient will be better off with a pair of end-ureterostomies than being dead.

If the ureter is dilated, then it may be treated exactly like the bowel: its end is spatulated, everted, and sewn to the skin (7.61).

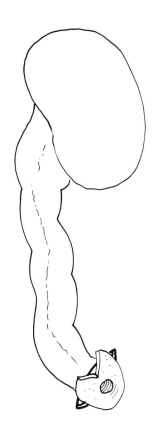

7.61. End-ureterostomy with a dilated ureter. The dilated ureter may be split and turned back as a cuff in the usual way.

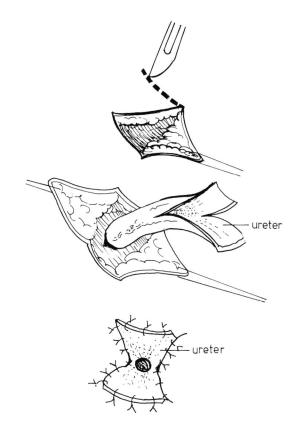

7.62. Z-plasty. This is a useful manœuvre to help to prevent stenosis of a ureter of nearly normal calibre. The two limbs of the 'Z' are let in to the slit-up ureter.

Unfortunately such grossly dilated ureters are rare, and one more often finds a ureter of almost normal calibre. To prevent it stenosing at its junction with the skin, the end is split, and sewn to the skin with a double-Z plasty to prevent subsequent narrowing (7.62).

Uretero-ureterostomy can be added to a permanent end-ureterostomy (7.63). This provides the patient with only a single stoma, and can be quite satisfactory when one of the ureters is very dilated. It is particularly useful after cystectomy, and of course minimizes the operating time.

Intubated ureterostomy should be borne in mind. It may be followed by infection in a high proportion of cases, but if a Gibbon's tube or a narrow Foley catheter is left in the ureter to obviate stenosis of its last few centimetres, one can buy time to get an ill patient over a major operation, and then, later on, consider revising the ureterostomy to an ileal conduit.

References

Boari A. (1894) *Chirurgia dell'uretere.* Societa Editrice Dante Alighieri, Rome.
Bowsher W.G., Shah P.J.R., Costello A.J., Tiptaft R.C., Paris A.M.I. & Blandy J.P. (1982) A critical appraisal of the Boari flap. *Brit. J. Urol.* **54**, 682.
Bricker E.M. (1950) Bladder substitutes after pelvic evisceration. *Surgical Clinics of North America*, **30**, 1511.

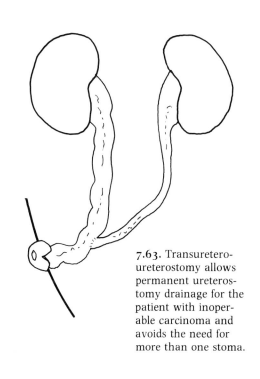

7.63. Transuretero-ureterostomy allows permanent ureterostomy drainage for the patient with inoperable carcinoma and avoids the need for more than one stoma.

Bright T.C. (1982) Emergency management of the injured ureter. *Urological Clinics of North America*, **9**, 285.

Cohen J. (1969) *A new method of vesicoureteric implantation*. Society of Paediatric Urological Surgeons, Oslo.

Dormia E. (1982) Dormia basket: standard technique, observations and general concepts. *Urology*, **20**, 437.

Cukier J. (1966) L'operation de Boari. *Acta Urologica Belgica*, **34**, 15.

Edwards D., Normand I.C.S., Prescod N. & Smellie J.M. (1977) Disappearance of vesicoureteric reflux during long-term prophylaxis of urinary tract infection in children. *Brit. Med. J.* **2**, 285.

Ehrlich R.M. & Skinner D.G. (1975) Complications of transuretero-ureterostomy. *J. Urol.* **113**, 467.

Flynn J.T., Tiptaft R.C., Woodhouse C.R.J., Paris A.M.I. & Blandy J.P. (1979) The early and aggressive repair of iatrogenic ureteric injuries. *Brit. J. Urol.* **51**, 454.

Hendren W.H. (1969) Operative repair of megaureter in children. *J. Urol.* **101**, 491.

Hodges C.V., Barry J.M., Fuchs E.F., Pearse H.D. & Tank E.S. (1980) Transureteroureterostomy: 25 years experience with 100 patients. *J. Urol.* **123**, 834.

Ockerblad N.F. (1936) Reimplantation of the ureter into the bladder by a flap method. *J. Urol.* **57**, 845.

Politano V.A. & Leadbetter W.F. (1958) An operative technique for the correction of vesicoureteric reflux. *J. Urol.* **79**, 932.

Ransley P.G. (1978) Vesicoureteric reflux: continuing surgical dilemma. *Urology*, **12**, 246.

Simon J. (1852) Ectropia vesicae. *Lancet*, **ii**, 568.

Smith I.B. & Smith J.C. (1975) Transureteroureterostomy: British experience. *Brit. J. Urol.* **47**, 519.

Tiptaft R.C., Costello A.J., Paris A.M.I. & Blandy J.P. (1982) The long-term follow-up of idiopathic retroperitoneal fibrosis. *Brit. J. Urol.* **54**, 620.

Walsh A. (1969) Ureterostomy in situ. *Brit. J. Urol.* **39**, 744.

Wallace D.M.A., Rothwell D.L. & Williams D.I. (1978) The long-term follow up of surgically treated vesicoureteric reflux. *Brit. J. Urol.* **50**, 479.

Weinberg R.W. (1976) Appendix ureteroplasty. *Brit. J. Urol.* **48**, 234.

Wells C.A. (1956) The use of the intestine in urology. *Brit. J. Urol.* **28**, 335.

Whitaker R.H. (1973) Methods of assessing obstruction in dilated ureters. *Brit. J. Urol.* **45**, 15.

Chapter 8
Benign conditions of the bladder

Approaches to the bladder

For most needs adequate access is obtained through Pfannenstiel's incision, which has the advantages of a sound scar, no risk of incisional hernia, and an excellent cosmetic result. More extensive abdominal operations require the midline incision which can be extended as far as necessary.

For most approaches to the bladder the patient lies in the supine position, but it is always worth considering whether there may be an advantage in having the patient in the cystoscopy position. A second assistant may stand between the patient's legs and have an excellent view of the operation and a good purchase for retraction, while access is provided to the vagina or perineum.

Pfannenstiel incision

The incision (8.1) begins a finger's breadth above the symphysis pubis in the skin crease and extends towards the anterior superior iliac spine on either side, its length being governed by the obesity of the patient and the exposure required by the underlying pathology.

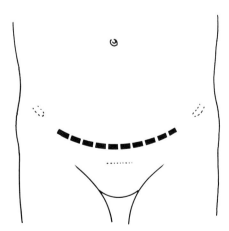

8.1. Pfannenstiel incision.

In dividing the skin and fat in the line of the incision two superficial veins are secured (8.2). The anterior layer of the rectus sheath is opened (8.3) and the incision carried

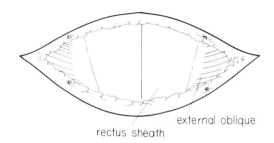

rectus sheath   external oblique

8.2. Exposure of the rectus sheath.

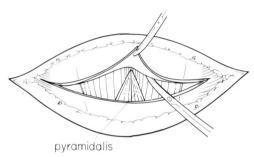

pyramidalis

8.3. Dissection of the upper flap of rectus aponeurosis.

laterally through the external oblique aponeurosis and muscle of the internal oblique in the line of its fibres. Dissect the linea alba with knife or scissors. Lift its sheath off the underlying rectus towards the umbilicus and take care to diathermize the two little arteries that enter the sheath, before they are torn. Start the inferior flap by picking up the apex of the triangle of pyramidalis and dissect it away from the rectus (8.4). Separate the

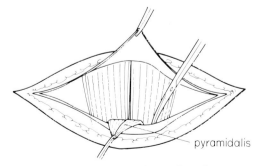

pyramidalis

8.4. Beginning with the apex of pyramidalis (when present) the lower flap of rectus aponeurosis is elevated.

bellies of the rectus muscle in the midline and retract them with Millin's self-retaining retractor (8.5).

After the operation is over the rectus muscle bellies should be loosely approximated with a few catgut sutures, one of which catches the apex of the pyramidalis to restore the original anatomy (8.6). A drain is always needed in operations on the bladder and lower ureter and it is brought out through a stab in the upper leaf of the aponeurosis and skin. The aponeurosis is closed with continuous or interrupted catgut in a single layer (8.7). The subcutaneous fat and skin are brought together with fine catgut to obliterate the dead space, and the skin is closed with clips or sutures according to the whim of the surgeon.

Vertical incisions

There is nothing unusual about a vertical midline incision for the bladder, and no advantage in making it paramedian. It is made and closed in the usual way standard to all abdominal operations except that when the urinary tract has been opened, non-absorbable sutures are never used for fear of causing a persistent and tiresome sinus.

Apron incision

With contemporary methods of radiotherapy this incision is almost never needed, but it should be kept in mind for the occasional patient whose lower abdomen has been given so much radiotherapy that the skin has become indurated and the underlying fat hard and avascular. Incisions, whether transverse or vertical, that transgress this unhealthy tissue will not heal. To avoid this danger, one may form the incision like an apron (8.8). The upper edge of the apron may go above or below the umbilicus according to the shape of the patient, the lateral limbs follow the direction of the external oblique muscle. Great care is taken when making this flap to preserve the inferior epigastric artery and vein on each side. In planning this incision, fortunately rarely needed nowadays, great care must be taken to site the urinary stoma to prevent placing it too near the suture line.

Closure of the bladder

The bladder is kept empty after any operation by an indwelling urethral or suprapubic catheter. The space outside the bladder is

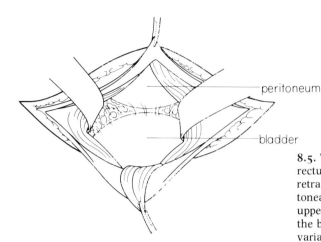

8.5. The bellies of the rectus muscles are retracted. The peritoneal fold covers the upper anterior part of the bladder to a variable extent.

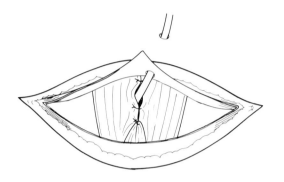

8.6. Closure of the Pfannenstiel incision: the rectus muscle bellies are approximated and the pyramidalis restored. The prevesical space is drained with a tube connected to a closed system.

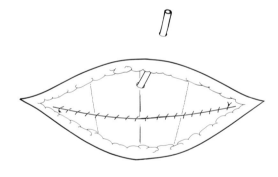

8.7. The rectus aponeurosis is closed with continuous catgut.

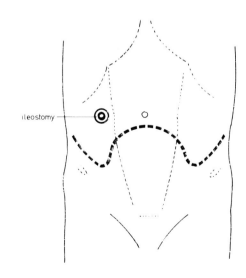

8.8. The 'apron' incision for use when the suprapubic region has been subjected to radiation damage.

drained so that urine and blood cannot accumulate. If it is convenient to close the bladder in layers, the mucosa is approximated with 3-0 chromic catgut (8.9) and a similar suture is used to bring the muscle layer together over it (8.10). Either or both these layers may be made with interrupted sutures if they seem easier to place. Non-absorbable sutures are never used near the bladder because they will inevitably give rise to stones at some future period.

When the wall of the bladder is very thin, it may be closed with interrupted figure-of-eight sutures that take in a full thickness of mucosa and muscle (8.11). Interrupted suture lines are not waterproof, but this does not matter providing the bladder is kept empty with a catheter and the suture line is drained.

Suprapubic cystostomy

Percutaneous suprapubic cystostomy

Indications

There are numerous indications for inserting a temporary suprapubic tube, mainly for retention of urine when a catheter cannot easily be passed through the urethra.

Position on the table

The patient is supine.

Anaesthetic

Using 1% lignocaine, a weal is raised in the skin one finger's breadth above the symphysis pubis (8.12). Using a longer needle, local anaesthetic is infiltrated as the needle is advanced towards the bladder, alternately injecting local and withdrawing, until urine is aspirated. Mark the depth at which urine is obtained by putting an artery forceps on the needle.

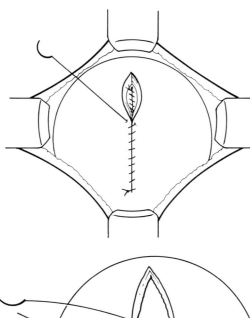

8.9. Closure of the bladder after cystostomy: the mucosa and inner layers of muscle are closed in one layer of catgut.

mucosa

muscle

8.10. The outer muscle layers are closed in a second layer of catgut.

8.11. If the bladder wall is very thin and atrophic, it may be closed with a series of cross-stitches.

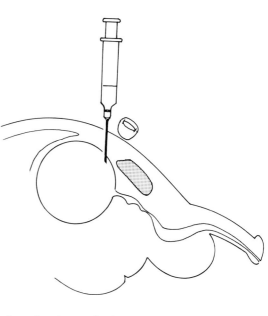

8.12. Local anaesthetic is infiltrated down to the bladder.

Inserting the catheter

Incise the skin through the weal of local anaesthetic for a few millimetres. Holding the catheter and introducer (8.13) firmly, thrust it into the bladder, aiming towards the patient's anus, that is a little caudally. Trochar and cannula are inserted beyond the depth indicated by the mark on the anaesthetic needle. The trochar is removed and the cannula advanced further into the bladder. If it is provided with a balloon, this is inflated and the catheter connected to sterile drainage. Fix the catheter to the skin with two silk sutures taking care to place them in the anaesthetized part of the skin (8.14).

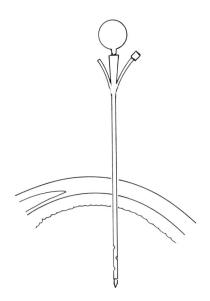

8.13. The trochar and plastic cannula are inserted into the bladder.

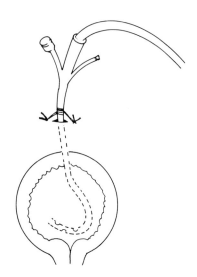

8.14. The cannula is attached to the skin.

Open suprapubic cystostomy

Indications

Occasionally the small catheter that can be introduced percutaneously will not suffice to drain a bladder full of thick pus, or previous surgery may have made it difficult and dangerous to place the cannula blindly lest small bowel and peritoneum are tethered in front of the bladder.

Precautions

The bladder should be full if this is to be an easy and safe operation. If the patient is not in retention already, have the bladder filled up with sterile saline until it can be unmistakably felt.

Position on the table

Supine.

Anaesthetic

A general anaesthetic should be used wherever possible. If the patient strains and coughs it is exceedingly easy to injure the peritoneum.

Incision

For most cases a straight midline incision will be used except when making a formal cystostomy at leisure when the bladder is approached through a short Pfannenstiel, and the suprapubic tube brought out well above the incision through a short tunnel (8.15).

Steps of the operation

After incising skin and fat the linea alba is divided in the midline and retracted. Wipe away the fold of peritoneum with a gauze-protected finger to reveal the characteristic woven texture of the bladder. When re-operating in this field, even the most experienced surgeon may be unsure of his

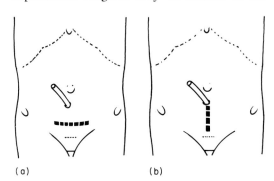

(a)   (b)

8.15. A suprapubic cystostomy tube should lie half-way between umbilicus and symphysis: either a vertical midline incision or a short Pfannenstiel may be used.

8.16. (a) The rectus muscle bellies are parted, revealing the criss-cross fibres of the bladder (b) which is opened between stay sutures.

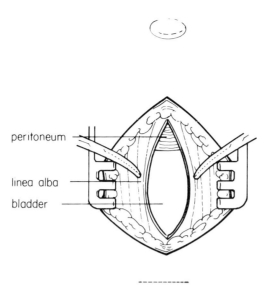

peritoneum

linea alba

bladder

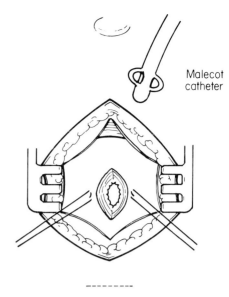

Malecot catheter

8.17. Bladder closed over Malecot catheter.

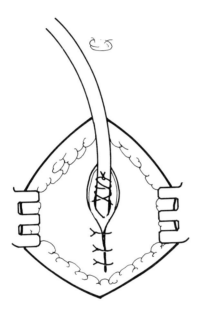

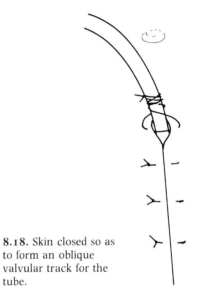

8.18. Skin closed so as to form an oblique valvular track for the tube.

whereabouts, and it is no shame to insert a fine needle on a syringe to make doubly certain that what you think is the bladder is indeed the viscus. Now insert two stay sutures and open the bladder between them just widely enough to allow a catheter to go in (8.16). A Malecot catheter has a large lumen and open tip and is useful if there is pus or blood in the bladder. Otherwise a Foley may be used. Close the bladder around the catheter and stitch the catheter to the bladder (8.17). The rectus and skin are now closed in a tunnel so that the catheter emerges at the upper end of the incision, at least half-way between symphysis and umbilicus (8.18).

If a Pfannenstiel incision has been used to insert the tube into the bladder, the catheter is made to come out through the upper flap of rectus again, as a tunnel, to emerge half-way between umbilicus and symphysis (8.19).

8.19. Pfannenstiel incision allows access to the bladder, into which the tube is placed and led through the upper leaf of the abdominal incision.

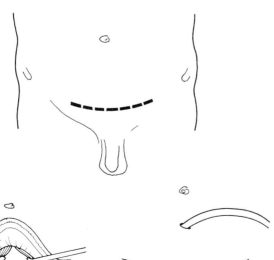

Rectus aponeurosis

Recti

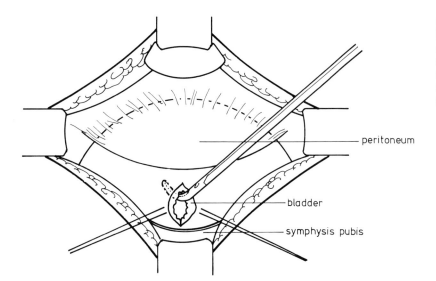

8.20. When there have been previous operations in the suprapubic region, approach the bladder as near to the symphysis as possible.

peritoneum

bladder

symphysis pubis

Too low a catheter makes it difficult to fit an appliance and uncomfortable for the patient, and it risks osteomyelitis of the symphysis pubis.

A suprapubic catheter is never closed with a spigot: always connect it to closed drainage.

Stone in the bladder

Suprapubic cystostomy

Indications

Large calculi in bladders with diverticula and saccules may need an open removal of the stones (Blandy 1976). Some foreign bodies cannot be removed through the cystoscope.

Position

Supine or cystoscopy.

Incision

Pfannenstiel or vertical.

Steps of the operation

Having retracted the peritoneum from the bladder and identified its muscle fibres, two stay sutures are inserted and the bladder opened between them (8.20, 8.21). The stone is lifted out, the bladder is inspected and if any suspicious places are noted, they are biopsied to exclude squamous cell carcinoma. Then the bladder is closed over a catheter.

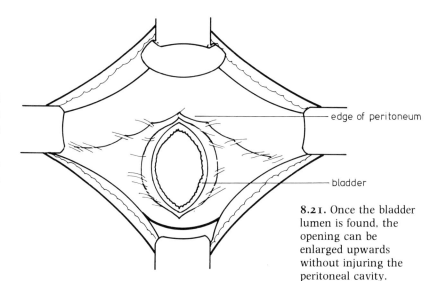

edge of peritoneum

bladder

8.21. Once the bladder lumen is found, the opening can be enlarged upwards without injuring the peritoneal cavity.

Litholapaxy

Indications

Nearly all stones in the bladder may be safely removed with the classical lithotrite (Swift-Joly 1929) and it is one of the instruments that every urologist must master. There are only a few contra-indications to its use: when the surgeon has never been taught how to use it; when there are multiple diverticula in the bladder and bits of stone may get stuck in them; when the prostate is so large that the lithotrite cannot be got over it and the bladder must be opened anyway at the time of the Millin's prostatectomy (see page 168).

A stone in the bladder in a boy can be removed with a child's lithotrite, but this may damage the urethra and suprapubic removal is safer. Similarly, if an adult has a severe stricture, it may be better not to make it worse by repeated passage of the lithotrite.

Position

As for cystoscopy.

Anaesthetic

The patient must be deeply relaxed. It is impossible to crush stones safely in a patient who is heaving and straining.

Steps of the operation

Urethrocystoscopy is performed to assess the urethra and bladder, and to make sure that the prostate is not so large that it will need a Millin's operation.

Leave about 200 ml of sterile fluid in the bladder, since it must be full enough to give you room to manoeuvre the blades of the lithotrite without catching a fold of mucosa.

Select a well-tried and well-lubricated classical lithotrite, and check that its lock is working smoothly. When passing it, note that its blades are set almost at a right-angle, a more sharp bend than is found on the ordinary urethral bougie (8.22).

Never try to pick up the stones with the jaws of the lithotrite by 'pecking' at them: this error of technique may lacerate the mucosa. The secret is to depress the female blade of the lithotrite onto the posterior floor of the bladder whilst opening the jaw, so that a stone can roll into the depression (8.23). As the female blade is firmly but gently held down onto the floor of the bladder, the male blade is moved up and down until one has the unmistakable sensation that the stone is within the jaws.

The next step is to make sure that the lithotrite has seized the stone and nothing but the stone. Lift it up off the floor of the bladder and move it from side to side so that it is obviously quite free from the bladder. (Occasionally a stone will be fixed to the bladder on a foreign body or a carcinoma and will probably need an open operation.)

Having made sure the stone is free, lock the screw, and tighten the knob. Most stones crack at once, but sometimes a calculus can be very hard. The secret here is patience: screw down as hard as you can, and wait. After a few seconds you may be rewarded by the crack of the stone, like a muffled pistol-shot.

One the main part of the stone is broken, each of its fragments must be broken again in the same way until nothing remains wider than the lumen of the resectoscope sheath through which all the bits are to be aspirated. Smaller fragments break easily by the merest pressure of the male against the female blade, but larger ones will need the force of the screw and its locking mechanism. Litholapaxy calls for patience and gentleness. It must not be hurried. Take time to make sure that all the bits are thoroughly broken up, and try to avoid repeated removal and reinsertion of the lithotrite.

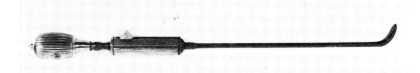

8.22. Freyer's 'blind' lithotrite.

8.23. Steps in litholapaxy: the instrument is put into the bladder with the jaws closed (a); the female blade is pushed firmly down on to the floor of the bladder and the male blade lifted up (b); the stone rolls into the depression in the floor of the bladder and is caught between the jaws and crushed (c).

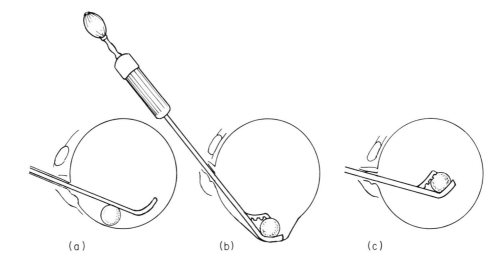

(a)   (b)   (c)

When at last it seems that there are no large bits left, remove the lithotrite, and pass a resectoscope sheath on its obturator. Attach Ellik's evacuator, and remove the bits (8.24). The object of the evacuator and bulb is to swirl the contents of the bladder around: no force is needed. Repeat the irrigation several times until all the cloudiness has been washed away, and then examine the interior of the bladder with the resectoscope and 30° telescope (Hadley *et al.* 1977; Smith & O'Flynn 1977).

Mauermayer's modification of the resectoscope is very useful at this stage (Mauermayer & Hartung 1976). It has a sturdy sheath and a strong 'loop' with which tiny fragments of stone can be caught and crushed against the beak of the 'resectoscope' (8.25). Equally useful if a few small bits remain at this stage is the Storz ultrasonic lithotriptor with which small fragments are shaken to bits by the oscillating teeth of the inner cylinder, and aspirated up its lumen (8.26). Also useful is a sturdy forceps (8.27) for breaking up small bits of stone.

Only when all the little bits have been removed should the sheath be removed and a catheter passed. The bladder is often rather bruised and sore, and a three-way irrigating catheter left in for twenty-four hours gives the patient a comfortable post-operative period.

Hazards of classical litholapaxy

The danger of litholapaxy is crushing or laceration of the mucosa of the bladder, from taking insufficient care to make sure that the stone caught in the jaws of the instrument is not completely free from the wall of the bladder. Since many of these stones are infected, one must watch out for post-operative bacteraemia, and if the urine is known to be infected, cover the procedure with an appropriate antibiotic.

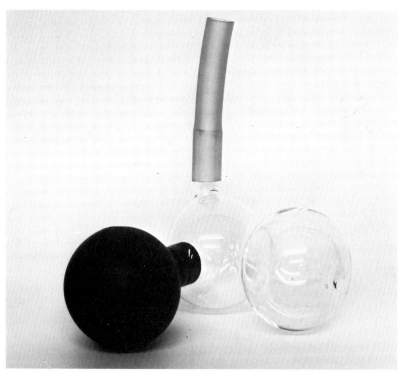

8.24. Ellik evacuator.

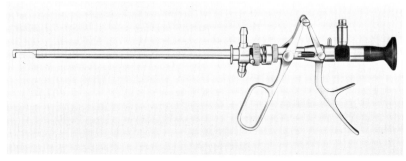

8.25. Mauermayer's stone punch (courtesy of Messrs Rimmer

Bros, UK Agents for Karl Storz A.G.).

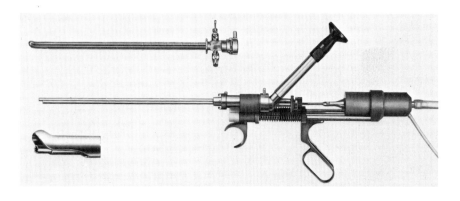

8.26. Storz ultrasonic lithotriptor (courtesy Messrs Rimmer Bros, UK Agents for Karl Storz A.G.).

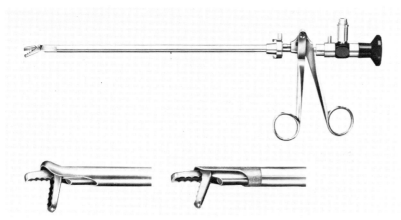

8.27. Heavy duty cystoscopic forceps ideally suited for breaking up small fragments of calculus remaining after classical litholapaxy (courtesy of Messrs Rimmer Brothers, UK Agents for Karl Storz A.G.).

Stories are told of lithotrites being fractured in the urethra, or of them becoming jammed. On one occasion I jammed the blades half-open, and had to dismantle the handle of the instrument to put things right. Since this particular lithotrite was more than a century old, it was hardly surprising that it needed a new retaining screw.

Visual lithotrites

They have a limited role: once the field has become cloudy with crushed stone, or has started to bleed, it is difficult to see anything, and their relative weakness compared with the strength of the classical instrument makes them suitable only for small fragments, for which Mauermayer's stone 'punch' is generally more useful.

Diverticulum of the bladder

Indications

Small saccules and diverticula can be left alone as long as the outflow obstruction which caused them has been corrected by transurethral resection. Large diverticula may need to be removed if they harbour persistent infection or cannot be inspected adequately, so that there is a risk of carcinoma going unnoticed (Gerridzen & Futter 1982).

The obstructing prostate which gives rise to diverticula so large that they need surgical excision is seldom big enough to warrant prostatectomy. It is best to begin by resecting the prostate in the usual way (page 150) and then open the bladder to deal with the diverticulum. This is better than trying to cope with both lesions through the open bladder, for the small fibrous prostates that usually accompany diverticula are notoriously difficult to remove transvesically, but easy to do transurethrally.

Special preparations

Many diverticula requiring excision are infected and there is a danger of post-operative bacteraemia. Make sure the urine microbiology has been studied and that adequate antimicrobial cover has been given.

Position on the table

The patient is in the cystoscopy position. The transurethral resection is performed in the usual way (page 151). Set up a three-way irrigating system.

Incision

Pfannenstiel (page 115).

Steps of the operation

Retract the rectus muscles and wipe the peritoneum from the side of the pelvis until the obliterated hypogastric artery is found, which leads down to the superior vesical vessels. Under-ligate and divide them (8.28). This is the key to easy exposure of the diverticulum because it allows the side of the bladder to be rolled towards the surgeon.

Open the bladder between stay sutures and pull the catheter up and out of the way. A ureteric catheter is placed in the ureteric orifice on the side of the diverticulum as a safety precaution (8.29). This catheter will not necessarily prevent inadvertent damage to the ureter, but makes it easier to recognize such an injury and avoids delay in reimplantation of the ureter.

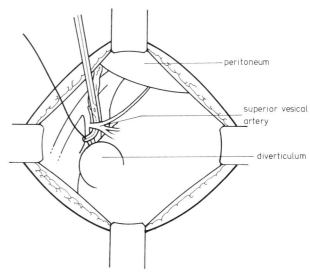

peritoneum

superior vesical artery

diverticulum

8.28. The first step in removing a diverticulum is to divide the superior vesical vessels on that side, in order to free the side of the bladder.

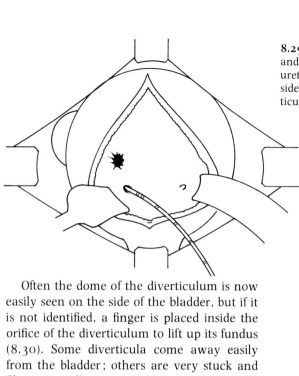

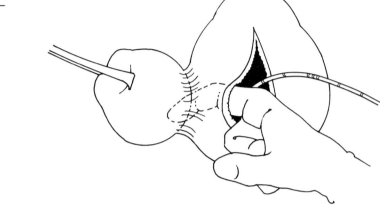

8.29. Open the bladder and catheterize the ureteric orifice on the side of the diverticulum.

8.30. A finger inside the lumen of the diverticulum helps in its dissection.

Often the dome of the diverticulum is now easily seen on the side of the bladder, but if it is not identified, a finger is placed inside the orifice of the diverticulum to lift up its fundus (8.30). Some diverticula come away easily from the bladder; others are very stuck and fibrous. In all cases tough strands of muscle that cross from the detrusor must be peeled away. Dissect down to the neck of the diverticulum and open it partially. Start a stitch in the neck of the diverticulum at this stage (8.31). Finish dissecting the neck of the diverticulum little by little, peeling its mucosa away from the surrounding muscle and fibrous tissue (8.32). Although this forms a thick layer, there is no need to remove it. While dissecting the neck, make sure the catheter can be felt in the ureter and that it is out of harm's way. Once the neck of the diverticulum is divided, pull it up into the wound and free its lining from the fibro-muscular coverings, delivering it like the sac of a hernia (8.33).

Sometimes operating on a diverticulum is not so easy: inflammatory oedema and fibrosis may convert the wall into a thick mass which bleeds freely, while the fundus seems to disappear somewhere right down behind the bladder, dangerously near the rectum. There is no need to take unnecessary risks in this dissection. It is sufficient to leave the sac *in situ* so long as the neck has been closed and the outflow obstruction has been dealt with. The residual fundus of the sac should, of course, be drained (8.34).

Finish closing the opening of the diverticulum with the stitch that has been started, and include a generous bite of bladder muscle to prevent relapse of the diverticulum. Close any defect on the inside of the bladder with a second suture (8.35). The wound is closed with drainage to the site of the diverticulum, and a catheter in the bladder.

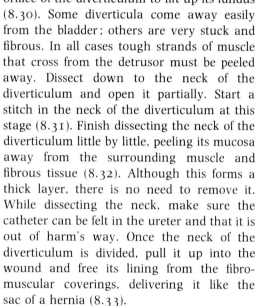

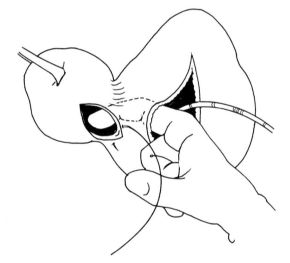

8.31. Open the diverticulum at its neck, and insert the suture with which it is going to be closed later on so that it may be used as a retractor.

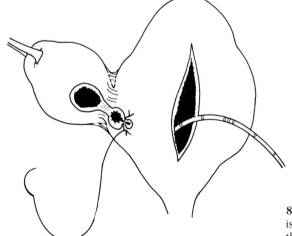

8.32. The diverticulum is dissected away at the neck first.

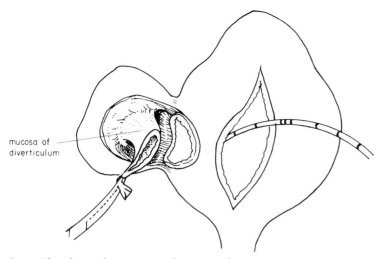

8.33. After the neck of the diverticulum is cut across, the lining may be removed leaving the fibro-muscular coat behind.

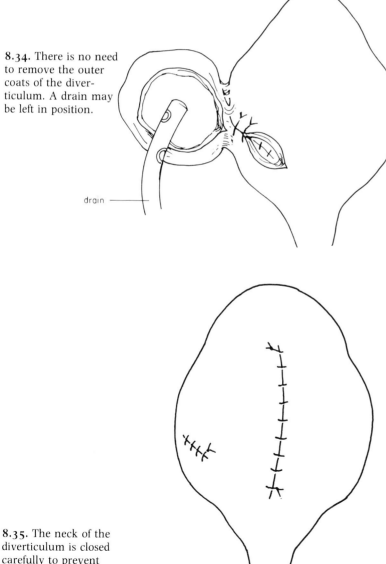

8.34. There is no need to remove the outer coats of the diverticulum. A drain may be left in position.

drain

8.35. The neck of the diverticulum is closed carefully to prevent recurrence.

Hazards of the operation

The main hazard is haemorrhage, and safety depends on good exposure of the side of the bladder and the orifice of the diverticulum. This is why it is important to divide the superior vesical vessels to allow the bladder to be rolled towards you.

Carcinoma may occur in the wall of the diverticulum, so when it is removed it is worth taking trouble to fill the specimen with cotton wool soaked in formalin to fix it, so that your pathologist can study it carefully.

The ureter is sometimes closely applied to the back of the diverticulum or may even enter it. If it is damaged—and the catheter makes this easy to detect—it must be reimplanted in the usual way with a tunnel-and-cuff technique.

Cystoplasty

Indications

If the bladder is shrunken, or a large part has had to be removed, it may need to be enlarged. Every part of the bowel from stomach to sigmoid has at one time or other been employed as a substitute for the bladder. Today the caecum seems to be the best of the alternatives (Dounis *et al.* 1980). It is used to enlarge the bladder after subtotal cystectomy for Hunner's ulcer, or tuberculosis, to replace it after necrosis from cyclophosphamide poisoning, and in helping to repair very severe post-partum vesicovaginal fistulae. The only indication about which I have regrets and reservations is replacement of the bladder after resection for cancer: whenever I have tried this, there has always been recurrence of the cancer sooner or later.

In many cases for which caecocystoplasty might be considered, the ureters are also damaged, or there will be uncertainty about continence. In these circumstances, Turner-Warwick's 'three-option' method is preferred. Here the terminal ileum is left on the caecum, the ureters are anastomosed to the ileum, and the patient can, if necessary, have the caecocystoplasty converted to an ileal conduit if the end-result of the caecocystoplasty is less than perfect. In this technique the ileocaecal valve may help to protect the upper tracts from the pressure of the caecal bladder (Turner-Warwick 1976).

Special precautions

In addition to the preparations used before any

major abdominal operation, the bowel is cleansed mechanically, and prepared with neomycin and metronidazole.

Position on the table

Supine.

Incision

To give plenty of room a long midline incision is used.

Steps of the operation

Usually the lower limit of the resection need to be no further down than the trigone. This gives a thick cuff to which the caecum may be anastomosed. Resection of the bladder wall is made in short lengths, and haemostasis is secured by suture-ligature, piecemeal, which prevents bleeding and keeps the field dry and clean.

Divide the peritoneal reflexion on the lateral aspect of the ascending colon and continue this incision round the corner of the caecum, along the left side, to mobilize the lower part of the ileum and caecum on a mesentery (8.36). By holding this loop up on its mesentery, and shining a light through it, the arcade of the ileocaecal artery and its branches can be identified (8.37). Divide the marginal artery of the ascending colon a little way below the right colic artery, ligating each vessel carefully with fine thread.

The length of the ileal segment is governed by the possible need to change it later to an ileal conduit. Divide the mesentery, taking care to have always two good branches of the mesenteric artery supplying the ileal loop.

Placing Doyen's intestinal clamps across the ileum and ascending colon, cut the bowel across and wrap the isolated ileocaecal segment in moist packs.

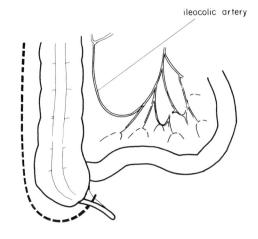

ileocolic artery

8.36. Caecocystoplasty: mobilization of the ileocaecal segment.

Slit the antemesenteric border of the ileum for 3 cm and anastomose it end-to-end to the ascending colon using an all-coats 3-0 chromic catgut layer and a seromuscular layer of 3-0 thread or silk. Close the defect in the mesentery and replace the bowel in the abdomen.

The caecum is now rotated to bring its cut end near the stump of the bladder (8.38). The anastomosis between the wall of the caecum and the bladder is made with catgut, since non-absorbable material will sooner or later form stones. It is generally easier to use interrupted sutures and put the posterior layer in first, getting good bites of caecum and the muscle of the bladder behind the trigone. Before completing the anastomosis arrange suitable drainage of the new bladder. A good place for a drain is the stump of the appendix.

If the terminal ileum has been removed, now is the time to trim it away, carefully closing off the entry of the ileum into the caecum with two layers of catgut. If the ureters are to be anastomosed to the ileum, they are put in by Wallace's method (page 145), first sewing the spatulated ureters to each other to make a common orifice, and then to the open end of the ileum. Nasogastric tubes make excellent splints for the ureters

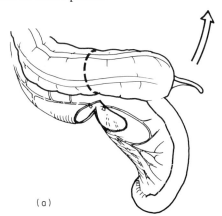

(a)

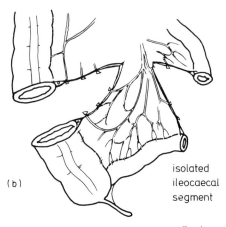

(b)

isolated ileocaecal segment

8.37. (a) The ileocaecal segment is held up and its blood supply examined with transmitted light. Select the site at which the marginal artery of the colon is to be divided below the right colic artery. (b) Ensure that there are at least two large branches of the ileocolic artery going to your segment.

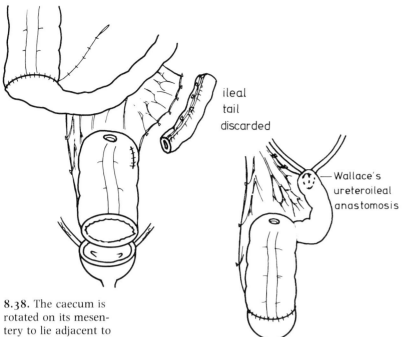

8.38. The caecum is rotated on its mesentery to lie adjacent to the bladder. The surplus ileal tail may be removed or left *in situ*, according to whether or not the ureters are to be implanted into it.

ileal tail discarded

Wallace's ureteroileal anastomosis

and these are led out through the appendix stump alongside the Malecot catheter used to drain the new bladder.

The caecum continues to form mucus, and for the first few days a large Malecot catheter is needed to allow this mucus to be irrigated from time to time. A second catheter drains the bladder via the urethra.

Hazards of the operation

Caecocystoplasty is a remarkably successful operation and its complications are few. The ileocolic anastomosis gives less post-operative ileus than an ordinary end-to-end anastomosis. Mucus formation may call for occasional irrigation of the suprapubic and urethral catheter, for which 1% sodium bicarbonate solution is particularly useful.

In addition to the ordinary hazards of any abdominal operation, after caecocystoplasty one must look out for hyperchloraemic acidosis, caused by absorption of urine from the caecal wall. It should not be troublesome unless renal function is already precarious. The other difficulty which is commonly seen with caecocystoplasty is incontinence of urine. Within a few weeks most of the patients are continent, but the tendency to wet the bed at night may continue for as long as three months.

One should check the system with an IVU in three months' time to make sure that the new bladder is emptying itself properly. If the operation has been performed in an elderly male, residual urine may call for trans-urethral resection of the prostate to reduce outflow obstruction.

Operations to make the bladder smaller

Previous operations to plicate the bladder have now almost entirely been replaced by intermittent self-catheterization. Rarely one may attempt to reduce the capacity of a really huge bladder. In such a case Hamilton Stewart's plication (8.39) is an easy and safe alternative to partial cystectomy, but its long term results are unpredictable: indeed I have not performed this operation for a decade.

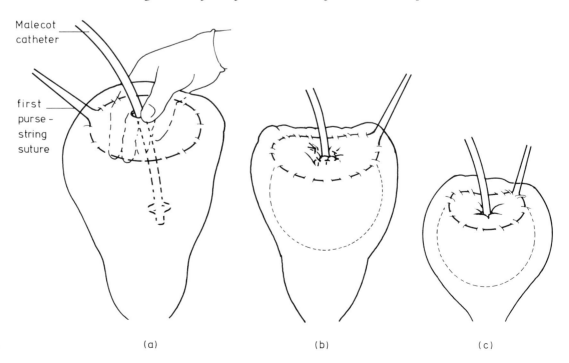

Malecot catheter

first purse-string suture

8.39. Bladder plication by the ink-pot method.

(a)   (b)   (c)

References

Blandy J.P. (1976) Stones and foreign bodies in the bladder. In *Urology* (ed. by Blandy J.P.), p. 753. Blackwell Scientific Publications, Oxford.

Dounis A., Abel B.J. & Gow J.G. (1980) Cecocystoplasty for bladder augmentation. *J. Urol.* **123**, 164.

Gerridzen R.G. & Futter N.G. (1982) Ten year review of vesical diverticula. *Urology*, **20**, 33.

Hadley H.L., Barnes R.W. & Rosenquist R.C. (1977) Tactile litholapaxy—safe and efficient. *Urology*, **9**, 263.

Mauermayer W. & Hartung R. (1976) Bladder stone punch—new principle of visual lithotripsy. *Urologe*, **15**, 164.

Smith J.M. & O'Flynn J.D. (1977) Transurethral removal of bladder stone: the place of litholapaxy. *Brit. J. Urol.* **49**, 401.

Swift-Joly J. (1929) *Stone, Calculous Disease of the Urinary Organs.* Heinemann, London.

Turner-Warwick R.T. (1976) Cystoplasty. *Urology* (ed. by Blandy J.P.), p. 840. Blackwell Scientific Publications, Oxford.

Chapter 9
Bladder tumours

Endoscopic assessment of a bladder tumour

Today it is axiomatic that every patient with haematuria needs an excretion urogram, which may show a filling defect in the bladder. In many instances it is only by cystoscopy that the tumour is discovered. The first cystoscopy for haematuria is therefore essentially a reconnaissance, but it is of immense importance, since it is at this examination that the Grade and Stage of the tumour are established, on which all treatment ultimately depends.

Special preparations

If a large filling defect has been seen in the urogram, then blood should be cross-matched. If the urine is infected, the microbiological sensitivities of the urinary organisms should be used to determine what antibiotic cover is given.

Anaesthetic

Cystoscopic evaluation of a bladder tumour calls for profound relaxation to allow bimanual palpation of the wall of the bladder. A deep biopsy of the tumour, to include muscle, is also necessary.

Position on the table

The patient is placed in the cystoscopy position, with an O'Conor drape to permit rectal examination without breach of asepsis.

Stages of the operation

The endoscope is introduced with the o° telescope so that the urethra is examined, the prostate evaluated, and extension of tumour into the prostatic urethra observed.

The o° telescope is exchanged for the 70° one, and every part of the interior of the bladder is examined. If clot and debris are present, evacuate them with the Ellik. Then empty the bladder, withdraw the cystoscope, and perform a bimanual examination to assess the T stage (9.1) of the tumour.

Small pedunculated or sessile papillary tumours

When the tumour is very tiny it is easier to seize it in the biopsy forceps (9.2) and remove it with its stalk, including muscle, and then coagulate the base with the ball electrode. This gives excellent material for histological examination as muscle is always present at the base of the tumour (9.3).

When the tumour is less than 3 cm in diameter, it can be easily removed with the resectoscope. Small ones may be cut off with a single stroke of the loop (9.4); larger ones need several bites. A separate section is taken from the muscle at the base of the tumour and sent in a separate pot for histology; the base is then thoroughly coagulated.

Larger pedunculated tumours

Larger growths need more skill and cunning. They will not come away in a single slice. They must be tackled in two distinct stages:

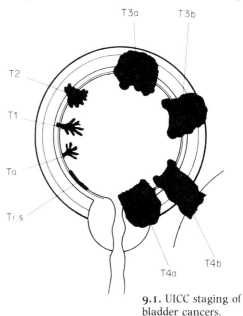

9.1. UICC staging of bladder cancers.

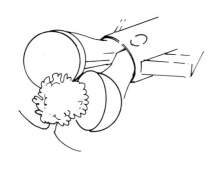

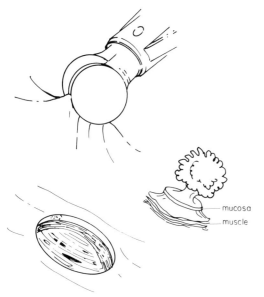

9.2. Removing a small bladder tumour with the cup forceps. Note that a portion of muscle will be included in its base.

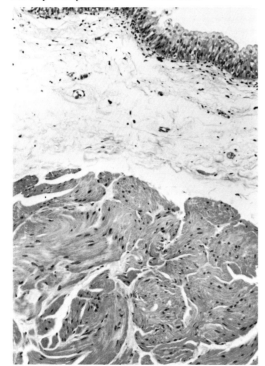

9.3. Photomicrograph of typical biopsy from bladder wall obtained with cold-cup forceps. Note the good layer of muscle which enables pT staging of a small tumour.

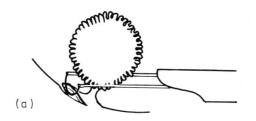

(a)

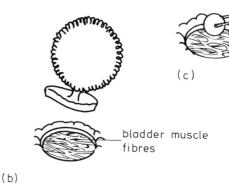

(b)

(c)

bladder muscle fibres

9.4. Transurethral resection of a small pedunculated bladder tumour. (a) The base and stalk are cut across with the cutting loop, exposing bladder muscle fibres (b) in the base, which is thoroughly coagulated with the rolling-ball electrode (c).

first the 'bush' is removed, and second the 'stalk' is taken out.

The real difficulty in resecting these tumours starts with the first cut, which makes the tumour bleed and obscures the view. The difficulties are compounded when more than one tumour is present. Keep two principles in mind: concentrate on one tumour at a time, and always find the stalk as soon as you can.

Before letting the loop of the resectoscope touch the tumour, make a very careful survey of it. Remember that most tumours are shaped like a mushroom (9.5). To reach the stalk it is first necessary to cut away part of the 'bush' of the tumour, but of course, as soon as this is cut, it starts to bleed. If you cut right in front of you, it will bleed straight into the objective lens of the telescope and you will be blinded. It is more cunning to take a series of slices from the side of the 'bush', continuing

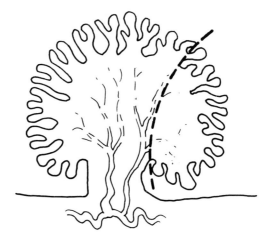

9.5. Larger bladder tumours are shaped like mushrooms. Large arteries run up in the stalk. The resection begins by cutting away part of the side of the mushroom so that the stalk may be reached and its vessels coagulated.

9.6. Transurethral resection of a larger papillary tumour begins by removal of the 'bush' (a) which is cut away until you identify the edge of the stalk (b). Work around the edge of the stalk (c) until the main part of the tumour is removed. (d) The base should be sent separately for section to determine how deeply the tumour has invaded.

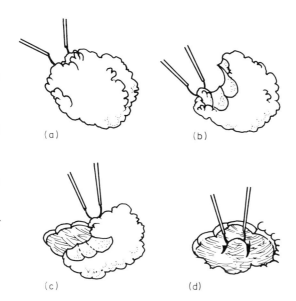

(a) (b) (c) (d)

until you come across the edge of the 'stalk' (9.6).

The bleeding comes from large arteries that pursue a serpentine course in the base of every tumour of the bladder. In a very large and very bloody tumour, as soon as an edge has been defined, and it is possible to know where the main trunk of the stalk is situated, a useful trick is to change the loop for the roly-ball electrode, and then plunge the ball into the stalk, coagulating for several seconds until all the tissue is blanched (9.7). By this manoeuvre the pedicle that brings blood to the outlying parts of the tumour will be coagulated, and the remainder of the resection of the mass will be relatively bloodless.

This same principle should be used when there are a large number of tumours in the bladder. Each one of them will start to bleed when the resectoscope touches it. Try to guess where the stalk of the tumour is situated, and using the roly-ball electrode, plunge the ball deeply into the middle of the fronds, and coagulate the stalk.

When the view is darkened, and orientation is lost, a terrible sense of despair overtakes the endoscopist. Now is the time to wash the bladder out thoroughly with the Ellik. Replace the loop with the ball-electrode. Keep to a definite system. Attack one growth at a time: where you see a frond, coagulate it, and follow the coagulation by plunging the electrode deep into the base of the 'bush' and stepping on the coagulating pedal. Ellik out the bladder. Try the next tumour; stop it bleeding, and so on to the next. The important principle is to deal with one tumour at a time, and get it thoroughly dry before tackling the next.

pT staging

During the first resection of a tumour of the bladder the surgeon has certain responsibilities. He must send the pathologist a representative section of the tissue in the base of the tumour: hence the need to be extra careful to evacuate all the 'bush' of the tumour and take separate slices from the 'stalk'. It is equally necessary for him to make sure that the various pieces of tumour are

9.7. Transurethral resection of large papillary tumours. (a) Cut away the 'bush' until you find the edge of the stalk (b) which is worth coagulating thoroughly to diminish bleeding during the subsequent resection of the remainder of the 'bush'. It is easier to work from healthy bladder mucosa towards the middle (d). Large vessels are often exposed in the base, especially when you resect deeply into bladder muscle; the rolling-ball electrode helps stop bleeding from the base (e).

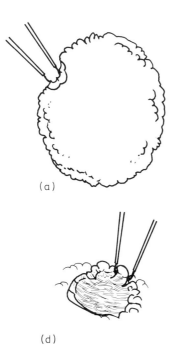
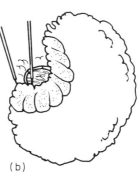
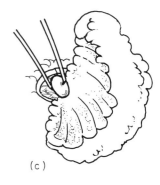
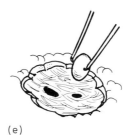

(a) (b) (c) (d) (e)

labelled correctly. I would add that in my practice it is just as important to see the sections in consultation with my pathologist colleague. Every urologist should be thinking in terms of the histological section each time he takes a chip with the resectoscope.

When TUR is impossible

From time to time even the most experienced resectionist will be daunted when he looks into the bladder and can find no normal mucosa at all: everywhere there are gigantic papillary tumours. Nowhere is there any sign of a stalk, and even introducing the resectoscope has made all of them bleed. In former days one was obliged to open the bladder, remove the tumours with a snare and diathermy (Dix et al. 1970) and perhaps follow this with radiotherapy of one sort or another. Today we have one additional shot in our locker—Helmstein's distension technique.

Helmstein's distension method

Helmstein (1966, 1972) described an orginal technique for dealing with tumours of the bladder. He distended the bladder with a balloon, inside which the pressure was kept higher than the diastolic pressure for more than six hours. As a result there was pressure necrosis of the tumour in the bladder, and the projecting parts of the tumour sloughed off.

The technique is simple but the details are important. The anaesthetist must be skilled in epidural anaesthesia, for the patient must be kept anaesthetized for six hours, and the nerves must be blocked as high as T8 if all afferent sensation from the bladder is to be cut off.

Special latex balloons are used, each of which has been tested to a three litre capacity. They are tied on to a Foley catheter (9.8). The bladder is emptied of urine; the balloon is filled from a reservoir of saline or 2% glycine at a height adjusted to 10 cm of water greater than the diastolic blood pressure which, with effective epidural anaesthesia, is always considerably depressed. Regular monitoring of the blood pressure and the pressure in the inflow tube to the balloon ensures a correct difference between them (9.9).

This is excellent for reducing the bulk of large tumours and for stopping bleeding (England et al. 1973). Today it is used in our unit perhaps two or three times a year.

Large solid tumours

All too often at the first cystoscopy a bladder tumour is found to be fixed, solid, ulcerating, and inoperable. A deep biopsy should be taken to confirm the diagnosis and establish the Grade of the tumour. Bimanual examination will establish the T stage. A separate slice through the prostate will reveal whether or not the prostate is involved (pT4b).

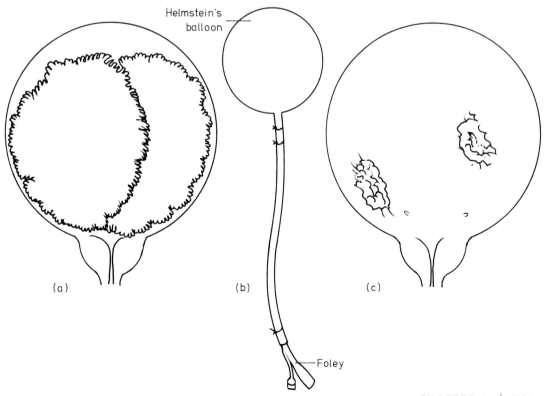

Helmstein's balloon

(a)   (b)   (c)

Foley

9.8. When there are very large papillary tumours the view may be impossible (a) but after distension with Helmstein's balloon (b) the bulk of the tumour undergoes necrosis leaving you with the relatively easy problem of a circumscribed 'stalk' to resect (c).

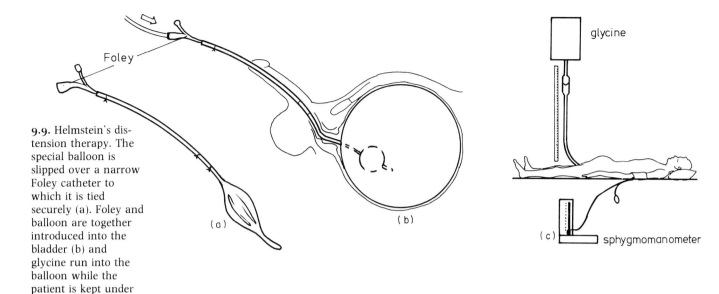

9.9. Helmstein's distension therapy. The special balloon is slipped over a narrow Foley catheter to which it is tied securely (a). Foley and balloon are together introduced into the bladder (b) and glycine run into the balloon while the patient is kept under continuous epidural anaesthetic. The reservoir containing glycine is kept at a height 10 cm of water greater than the diastolic blood pressure (c).

Carcinoma *in situ*

Frequently a patient is referred with symptoms of 'cystitis' but has no organisms in the urine. The Papanicolaou cytological test of the urine may suggest that malignant cells are present. Other investigations are normal.

Cystoscopy often shows nothing amiss—perhaps a hint of redness here and there in the bladder.

In such cases it is essential to regard the patient as having carcinoma *in situ* until proved otherwise. Using cup forceps, biopsies are taken in each of the four quadrants of the bladder. If any of these are positive, the patient is returned to the operating room, and a slice is taken from the prostate. Involvement of the prostatic ducts in carcinoma *in situ* materially worsens the prognosis and calls for radiotherapy and/or salvage cystectomy.

Flat mossy areas

After taking adequate material for biopsy with the cup forceps and perhaps the resectoscope loop, these wide flat velvety areas may be rolled over with the diathermy electrode using the coagulating current.

Adjuvant chemotherapy

For multiple and rapidly recurring tumours of the bladder there is ample evidence today that adjuvant chemotherapy is valuable in diminishing the number and frequency of recurrences (England *et al.* 1981). We use Oravisto's regime (Oravisto 1972) which gives 30 mg of Thiotepa dissolved in about 50 ml water on alternate days for three doses. Once the tumour has been controlled, a further 30 mg Thiotepa is instilled at every check cystoscopy for an indefinite period. A full blood count and platelet count are performed between every instillation of Thiotepa.

For patients who fail to respond to Thiotepa there are many alternatives, of which Mitomycin is the most effective to date.

Hazards of endoscopic resection of tumours of the bladder

The main risk of resecting a small bladder tumour is perforation of the wall of the bladder. This is fortunately of little consequence if the perforation is extraperitoneal, and it must happen nearly every time a bladder tumour is removed. It is important to make sure that the bleeding is stopped and that the bladder is drained with a catheter.

Rarely, there is a perforation into the peritoneal cavity. A swelling may be noted in the suprapubic region, or the irrigating fluid fails to return freely. Do not hesitate to perform a suprapubic exploration, preferably through a Pfannenstiel incision. Open the peritoneum. If there is free fluid, lift out the adjacent loops of bowel and examine them to make sure none of them have been burnt by the diathermy. Examine the bladder; oversew a hole if there is one, and stop the bleeding with suture-ligature. Close the wound with an extravesical drain.

Obturator spasm

The common cause of perforation of the bladder during resection of a tumour is jumping of the leg from stimulation of the obturator nerve by low-frequency currents induced from the diathermy (9.10). It may be avoided partially by reducing the voltage of the cutting current, until the loop only just cuts cleanly. If this does not stop the leg jumping, have the patient curarized, intubated and ventilated. If you insist on this, then you must also be prepared to wait while your anaesthetic colleague makes the necessary arrangements. To continue with the resection while the leg keeps jumping is reckless.

Partial cystectomy

Indications

Partial cystectomy is almost never indicated for cancer of the bladder. Endoscopic resection can remove almost everything that can be removed by open partial resection (Barnes *et al.* 1977) and in most other cases it is better to offer the patient radiotherapy with or without salvage cystectomy.

There is an exception. A tumour at the air-bubble or urachus is just as well treated by partial as by total cystectomy.

For a tumour arising in a diverticulum, partial cystectomy may be needed when combined with radiation therapy.

Finally, we must note the astonishing results obtained by Socquet (1980) who uses partial cystectomy in combination with large doses of Methotrexate, and claims results in invasive cancer of the bladder that are unequalled anywhere else in the world. If confirmed, they provide an additional reason for continuing to describe the operation in this handbook.

Special precautions

There is a real risk that tumour will be implanted into the wound during partial cystectomy. To prevent this the bladder is first filled up with distilled water or some other equally cancericidal fluid.

Anaesthesia

Moderate controlled hypotension provides a dry operating field and may speed the operation.

Position on the table

Supine.

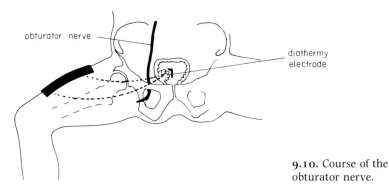

9.10. Course of the obturator nerve.

Incision

A vertical incision may be used in thin patients, and for carcinoma of the urachus. It should include and excise the umbilicus, so that the lymphatics of the urachus can be removed *en bloc* (9.11).

Steps of the operation

Since the tumours are near the fundus, when the wound is opened, one begins by carefully circumcising the umbilicus and urachus. Start the dissection by defining a triangle of potentially cancer-infected tissue on either side of the urachus, along the line of the obliterated hypogastric arteries. A strong tissue forceps is placed on the umbilicus to lift the dome of the bladder right up (9.12). When the bladder has been drawn into the wound, and separated from the back of the rectus on either side, it is incised between stay sutures, well clear of the tumour as mapped out by previous cystoscopy. Make the incision with the diathermy needle, and catch up all the little arteries with suture-ligature to prevent unnecessary loss of blood (9.13).

When the limit of the resection gets near the trigone, insert a catheter into each ureter to

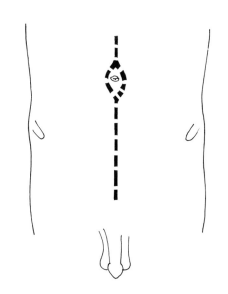

9.11. Incision for partial cystectomy for carcinoma at the fundus of the bladder.

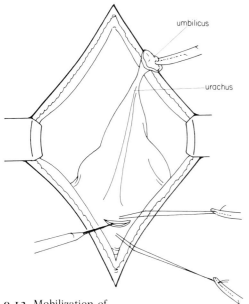

9.12. Mobilization of the bladder. It is incised between ligatures well away from the tumour.

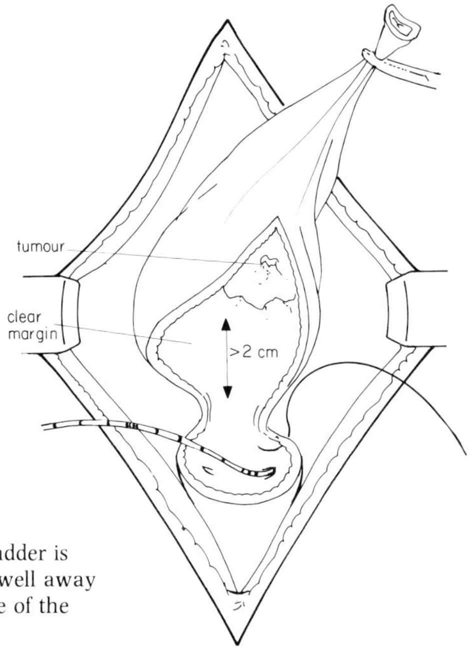

9.13. The bladder is cut through well away from the edge of the tumour.

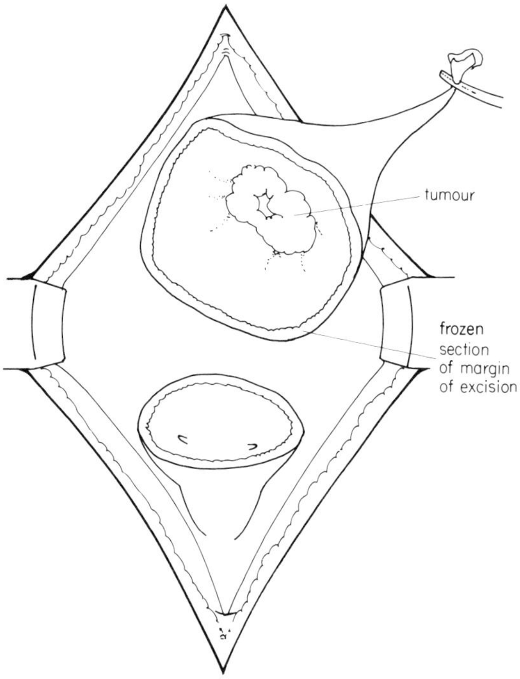

mark and protect it. The limit of resection should go at least 2 cm around the visible tumour, and a frozen section should confirm that you are clear of growth (9.14).

Removing the ureter

When the lower end of the ureter must be taken with the tumour in the bladder, divide the superior vesical vessels on the side of the tumour to bring up the ureter and the bladder. Follow down behind the ureter, under the trigone, so that an ellipse of trigone may be removed *en bloc* with the ureter (9.15).

Close the defect in the bladder in layers with catgut in the usual way. Do not be alarmed to see how little bladder is left behind. Unless the residual bladder is already diseased, as in bilharziasis or Hunner's ulcer, it can be relied upon to regenerate. Make sure that inadvertent injury does not occur to the good ureter. When it is necessary to remove the lower end

9.14. Frozen section confirms that the edge of the excision is tumour-free.

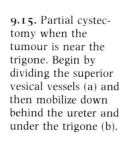

9.15. Partial cystectomy when the tumour is near the trigone. Begin by dividing the superior vesical vessels (a) and then mobilize down behind the ureter and under the trigone (b).

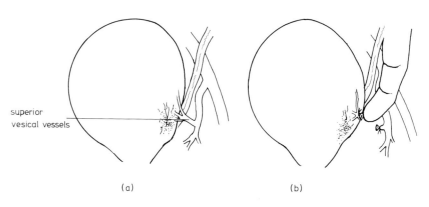

(a)   (b)

of the ureter on the affected side it must be reimplanted with the usual tunnel-and-cuff technique (9.16). The wound is closed with drainage and a urethral catheter. Since there is little room left in the bladder, use a whistle-tip catheter, and secure it in the bladder with a nylon retaining suture fixed to a Morson button.

Hazards of the operation

Blood loss, clot retention, wound infection and late implantation of carcinoma into the wound are the most serious consequences of partial cystectomy but the main reason why it was given up for cancer is that recurrence in the edge of the excision was so common in former times.

Total cystectomy

Indications

The indications for total cystectomy in carcinoma of the bladder are among the most vexing questions in the whole of urology. In our unit the indications have been crystallized by a retrospective analysis (Blandy *et al.* 1980) which has shown that: (a) in our hands, cystectomy did no good in patients whose tumours were completely unresponsive to radiation therapy; (b) if they were responsive to radiation, and stayed in response, then there was no point in adding cystectomy; and (c) if the tumour only responded partially, or came back after an initial response to radiation therapy, then one ought to perform a cystectomy. Critical to the interpretation of these studies is the type and dosage of radiation that these patients received. Many other studies have also shown that good results of cystectomy only occur in tumours that are radiosensitive (Bloom *et al.* 1982; Genster *et al.* 1979). At the London Hospital the aim has been to irradiate only the bladder and a 1–2 cm margin of tissue around it, the aim being guided by a cystogram (Hope-Stone *et al.* 1981).

Patients with pT1mG1—multiple superficial well-differentiated tumours that resist intravesical medication with Thiotepa, Mitomycin, Adriamycin or Epodyl—are candidates for radiotherapy, but in practice usually relapse and so frequently end up having to undergo cystectomy that one may consider the operation in young patients without a trial of radiation. In such cases it is wise to remove the urethra *en bloc* with the bladder.

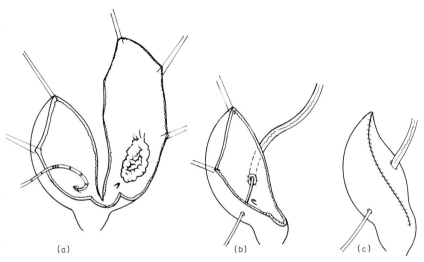

(a)   (b)   (c)

9.16. Partial cystectomy for tumour near the trigone—having mobilized the trigone and divided the ureter (a) the ureter is reimplanted through an anti-reflux tunnel (b) splinted with a Gibbon catheter. The bladder is closed in layers in the usual way (c).

Special preparations

Cystectomy carries such a high mortality that every effort must be made to prepare the patient beforehand. Many of the preventable complications of cystectomy are pulmonary, and to avoid them, time is well spent in a period of breathing exercises, giving up smoking, attending to septic gums and decayed teeth, culturing the sputum and treating infection. Anaemia is common in these patients, and should be corrected by appropriate transfusion well ahead of the operation. Many patients have cardiac disorders and need digitalis and diuretics; others are malnourished, and need feeding-up and rehydration (Bracken *et al.* 1981).

Preparation of the bowel is important. Today the patient is subject to intensive fluid loading, that clears the bowel mechanically, and leaves it empty of solid faeces; this is supplemented by oral antibiotics—neomycin and metronidazole.

The choice of urinary diversion needs thought, and should be discussed with the patient. If radiotherapy has been omitted, one may offer the alternatives of an ileal conduit, ureterosigmoidostomy, or the Mauclaire bladder. If the pelvis has been heavily irradiated, failure of healing between ureter and sigmoid colon is almost inevitable and rules this out as a method of diversion. Hence one must choose between cutaneous ureterostomy or an ileal conduit. Facing such an ordeal, many a frightened patient draws strength from contact with another who has been through the experience, and who is willing to discuss the practical problems of life with a urinary stoma. This can give more reassurance than anything which the surgeon can say.

An ileal conduit is often the only practicable diversion, so one must spend time in making sure where the stoma should be sited. It is not enough to fit the bag a few hours before the operation: it should be filled with water and worn around the ward to make sure that the site will not overlie the iliac spine or chafe under the belt.

Anaesthesia

To have the blood pressure lowered gives many advantages to the surgeon, for the pelvic dissection is done in a dry field and haemorrhage is controlled with precision. In return this requires meticulous haemostasis, for what seems to be a trivial vessel when the blood pressure is lowered, may bleed like the radial artery at the wrist when the blood pressure returns to normal. Lost blood should be accurately and synchronously replaced during the operation.

With these precautions hypotensive anaesthesia can make cystectomy easier for the operator and safer for the patient. Careless haemostasis or failure to replace lost blood may be followed by disaster.

Position on the table

If the urethra is to be removed *en bloc* the patient is placed in the cystoscopy position with legs on Lloyd-Davies supports so that the perineum is accessible. Even when there is no need to remove the urethra, this position has the advantage of allowing an assistant to stand between the legs in an ideal position for retracting. After cleaning the skin and putting on the drapes, a small Foley catheter is passed and connected to closed drainage.

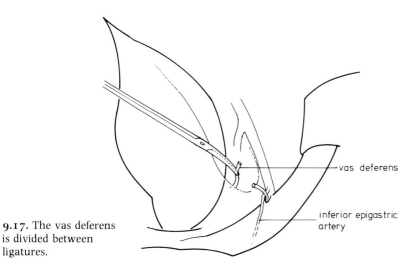

9.17. The vas deferens is divided between ligatures.

Incision

A long midline incision is used unless there has been heavy radiation therapy resulting in induration of the lower part of the abdominal wall—common a decade ago. In such patients the apron incision (page 116) avoids cutting into ischaemic tissue that will not heal.

Simple cystectomy

Open the peritoneum and divide all the adhesions that tether the bowel in the pelvis so that the bowel can be safely packed away. Pull up the urachus and divide the peritoneum down to the external iliac vessels, taking care not to injure the inferior epigastric artery. This opens up the retropubic space. As this incision is made, the vas deferens will be found and should be divided between ligatures (9.17). In a female the round ligament is similarly divided. The side of the bladder is mobilized down to the external iliac artery.

Now trace the common iliac artery down to its bifurcation and follow the internal iliac down until it gives off the superior vesical leash of vessels. These are carefully divided between ligatures (9.18).

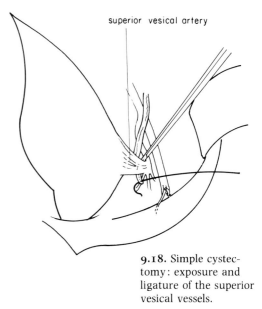

9.18. Simple cystectomy: exposure and ligature of the superior vesical vessels.

Putting traction on the bladder, and working down both from the front and the side, define the middle leash of vessels that spring from the internal iliac artery (9.19). The ureter should be divided at this stage, a ligature being placed on the distal end, but the proximal end left to drain freely (9.20). The middle leash of vessels is now divided between ligatures or ligaclips. Firm traction on the

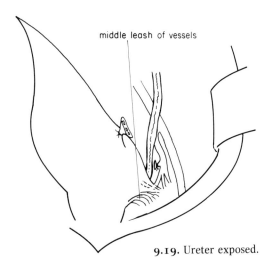

9.19. Ureter exposed.

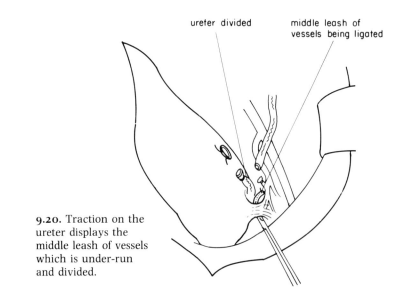

9.20. Traction on the ureter displays the middle leash of vessels which is under-run and divided.

bladder, and finger dissection in front and at the side will now identify the third or inferior ribbon of connective tissue which must be divided (9.21).

Exactly the same process is repeated on the other side, for which it is often more easy if the surgeon crosses to the opposite side of the table.

The next step is to complete the incision in the peritoneum along the front of the rectum, about 1 cm above the peritoneal recess between bladder and rectum. Develop the plane between the anterior wall of the rectum and the bladder with scissors until, pulling firmly upwards on the bladder, direct the tip of the scissors a little anteriorly; they enter the cleft between the two embryological layers of peritoneum that constitute Denon-villiers' fascia (9.22). In a favourable, unirrad-iated case, this plane opens out like the pages of a book. If the third, inferior ribbon of tissue has not already been divided, now is the time to define and cut each one (9.23).

The last step in a simple cystectomy is to separate the urethra from the symphysis. Peel the bladder back from the symphysis until you feel a firm band of fibrous tissue tethering the prostate to the bone. This contains large veins, and if possible, they should be defined and secured by suture-ligature or ligaclips before they are cut (9.24), so opening up a distinct gap between the fibrous band and the urethra. On either side is the superior layer of the pelvic fascia in which run other veins. The fascia and these veins are now secured and divided bit by bit. The finger now easily feels the urethra and the catheter within it. The finger-tip can be wriggled around the urethra until it lies in the crook of the finger. Seizing the urethra with a long forceps, cut it through,

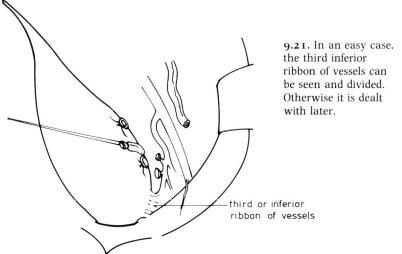

9.21. In an easy case, the third inferior ribbon of vessels can be seen and divided. Otherwise it is dealt with later.

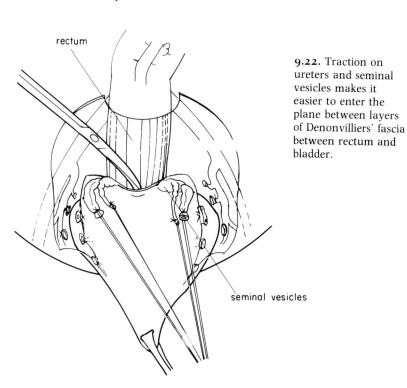

9.22. Traction on ureters and seminal vesicles makes it easier to enter the plane between layers of Denonvilliers' fascia between rectum and bladder.

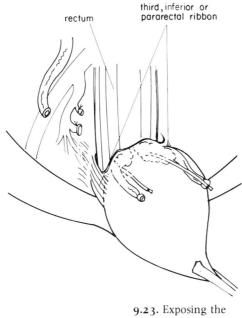

9.23. Exposing the plane between prostate and rectum defines the inferior 'ribbons' if they have not already been divided.

allowing the severed lower end to sink back into the depths, oozing sullenly.

Pull the proximal urethra up into the wound. This will show clearly the ribbons of pararectal tissue that remain on either side if they have not already been divided. They should be clamped and cut (9.25). The specimen should now be free. Make sure that it is distended with formalin before it is fixed; otherwise it is difficult for the pathologist to evaluate the stage of the tumour.

Residual bleeding may now arise from the cut end of the urethra, or the pararectal ribbons. If the bleeding is severe, put in a pack and wait five minutes. A good way of securing the bleeding from the lower urethra is to catch it up with a 2-0 chromic catgut suture, and sew it to the tissue behind the symphysis, thus angulating and squeezing the veins that are bleeding (9.26). Similarly, bleeding from the pararectal tissue is best controlled by a running suture on either side of the rectum. Finally, if the bleeding is still daunting, pass a large Foley catheter, inflate the balloon with about 50 ml of water, and apply firm traction

9.24. Separating bladder and prostate from symphysis displays the prevesical and preprostatic veins (a) which are sutured, ligated, and divided (b) in their strands of fibrous tissue. Under the veins lies the superior layer of pelvic fascia which is divided to allow you to dissect around the urethra.

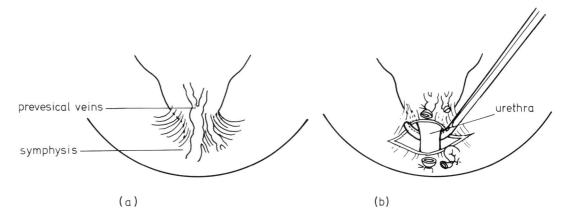

(a)

(b)

9.25. Divide the pararectal ribbons first on one side and then on the other.

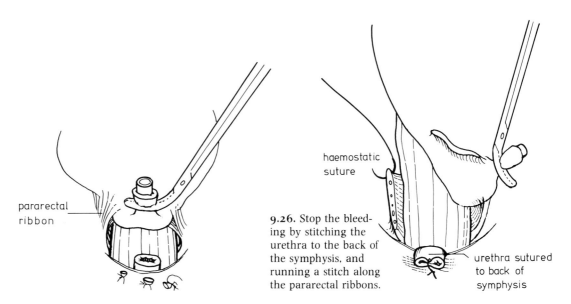

9.26. Stop the bleeding by stitching the urethra to the back of the symphysis, and running a stitch along the pararectal ribbons.

to squeeze flat the veins around the lower end of the urethra. It only remains to perform the urinary diversion (page 144).

Urethrectomy in the male

With the patient in the cystoscopy position, begin the dissection in the perineum as soon as the pelvic dissection has been completed, and the plane between rectum and prostate has been opened up.

A midline incision is made behind the scrotum and held open with a self-retaining catheter. Feeling for the catheter in the urethra, display the urethra in the mid-line (9.27). Reflect the bulbospongiosus muscle by lifting it off the urethra, and dividing it along the median raphe. Picking up urethra and catheter together, dissect the corpus spongiosum from its attachments to the underside of the corpora cavernosa, and as soon as possible, pass a tape around the urethra to retract it firmly (9.28). The urethra is now dissected away from the corpora cavernosa until, little by little, it begins to turn the penis inside out like the finger of a glove (9.29). When the glans penis is recognized, cut the urethra across, and sew over the divided spongy tissue with a 3-0 chromic catgut suture (9.30). Make sure that all the little bleeding points along the exposed corpora cavernosa are sealed with diathermy or closed with a suture before replacing the inside-out penis.

It is helpful, during the operation of cysto-urethrectomy, to leave the Foley catheter in position as a means of traction, so

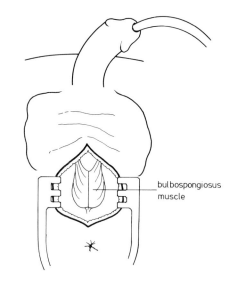

9.27. Urethrectomy in the male. A midline perineal incision is made over the bulb.

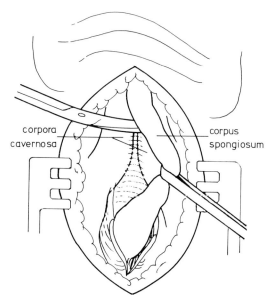

9.28. The corpus spongiosum is separated by sharp dissection from the underside of the united corpora cavernosa.

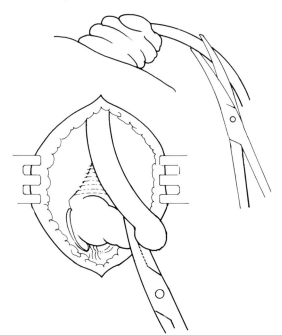

9.29. After clamping the urethra, the catheter is cut through.

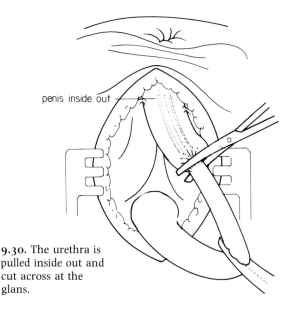

9.30. The urethra is pulled inside out and cut across at the glans.

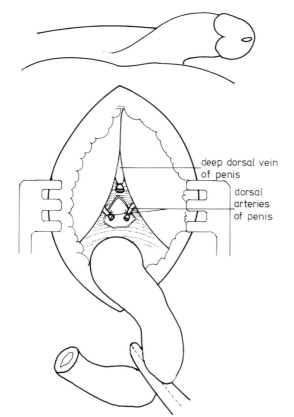

before cutting across the urethra, apply a strong forceps to both urethra and catheter, to prevent the Foley balloon from deflating.

Drawing the urethra firmly down, continue dissecting the bulbar urethra from the corpora as they diverge on either side. As you draw the urethra firmly down, it is possible to see the two stout dorsal arteries of the penis: they should be secured before they are torn. Similarly, the dorsal vein of the penis should be sutured and divided (9.31). The fascial membrane which fills the triangle between the divergent corpora cavernosa and the back of the symphysis is now cut, keeping the scissors close to the underside of the bone (9.32).

A finger in the pelvis is thrust down behind the symphysis into the gap that has been opened, and the fascia is swept down on either side of the bulb, leaving it attached on either side to a firm strand of fascia containing the bulbar arteries, and to the perineal body behind (9.33).

Lift the bulb up and pull it forward with the catheter. Cut its posterior attachment to the perineal body, protecting the rectum which lies very close, with a finger on either side of the midline to push the rectum down. On either side of the bulb there only remains a strand of fibrous tissue: it is remarkably strong, and contains a vessel that is often quite large. Make a pedicle of this strand on

9.31. The dorsal vein of the penis and dorsal arteries of the penis are ligated and divided.

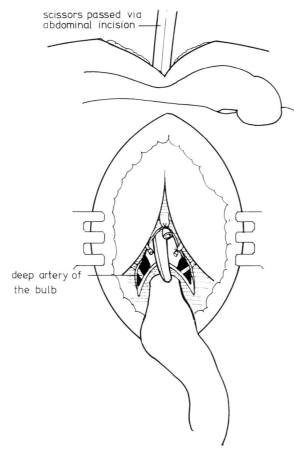

9.32. The inferior layer of pelvic fascia is divided around the urethra. The deep arteries of the bulb will need to be ligated. A scissors or finger can now be passed down behind the symphysis and around the front of the urethra.

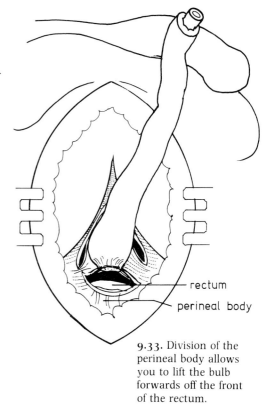

9.33. Division of the perineal body allows you to lift the bulb forwards off the front of the rectum.

either side: ligate and cut it deliberately (9.34), for if torn this vessel slips into the depths and is a nuisance to secure.

Radical cystectomy

Indications

To debate the place for radical, as opposed to simple, cystectomy, would occupy most of this book. It is very much a matter for controversy. I confess that I continue to practise the radical operation, not so much because of a firm conviction that it necessarily cuts away more of the cancer, but because: (a) it is technically a little easier, when the pelvis has been heavily irradiated, to get into a good tissue plane by defining the great vessels; (b) examination of the lymph nodes gives a useful prognostic index; and (c) just once in a while it might do good (Skinner 1980; Skinner *et al.* 1980; Skinner, 1982).

Steps of the operation

In radical cystectomy the lymph nodes of the pelvis are taken *en bloc* with the bladder, and the plane of dissection behind the bladder lies, not between the layers of Denonvilliers' fascia, but behind it.

A generous midline incision is made, adhesions divided and the omentum separated from the back of the peritoneum when stuck by previous abdominal surgery. A routine examination of the contents of the abdomen is performed, to search for other important pathology and to exclude hepatic metastases.

The reflexion of the peritoneum on the lateral side of the caecum is incised, carried round the lower end of the caecum and up along the medial edge of the mesentery of the small bowel, to display the bifurcation of the aorta (9.35). On the left side, the sigmoid and lower end of the descending colon are mobilized medially (9.36). The small bowel is lifted up and out of the abdomen and packed in moist towels or a plastic bag.

Beginning on one side, the great vessels are cleaned from lateral to medial, sweeping all the surrounding fibrofatty and lymphatic tissue towards the midline and towards the bladder. I prefer to begin on the left side, and after incising the fascial sheath on the lateral aspect of the left common iliac artery, develop the plane between sheath and vessel until the artery can be taped and lifted up. The same thing is done with the common iliac vein, and

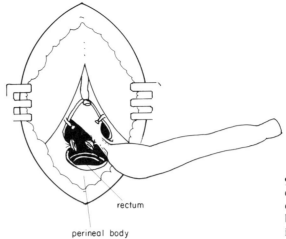

9.34. Make a pedicle of the strand of tissue on either side of the bulb; ligate and divide it.

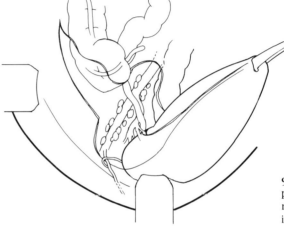

9.35. Incision of the peritoneum on the right side: the caecum is mobilized upwards.

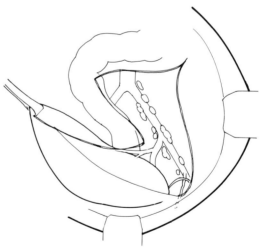

9.36. Radial cystectomy: the incision in the peritoneum. The sigmoid is mobilized up and medially to display the bifurcation of the aorta.

as the dissection proceeds, both great vessels are cleaned naked, as the lymphatic tissue is swept downwards and medially (9.37). As the division of the common iliac artery is displayed, the ureter is lifted up, and its lower end ligated and divided. The upper end is marked with a suture. The internal iliac artery is cleaned in the same way, and all the branches that spring off the anterior division of the internal iliac artery are in turn ligated and divided.

At this stage it makes matters easier if the urachus is lifted up, and the front of the bladder separated from the symphysis. When there has been much previous irradiation, there may be no clear plane of cleavage here, and it is necessary to cut the dense white

tissue with a diathermy needle until the periosteum on the back of the symphysis is found, and a finger is forced into the plane outside the pelvic fascia.

The peritoneum is divided along the line from the urachus to the external iliac artery, taking care not to injure the inferior epigastric vessels (9.38). As this peritoneum is divided, the vas deferens is discovered in a male and the round ligament in a female, and each is ligated and cut. Finally this peritoneal incision is made to join the incision made at the beginning of the operation, and the entire mass of bladder and fibrofatty tissue is retracted medially.

Now it is easier to clean the triangle bounded by the external and internal iliac arteries, at the bottom of which runs the obturator nerve, inside its firm sheath of fibrous and lymphatic tissue. This sheath must be deliberately slit open, and drawn out from behind the obturator nerve, taking care not to injure the nerve. It is even more important to take care to avoid tearing the obturator vein or artery, and to tie them if they are in the way (9.39).

The same dissection is repeated on the other side, and then the specimen is lifted forwards, so that the peritoneal cul-de-sac can be seen clearly. Pulling up the sigmoid firmly, continue the incision in the peritoneum across the front of the rectum, and carefully

9.37. The lymph nodes are swept downwards and medially leaving the iliac vessels dissected completely clean.

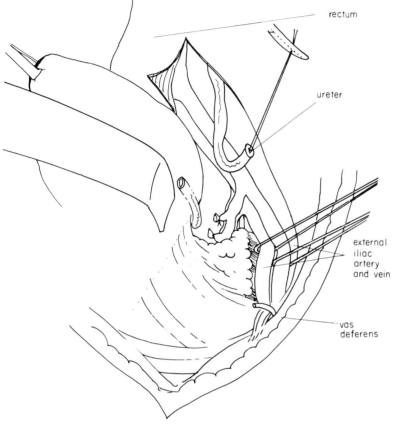

9.38. The inferior epigastric vessels are preserved as the peritoneum is divided from the urachus down to the iliac vessels.

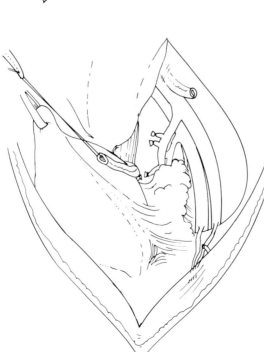

9.39. The nodes along the obturator nerve are slit up to expose the nerve, and then removed like a sleeve.

open the plane behind the peritoneum and in front of the longitudinal muscle of the rectum (9.40). After radiotherapy it is rarely possible to open up the layers of Denonvilliers' fascia, and not worth trying. Once in the right layer, the finger finds the space behind the prostate and urethra in front of the rectum, and it is possible to define the pararectal ribbons on either side which are carefully divided one by one to liberate the bladder. When the specimen is removed, the pelvis is cleaned like an anatomical specimen, the bladder and all its lymphatic drainage system having been removed *en bloc* (9.41). Diversion after this procedure is by means of an ileal conduit.

Ileal conduit

Examine the terminal ileum for evidence of radiation damage and avoid areas that seem suspiciously thickened or white. Carefully divide any adhesions. Lift up the loop of ileum, and let a light shine through it (9.42) to make sure that at least two large branches of the superior mesenteric artery supply the segment that has been chosen. Make a delicate incision, just through the peritoneum on each side of the mesentery, not deep enough to catch the vessels: this makes it easier to pick up the mesenteric vessels without tearing them (9.43). Each leash of vessels is doubly clipped

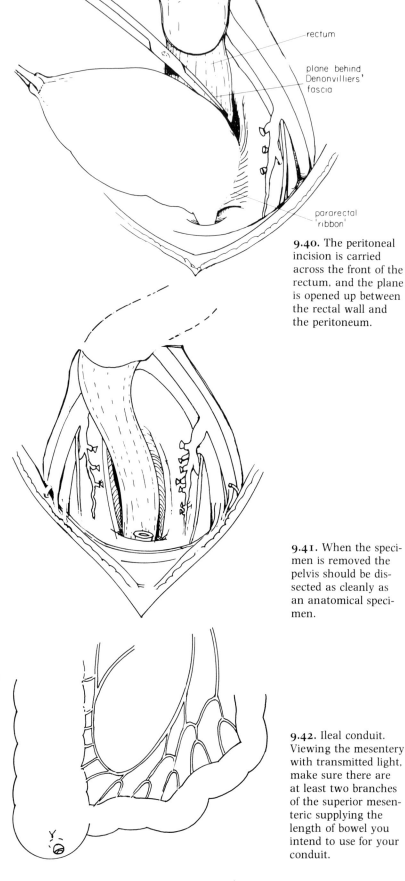

9.40. The peritoneal incision is carried across the front of the rectum, and the plane is opened up between the rectal wall and the peritoneum.

9.41. When the specimen is removed the pelvis should be dissected as cleanly as an anatomical specimen.

9.42. Ileal conduit. Viewing the mesentery with transmitted light, make sure there are at least two branches of the superior mesenteric supplying the length of bowel you intend to use for your conduit.

(a)

9.43. Incise only the peritoneum, sparing the vessels (a), which are picked up and ligated individually (b).

(b)

with mosquito forceps, divided, and ligated with 3-0 silk. The incision in the mesentery is continued right out to the muscle of the wall of the bowel.

Measure the distance from the promontory of the sacrum (where the ureters will be lying comfortably) to the site chosen for the abdominal stoma and marked on the skin by the ward staff ahead of the day of operation. This is the right length for the ileal conduit. Make the second incision in the mesentery just big enough to allow an easy anastomosis. The distal end should be free to reach the chosen site for the stoma without any tension, and it may be necessary to divide one or two arcades (9.44) to make it long enough.

Place a Doyen's intestinal clamp on either side of the bowel before it is divided. Wrap the isolated loop in a moist pack and put it aside while the end-to-end anastomosis is performed to restore continuity to the bowel (9.45). My preference is for an outer sero-muscular layer of interrupted 3-0 silk or thread, and an all-coats layer of 3-0 chromic catgut on the inside. The mesenteric defect is closed with a few interrupted sutures of 3-0

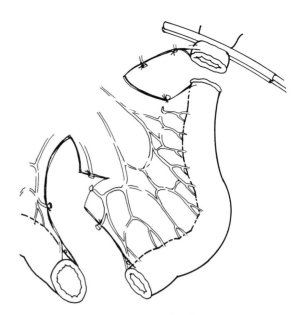

9.44. The appropriate length of ileum is isolated on its mesentery.

chromic catgut. No doubt a stapling instrument could do the work more quickly and just as well.

The isolated loop is now thoroughly irrigated with saline or 1% neomycin solution, taking care to allow none of the neomycin to spill into the peritoneal cavity. A well-lubricated Jaques catheter is passed along the loop, and used to draw through two naso-gastric or infant feeding tubes of 6 or 8 Ch (according to the calibre of the ureters).

The left ureter is brought behind the meso-sigmoid taking care that it does not snag on a mesenteric vessel (9.46). The ureters must lie

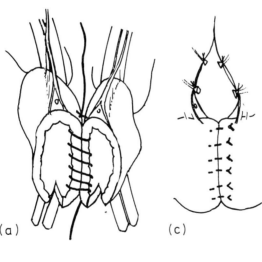

(a)   (c)

9.45. The continuity of the bowel is restored by end-to-end anastomosis. An all-coats 2-0 chromic catgut suture (a) inverts the bowel, using a Connell stitch (b) on the front of the anastomosis. This is reinforced with a series of sero-muscular 3-0 thread sutures (c) and the defect in the mesentery is closed with similar sutures (d).

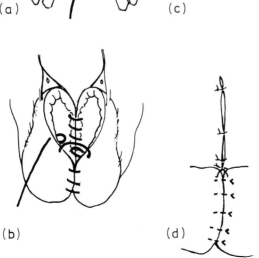

(b)   (d)

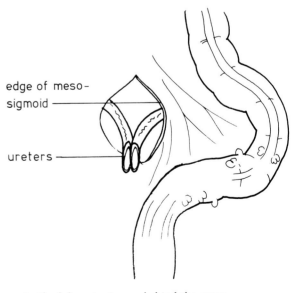

edge of meso-sigmoid

ureters

9.46. The left ureter is brought to the right behind the meso-sigmoid.

together without any kink or tension. Of the
several methods of making an ureteroileal
anastomosis, the technique described by
Wallace (1966) is least prone to complications and easiest to do. Lay the two ureters
alongside each other. Spatulate their lower
ends, and sew the medial edges together to
form a common oval stoma (9.47). This is
then anastomosed to the proximal end of the
isolated ileal loop over the two nasogastric
tubes, serving as splints. The ureters are
sewn to the bowel with 4-0 chromic catgut,
reinforced with a few interrupted sutures
between the connective tissue alongside the
ureter and the serosa of the bowel. The splints
are sutured to the ureters with a 3-0 chromic
catgut suture to prevent them being inadvertently dislodged. When the anastomosis is
complete it is buried under the mesosigmoid
on the left, and the ileal mesentery on the
right.

Close all potential holes in the mesentery,
and all gaps between the loop, the caecum
and the terminal ileum, to prevent subsequent volvulus and obstruction.

The stoma is made by cutting a circular
hole through all layers of the abdominal wall
at the site previously marked after careful
testing in the ward (9.48). (Note that this
site must be chosen after trial of a bag, half-
full of water, worn in the standing and sitting
position, with and without trousers.)

The free distal end of the loop is brought
through the hole together with the splinting
tubes. Close the dangerous little space lateral to
the loop, and attach it to the anterior wall of the
caecum with a few 3-0 sutures to prevent
subsequent volvulus (9.49).

Having restored the rest of the bowel to the
abdomen, check again that all bleeding has
been stopped. In recent years I have come to
add a simple gastrostomy before closing the
abdomen, having been taught by my patients
that this is far more comfortable than prolonged nasogastric intubation.

Gastrostomy

Lifting up the abdominal wall, draw the
stomach down into the wound. Hold the
stomach wall between two Allis forceps and
incise between them (9.50). Insert a 20 Ch
Foley catheter through the abdominal wall,
and pass it right inside the stomach. Insert a
2-0 catgut purse string suture. Inflate the
balloon of the Foley with 20 ml. Put in a
second purse string suture, and having tied it,
pull the Foley and the stomach up against the

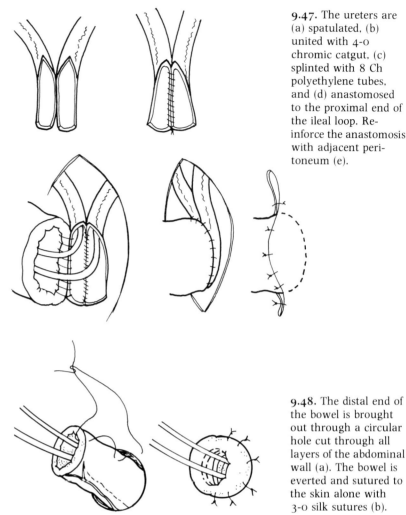

9.47. The ureters are
(a) spatulated, (b)
united with 4-0
chromic catgut, (c)
splinted with 8 Ch
polyethylene tubes,
and (d) anastomosed
to the proximal end
of the ileal loop. Re-
inforce the anastomosis
with adjacent peri-
toneum (e).

9.48. The distal end of
the bowel is brought
out through a circular
hole cut through all
layers of the abdominal
wall (a). The bowel is
everted and sutured to
the skin alone with
3-0 silk sutures (b).

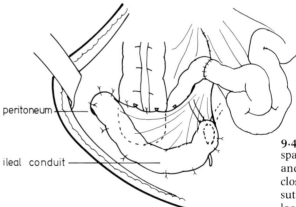

peritoneum

ileal conduit

9.49. The lateral
space between bowel
and peritoneum is
closed with interrupted
sutures which fix the
loop to the caecum
and peritoneum.

abdominal wall, and secure them there with
the same suture. Finally stitch the Foley
catheter to the skin.

The gastrostomy is allowed to drain freely
into a closed drainage system, and is not
removed until the patient recovers completely
from his post-operative ileus, has had a bowel
action, and is back on a normal diet. It is
removed not before the tenth post-operative
day.

![Gastrostomy illustration with 20 ch Foley catheter, purse-string suture, stomach labels]

9.50. Gastrostomy.

![Ureterosigmoidostomy illustration with suture attached to parietal peritoneum]

Ureterosigmoidostomy

Occasionally there is good reason to prefer ureterocolic anastomosis rather than an ileal loop (see page 144), but it is dangerous and unwise when the pelvis has been irradiated.

The left ureter is led through the meso-sigmoid (9.51), which forms a convenient tunnel for it. The ureter emerges just near the border of the bowel and, where it lies comfortably against the wall of the sigmoid, make a tunnel for it by incising the muscular wall of the bowel down to the muscularis mucosae (9.52). There is no special virtue in making the tunnel along a taenia. Hold the bowel with Allis forceps, stroke with a knife through the muscularis, until the unmistakable appearance of the muscularis mucosa is seen. Gently part the muscle coat, using a dissecting swab. Cut a hole in the mucosa at the lower end of the tunnel, and anastomose it to the ureter with 4-0 catgut (9.53). Then close the muscle over the ureter with 3-0 catgut, making sure that these sutures are not tied too tightly by laying a little rubber tube

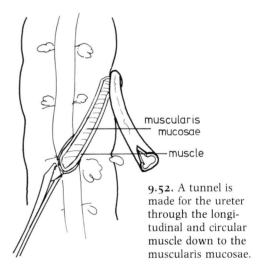

9.52. A tunnel is made for the ureter through the longitudinal and circular muscle down to the muscularis mucosae.

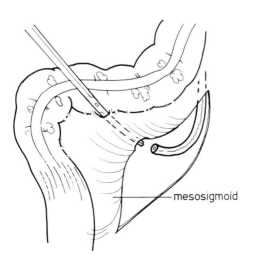

9.51. Ureterosigmoidostomy: the left ureter is led through the mesosigmoid.

9.53. The spatulated ureter is anastomosed to a circular hole in the mucosa.

alongside the ureter in the tunnel (9.54) until the sutures are tied, and then withdraw it (9.55). The right ureter is anastomosed in the same way. Bring it through a tunnel in the mesosigmoid if there is enough ureter, but anyway make sure there is no tension or kinking in the ureter.

So notorious is the hazard of leakage of urine after ureterosigmoidostomy that it is worth taking trouble to wrap the anastomoses up in omentum. Finally, stretch the anal sphincter and leave in a rectal drainage tube, connected to a closed drainage system.

6 Ch rubber tube

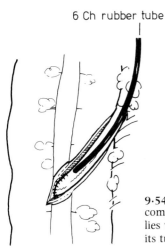

9.54. The anastomosis completed, the ureter lies without tension in its tunnel.

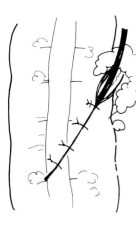

9.55. The muscle is approximated over the ureter. The fine rubber tube is withdrawn when the last stitch is tied: it prevents you from making the tunnel too tight.

Hazards of the operation

In the list of possible complications of cystectomy are included all the risks of major abdominal surgery (Skinner *et al.* 1980; Bracken *et al.* 1981). Wound dehiscence and infection, burst abdomen, adhesion-obstruction, ileus, pulmonary embolism—all these and many others occur after this operation with distressing frequency. Most lethal is leakage of urine from the uretero-ileal anastomosis, and for this reason I do not regret my routine use of a splint.

Paralytic ileus occurs after any major operation involving the intestine, but after cystectomy it is particularly severe and prolonged. Beware of discontinuing nasogastric suction too early: indeed, this is perhaps the chief advantage of a gastrostomy—one is not impelled by reasons of false pity to remove the distressing nasogastric tube too early. Gastrostomy allows the patient relief from the torture of thirst and at the same time allows swallowed fluids to escape without distending the abdomen.

The stoma

The patient must be able to manage the stoma before leaving hospital, be able to put on the bag and take it off, and know what to do when there is a leak. The patient should be put into touch with the local branch of the Ileostomy Association* and, if your hospital is so fortunate as to employ one, the stoma therapist. Nothing is more cruel than to think that the operation is over when the patient leaves hospital: for the patient, life with an ileal conduit has just begun.

References

Barnes R.W., Dicks A.L., Hadley H.L. & Johnston O.L. (1977) Survival following transurethral resection of bladder carcinoma. *Cancer Res.* **37**, 2895.

Blandy J.P., England H.R., Evans S.J.W., Hope-Stone H.F., Mair G.M.M., Mantell B.S., Oliver R.T.D., Paris A.M.I. & Risdon R.A. (1980) T3 bladder cancer—the case for salvage cystectomy. *Brit. J. Urol.* **52**, 506.

Bloom H.J.G., Hendry W.F., Wallace D.M. & Skeet R.G. (1982) Treatment of T3 bladder cancer: controlled trial of pre-operative radiotherapy and radical cystectomy versus radical radiotherapy. *Brit. J. Urol.* **54**, 136.

Bracken R.B., McDonald M. & Johnson D.E. (1981) Complications of single-stage radical cystectomy and ileal conduit. *Urology*, **17**, 141.

Dix V.W., Shanks W., Tresidder G.C., Blandy J.P., Hope-Stone H.F. & Shepheard B.G.F. (1970) Carcinoma of the bladder: treatment by diathermy snare excision and interstitial irradiation. *Brit. J. Urol.* **42**, 213.

England H.R., Rigby C., Shepheard B.G.F., Tresidder G.C. & Blandy J.P. (1973) Evaluation of Helmstein's distension method for carcinoma of the bladder. *Brit. J. Urol.* **45**, 593.

England H.R., Flynn J.T., Paris A.M.I. & Blandy J.P. (1981) Early multiple dose adjuvant Thiotepa in the control of multiple and rapid T1 tumour neogenesis. *Brit. J. Urol.* **53**, 588.

*Address: The Ileostomy Association, 149 Harley Street, London W1.

Genster H.G., Mommsen S. & Hojsgaard A. (1979) Post-irradiation total cystectomy for bladder cancer. *Urological Research*, **7**, 79.

Helmstein K. (1966) Hydrostatic pressure therapy —a new approach to the treatment of carcinoma of the bladder. *Opuscula Medica* (Stockholm), **7**, 238.

Helmstein K. (1972) Treatment of bladder carcinoma by a hydrostatic pressure technique. *Brit. J. Urol.* **44**, 434.

Hope-Stone H.F., Blandy J.P., Oliver R.T.D. & England H.R. (1981) Radical radiotherapy and salvage cystectomy in the treatment of invasive carcinoma of the bladder. In *Bladder Cancer, principles of combination therapy* (ed. by Oliver R.T.D., Hendry W.F. & Bloom H.J.G.), p. 127. Butterworths, London.

Oravisto K.J. (1972) Optimal intravesical dosage of Thiotepa in the prophylaxis of recurrent bladder papillomatosis. *Scandinavian Journal of Urology and Nephrology*, **6**, 26.

Skinner D.G. (1980) Current perspectives in the management of high-grade invasive bladder cancer. *Cancer*, **45**, 1866.

Skinner D.G., Crawford E.D. & Kaufman J.J. (1980) Complications of radical cystectomy for carcinoma of the bladder. *J. Urol.* **123**, 640.

Skinner D.G. (1982) Management of invasive bladder cancer: a meticulous node dissection can make a difference. *J. Urol.* **128**, 34.

Socquet Y. (1981) Combined surgery and adjuvant chemotherapy with high dose methotrexate and folinic acid rescue (HDMTX-CF) for infiltrating tumours of the bladder. *Brit. J. Urol.* **53**, 439.

Wallace D.M. (1966) Ureteric diversion using a conduit: simplified technique. *Brit. J. Urol.* **38**, 522.

Chapter 10
Transurethral resection of the prostate gland

Indications

For every urological surgeon, no matter how experienced, there is a limit to the bulk of tissue which he can resect. Where he draws the line is a matter for individual judgement, which may change with time, fatigue, and skill. Transurethral resection is such an individual, such a solo, and such a virtuoso performance that it is futile to offer anything other than advice based on personal experience. In my practice really enormous glands are still dealt with by retropubic prostatectomy, but more than 95% of cases are resected transurethrally. Each case is assessed on its merits: the extra safety of transurethral resection justifies some extra time and difficulty until a limit is reached when the sheer difficulty of controlling bleeding, and of removing all the adenoma, must be weighed against the ease with which a large ripe adenoma can be shelled out of its capsule in minutes, via the retropubic approach.

The futile debate of a former generation between proponents of endoscopic resection and of open prostatectomy has now largely died away. A new generation of urological surgeons are familiar with instruments through which they can see what they are doing and recognize that each type of operation has its place. At one extreme the majority of prostates which cause symptoms and lead to outflow obstruction can be readily managed by transurethral resection. At the other extreme are really large adenomas, over which the resectoscope passes only with difficulty, and for which resection will be obscured by continual bleeding, and will be dangerous because it is difficult to keep orientated.

A benign prostate needs to be removed when it causes significant obstruction to the outflow of the bladder, not merely because prostatic enlargement is felt per rectum, or because the patient complains of frequency and a poor stream. In most patients the diagnosis of significant outflow obstruction is demonstrated by a large residual urine in the urogram, a thick and sacculated bladder wall, diverticula, ureteric obstruction, or acute or chronic retention of urine. When in doubt, a flow-rate measurement will show a poor stream, and when one has a high index of suspicion that there is an alternative diagnosis —as in the younger man with severe frequency—it is prudent to make a complete urodynamic evaluation to confirm that there is indeed outflow obstruction. It is important not to be deceived by a severely unstable bladder, in which prostatectomy may actually be contra-indicated (Blandy 1977).

Although the size of the adenoma is not the factor which decides whether or not an operation is needed, it does very largely determine whether the prostatectomy can be done transurethrally or will need an open operation. Ultrasound measurement of the size of the gland will probably in the future come to be a routine investigation. I do not enjoy this facility, and therefore make sure that the patient understands that there is always a slight chance that the operation may not be feasible transurethrally.

Two kinds of prostatic outflow obstruction absolutely require transurethral resection. The first is the small fibrous gland in which there is no distinction between adenoma and capsule, where an open operation is bound to require sharp dissection in a field without visible landmarks, let alone any distinction between what must and what must not be removed. Second, obstructing cancers, where there is also no clear plane of cleavage, are impossible to enucleate. In both of these types of prostatic obstruction, transurethral resection is especially indicated.

Special preparations

Make sure of the sensitivities of the organisms in the urine, and if the urine is *infected*, provide adequate pre-operative antibiotic cover. *Haemorrhage* may be sudden, severe, and unexpected, so that it is essential to make provision against it. If your laboratory guarantees to provide plenty of blood with minimum delay, it may be safe to do without cross-matching two units prior to the operation. Today, blood transfusion is very seldom necessary, except when the gland is very big; nevertheless it is my practice to insist on cross-matching two units before every TUR, a practice which may change in the future.

There is no need to have the patient shaved before prostatectomy by the endoscopic route. Today, when barely one in fifty patients undergoes an open procedure in my practice, none are shaved preparatory to prostatectomy. The choice of method is left to the last minute, but the nursing team always understand that transurethral resection may, unforseeably, become an open operation if uncontrollable bleeding, perforation, or some other preoperative complication occurs. For the same reason, any surgeon embarking on transurethral surgery, must make sure he knows how to perform the rare procedure of open prostatectomy.

Anaesthesia

Anaesthesia must be expert and profound. Transurethral resection is not a minor operation to be delegated to an inexperienced anaesthetist. Whether spinal, epidural, or inhalational anaesthesia is chosen, three major calamities must be avoided: erection, coughing, and obturator spasm.

Erection is a curiously neglected hazard of anaesthesia in transurethral surgery. It is exceedingly dangerous. As the penis imperceptibly becomes elongated, the inexperienced surgeon may find his resectoscope pushed out beyond the sphincter, and as there is often increased bleeding at the same time, the view becomes obscured. These are the times when sphincters are cut and patients rendered permanently and incurably incontinent. Erection is a very sound reason for stopping the operation. Sometimes the erection will subside spontaneously; sometimes it persists, defying every trick of pharmacology and anaesthesia.

Coughing may occur when the patient is allowed to become too light and the endotracheal tube irritates his trachea. It can be very dangerous and has been occasionally responsible for perforations of bladder or capsule.

Equally dangerous is the *'obturator jump'*. If the current pathway crosses the obturator nerve, induced currents may stimulate the adductors to contract. The only remedy for this is to block the motor end-plates at the neuromuscular junction, or to infiltrate the obturator nerve with local anaesthetic. It is fortunately rare in prostatectomy, but should always be anticipated when resecting a tumour on the trigone.

I am often informed that one or other anaesthetic method is superior for transurethral surgery but this has not been my experience. It has been my privilege over the years to work with several expert anaesthetists whose techniques have varied considerably, and each has provided perfect conditions for the operation. Leave the choice of method to your anaesthetic colleague: there is no sense in buying a dog and barking yourself. Nevertheless, make certain that the anaesthetist appreciates the dangers of coughing and of an erection, and is prepared to paralyse and intubate the patient if he develops obturator spasm.

Position on the table

Put the patient in the cystoscopy position (10.1) on a table which can be lowered, raised, and tilted at will. Power-assisted

10.1. Position of patient for transurethral resection of the prostate: note that the hips are not fully flexed.

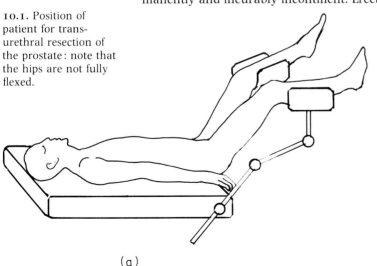

(a)

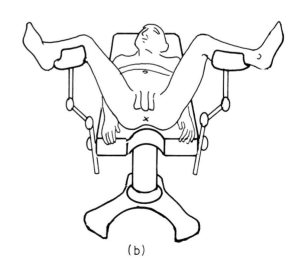

(b)

operating tables, purpose-built for endoscopic surgery are the best, but not essential. Avoid excessive flexion of the hips and knees, and make sure that the leg-rests (I prefer the standard Lloyd-Davies supports) put no strain on hips or knees. Clean the skin of the penis and scrotum with sterile hibitane or betadine. Put on sterile drapes (10.2).

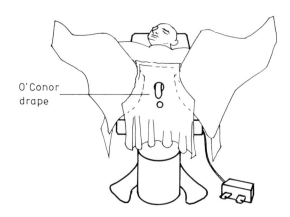

10.2. Patient draped ready for TUR.

Cysto-urethroscopy

After filling the urethra with sterile lubricant-antiseptic gel, examine the urethra from end to end with the 0° telescope and then the bladder with the 70° instrument, checking carefully for other pathology in the bladder, notably unsuspected carcinoma, diverticula and stones. Estimate the size of the prostate, and then decide whether or not to proceed to a transurethral operation.

Cutting tissue

The first skill to master in transurethral surgery is that of cleanly cutting a chip. The cutting current must strike an arc, and cut the chip off cleanly. Diathermy instruments of insufficient power merely fry the tissue, and coat the loop with charcoal. Always check that the loop stays bright and clean, and when examining the chips microscopically, check that the edge of each chip is only burnt one or two cells deep. To cut out a chip cleanly the loop is swung in, along, and out so that a boat-shaped piece of tissue is removed (10.3).

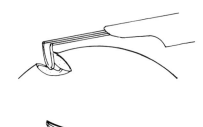

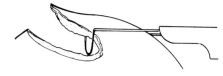

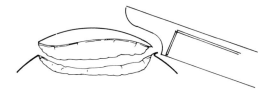

10.3. Cutting a chip.

One difficulty many inexperienced operators complain of is failure to detach the distal end of the chip. The reason for this is simple: the loop is not matching the end of the sheath (10.4). If the loop has been bent outwards, it may fail to engage the sheath. If it has been bent upwards, it may leave a gap between wire and sheath. If the sheath has become worn through use the loop may no longer go inside it. Temporary remedies include bending the loop back or bending it downwards. In simpler designs of cutting-loop, it is also quite easy to nip a millimetre off the end of the loop to shorten it but in doing this, make sure that the loop cannot touch the end of the telescope. A new loop costs only a few pounds; a new telescope costs hundreds, and if the arc is close to the lens it may be ruined.

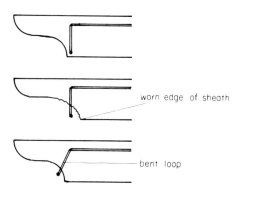

worn edge of sheath

bent loop

10.4. If the chip is not cut off cleanly, the loop is not engaging in the resectoscope sheath. This may be because the sheath has become worn away, or the loop has bent.

Haemostasis

Bleeding during transurethral resection may be arterial or venous. Arteries are easily identified, and are best sealed off using the loop and coagulating current. For very small vessels the loop is brought just to the opening from which the blood is issuing. For larger arteries, which are often atheromatous and rigid in the prostate, the trick is to indent the tissue on one or other side of the offending vessel to appose its walls, which are then sealed together with the diathermy current (10.5).

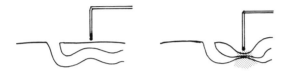

10.5. To coagulate a larger artery, indent the tissue a little way away from the spurter.

Failure to cut

If the cutting current does not slice cleanly through the tissues, or does not cut at all: (1) check that the patient is attached to the earth plate; (2) check that the earth is attached to the diathermy terminal; (3) check that you have been given water or glycine, not saline, as irrigating fluid; (4) make sure that the electrical contacts between diathermy machine and resectoscope, and between electrode and resectoscope, are all correctly made; (5) have the current increased.

Never call for more current without checking these simple safety precautions first.

Failure to coagulate

If the diathermy seems to be working, but the bleeding does not stop, it may be because the current is too strong, and instead of cooking the tissue, it is forming an arc, that is cutting. Turn the current strength down. Venous bleeding may continue when the side has been taken out of a vein, and the area to be coagulated is simply too large for the edges of the breach in the vein to close off. In such a situation it may be necessary to stop the operation and control the bleeding by firm traction on an over-inflated Foley balloon.

Steps of the operation

Transurethral resection of the prostate may be performed in many styles (Barnes 1943; Nesbit 1943), but the one described here is the sequence I was taught, and have practised ever since. When beginning, always stick to one pattern so that if trouble is encountered, another surgeon knows exactly how far you have got and what problems are likely to have been engendered (Blandy 1978). The sequence that I prefer falls into three distinct stages.

1 Finding the landmarks (removal of the middle lobe).
2 Removing the bulk of the lateral lobes.
3 Tidying up.

1 Finding the landmarks

The worst sin in transurethral surgery is to make the patient *incontinent*. To avoid this disaster, begin by identifying the external sphincter and the verumontanum. The external sphincter has two parts: one is visible, and appears like an anus, just downstream of the veru; the other is invisible, 'supramembranous', and lies in the tissue somewhere in the vicinity of the veru upstream of the visible contracting 'sphincter' (10.6). It is clearly an error to cut through the visible sphincter, but it is equally dangerous to cut too deeply into the tissue adjacent to the veru, or to use heavy coagulation in this area, lest the upper supramembranous element of the sphincter is injured (10.7).

The next sin, which alas, is not always

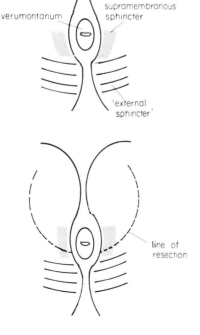

10.6. Proximal to (that is upstream of) the 'sphincter' lies the supramembranous sphincter in which resides an important part of the continence mechanism.

10.7. If the tissue resected includes the supramembranous sphincter then the patient may be left incontinent.

preventable, is to give the patient a *stricture*. Some post-TUR strictures are caused by chafing of too large a resectoscope sheath against too narrow a urethra, and may be prevented by preliminary urethrotomy with the Otis or a similar urethrotome, and this should certainly be done whenever the 24 Ch sheath is gripped by the urethra.

The third sin is to injure the *trigone* by 'climbing up' past the neck of the bladder; this gives rise to much unnecessary post-operative discomfort and may scar and stricture the ureters.

To avoid these three sins, begin by defining the three landmarks—the sphincter, the veru, and the bladder neck. The first two of these are easily identified. The sphincter has a characteristic appearance and feel, the sheath becoming loose in a quite unmistakable way as it emerges out of the grip of the sphincter. The verumontanum is usually easy to identify, though in a big prostate it is often pushed backwards, and obscured by a little clot of blood, and must be searched for. Do not make the error of mistaking the downward tail of the verumontanum for the prominence itself: always make sure the utriculus masculinus has been identified (10.8).

The bladder neck is not so easily seen. It is hidden behind and under the adenomatous tissue of the middle lobe which may stick up for a centimetre or more, and must be cut

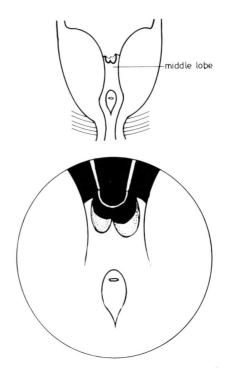

away until the transverse striations of the inferior fibres of the bladder's internal sphincter can be plainly seen (10.9). In a tiny prostate it takes only one or two chips in the midline at 6 o'clock to display these transverse fibres; in a large gland it may be necessary to remove many grams of adenoma before the bladder neck is identified. Once found, it should be respected as the *upper boundary*, above which the resection will not be taken (10.10).

The first step of the operation may therefore take only a second or two, or occupy several minutes. In a larger prostate, one must take

10.9. TUR first stage, resect the middle lobe at 6 o'clock to expose the muscle fibres of the bladder neck.

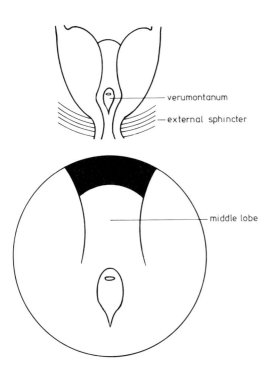

10.8. TUR first stage, defining the landmarks. The veru lies just proximal to the external sphincter.

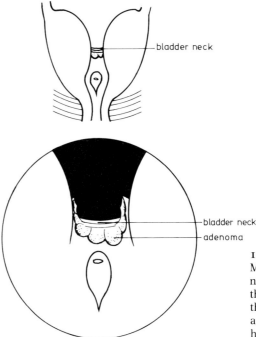

10.10. TUR first stage. Muscle fibres of bladder neck exposed. Now the two landmarks, the verumontanum and the bladder neck have been located.

care to remove the chips from the dome of the middle lobe in an even way, otherwise it is all too easy to cut a deep trench that bisects the middle lobe and forms two extra and very confusing 'lobes'. When the middle lobe is of any size, trim it away evenly along its bump (10.11). This is also the moment, when the middle lobe is large, to take a little extra time to seal off the large vessels that enter the prostate from the edge of the bladder neck at 5 and 7 o'clock (10.12).

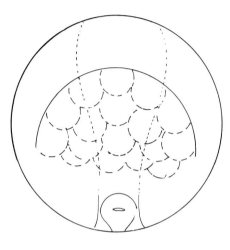

10.11. When the middle lobe is bulky, trim it evenly across the bump.

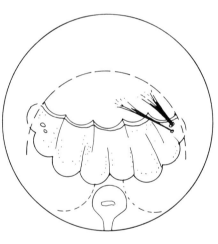

10.12. Seal off the large vessels at 5 and 7 o'clock.

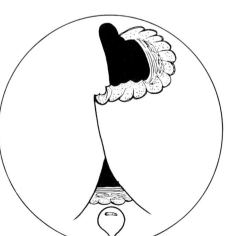

10.13. Second stage: take chips evenly from the inner edge of the lateral lobe.

2   Removing the lateral lobe adenoma

The next step is to remove the lateral lobes, shelling the adenoma out from the inner surface of the capsule. First check the position of the veru and the bladder neck since no cut must extend upwards or downwards of these two landmarks. Then, without pulling it out, rotate the resectoscope sheath to the 12 o'clock position to show the anterior commissure (10.13). Sink the loop in at 1 o'clock, just to one side of the anterior commissure, where the adenoma is usually very thin. This will reveal the bladder neck fibres (10.14). Continue to deepen this trench for the full length of the prostate, checking from time to time that the trench never goes further distal than the level of the veru. When this trench has been cut, the inner aspect of the capsule can be seen: it has a lacy texture, and looks distinctly different from the bread-like adenoma. As a rule the trench cuts through two or three arteries—the anterior arteries of Flocks— which must be carefully sealed off at this stage (10.15).

If the resectoscope sheath is now withdrawn, and rotated back so that the loop is once more at 6 o'clock, the lateral lobe is seen

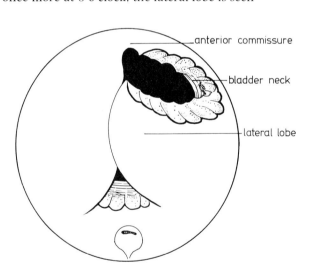

10.14. TUR second stage. The trench is cut down to the capsule, exposing the bladder neck at 11 o'clock and allowing the main bulk of the lobe to fall backwards and medially.

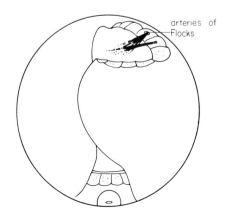

10.15. The arteries of Flocks are exposed in the base of the trench.

to have fallen backwards, as if detached from the capsule (10.16). Its main blood vessels, those that enter the lateral lobe at 5 o'clock and at 1 o'clock, have been diathermized, so removing the bulk of the adenoma is relatively bloodless. It is done as quickly as possible, taking long deep bites with the loop. The technique is like eating a boiled egg or hollowing out an avocado—spoonful by spoonful—leaving the capsule intact. In doing this, make a row of furrows in the projecting lump of lateral lobe, and then take a second row from the projecting ridges (10.17). Avoid hollowing out the middle of the lateral lobe without at the same time taking away its medial mucosal surface, or there will be a tiresome flap of tissue (10.18) that may confuse the inexperienced operator.

Continue until the ring of bladder neck is exposed all the way round from anterior commissure to midline posteriorly. Eventually the only part of the lateral lobe to be left is a little apical part just adjacent to the verumontanum: leave it at this stage (10.19).

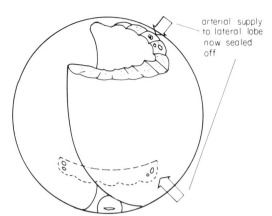

arterial supply to lateral lobe now sealed off

10.16. Once the 1 o'clock and 5 o'clock vessels have been sealed off, the bulk of the lateral lobe is virtually bloodless.

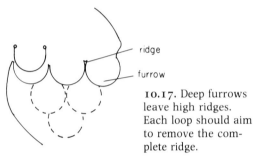

ridge

furrow

10.17. Deep furrows leave high ridges. Each loop should aim to remove the complete ridge.

Take time to secure perfect haemostasis of the hollowed-out capsule before proceeding to the right lateral lobe, and deal with it in exactly the same way, with a deep trench just to the side of the anterior commissure (10.20) sealing off Flocks' arteries, and rapid removal of the bulk of the lateral lobe adenoma (10.21).

3 Tidying up

The residual apical tissue either side of the veru is most easily resected if a finger is placed in the rectum to lift up the adenoma and veru (10.22). Taking very small bites, and using the pure cutting current (to avoid heat-injury to the supramembranous sphinc-

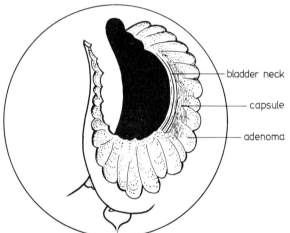

bladder neck

capsule

adenoma

10.18. TUR second stage. The error which results from hollowing the lateral

lobe like a boiled egg —a shell of lateral lobe tissue then flops down and obscures the veru.

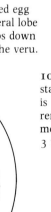

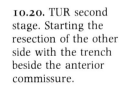

10.19. TUR second stage. The lateral lobe is almost completely removed; only the more distal tissue at 3 to 6 o'clock remains.

10.20. TUR second stage. Starting the resection of the other side with the trench beside the anterior commissure.

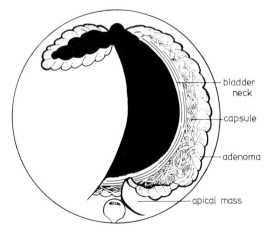

bladder neck

capsule

adenoma

apical mass

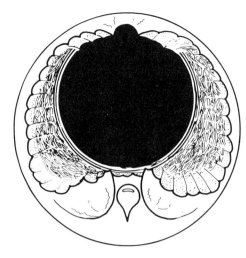

10.21. TUR second stage. The second stage is completed and both lateral lobes are removed except for tiny remnants beside the verumontanum and (perhaps) near the anterior commissure.

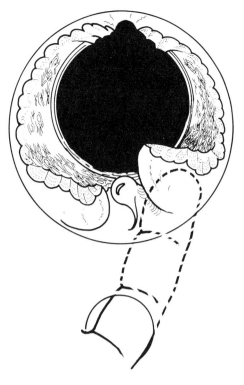

10.22. TUR third stage. A finger in the rectum helps to lift up the apex of each lateral lobe which is resected in very small bites to avoid going distal to the verumontanum.

ter), these little pyramidal pieces are trimmed away. There is a distinct semilunar line marking the lower edge of the adenoma, and it may help to cut from this line towards the bladder rather than downwards, a manoeuvre the beginner should avoid.

In very large adenomas the apical masses project past the verumontanum, and it is tempting to go on cutting away all the adenoma to expose the capsule. Err on the side of safety. It is far better to return the patient to the operating theatre the next week to trim away some apical tissue, than to make him incontinent. The patient (and his lawyers) will not forgive you if you have made him wet.

Check at this stage that there is no residual tissue just adjacent to the anterior commissure; withdraw the resectoscope to the sphincter, and empty the bladder. If there is a significant amount of tissue left here it will fall down into the lumen, and can be trimmed away using the same precautions as for the apical tissue, and when in doubt, erring on the side of caution (10.23).

Throughout the operation chips accumulate in the bladder and should be evacuated when they begin to make it difficult to see. Use the Ellik evacuator, having made sure that all the air is evacuated first (10.24). The

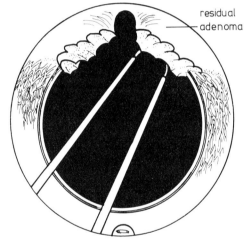

residual adenoma

10.23. TUR third stage. Removing any remaining tissue in the region either side of the anterior commissure.

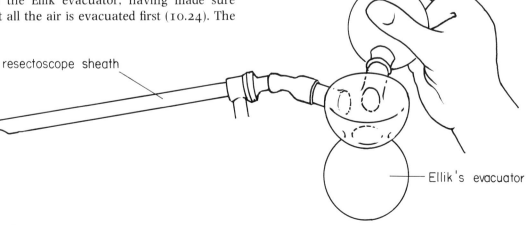

resectoscope sheath

Ellik's evacuator

10.24. Using the Ellik evacuator to remove all the remaining chips of prostate accumulated in the bladder.

purpose of the Ellik is to swirl the irrigation fluid round the bladder and suck out chips and blood clots: force is never necessary.

Finally, go round the capsule once more, sealing off all the bleeding vessels that can be found. Always check the sites of the major prostatic vessels, at 2, 5, 7, and 10 o'clock (10.25). Try to seal them with the loop, using pinpoint coagulation; only resort to the roly-ball electrode when there is a diffuse ooze. The more coagulation damage to the capsule, the greater the risk of subsequent secondary haemorrhage.

One source of confusion may baffle the beginner: a big spurting vessel may bounce back from the opposite wall of the prostatic cavity (10.26). Another difficulty arises when the vessel points straight at you, blinding your vision. Here the trick is to rotate the resectoscope, press it up against the capsule to angulate the artery and temporarily occlude it, and approach it from the side.

Large veins continue to bleed if a slice has been taken from their side, especially when one has resected too deeply into the capsule (10.27). A brief attempt to coagulate them may be made with the roly-ball, but more often than not this proves useless. Avoid spending time on such bleeding, for the irrigation fluid runs into the open veins as freely as blood runs out, and the longer you persist, the greater the risk of the TUR syndrome. Cut your losses, insert a Foley catheter, overinflate the balloon to 40 ml, and pull it down firmly to squeeze shut the opened veins long enough to give them time to seal with a clot (about twenty minutes) (10.28). Firm traction may

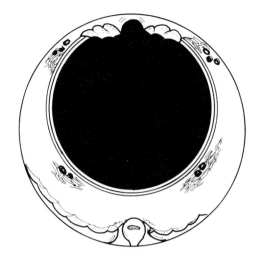

10.25. TUR third stage. Site of the main arterial bleeding in the prostatic bed, at the four quadrants.

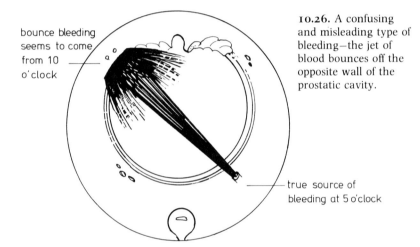

bounce bleeding seems to come from 10 o'clock

true source of bleeding at 5 o'clock

10.26. A confusing and misleading type of bleeding—the jet of blood bounces off the opposite wall of the prostatic cavity.

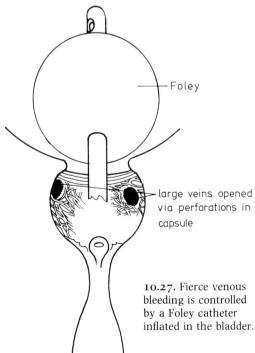

Foley

large veins opened via perforations in capsule

10.27. Fierce venous bleeding is controlled by a Foley catheter inflated in the bladder.

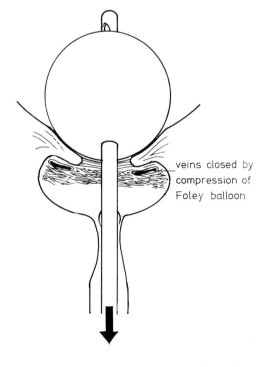

veins closed by compression of Foley balloon

10.28. The catheter is pulled down so that the balloon compresses the veins around the bladder neck.

10.29. Tension may be kept up on the balloon catheter by a swab tied round the catheter.

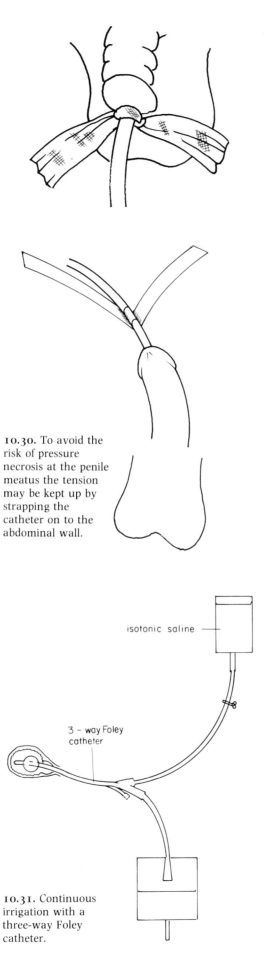

10.30. To avoid the risk of pressure necrosis at the penile meatus the tension may be kept up by strapping the catheter on to the abdominal wall.

isotonic saline

3 - way Foley catheter

10.31. Continuous irrigation with a three-way Foley catheter.

be kept up with a swab tied round the catheter (10.29), or attached to sticking plaster on the abdominal wall (10.30). If the Salvaris penile swab method is used for this tamponade, make sure that it is removed within twenty minutes, or there is a risk of a slough at the tip of the penis.

Keeping your bearings

The main difficulty in transurethral resection is to keep orientated throughout the operation. As in all other surgery, never cut unless you can see what you are cutting; always keep control of bleeding as you go; and constantly refer to the landmarks—the bladder neck fibres and the verumontanum. These are your sure reference points: keep referring to them, and you will stay orientated.

Above all, keep aware of the risk of erection. It may develop insidiously during the operation, and unless you appreciate what is happening, the resectoscope sheath will be pushed out as the penis elongates, and you may find yourself making the disastrous error of resecting the external sphincter instead of the lateral lobe.

Post-operative management of transurethral resection

In most cases a three-way irrigating catheter (size 20–22 Ch) is left in the bladder, and after the glycine used for irrigation has run through, physiological saline is used thereafter. To start with the saline runs in briskly, but after twenty minutes or so the rate of inflow is adjusted to keep the colour of the outflow pale pink. Small clots or chips that block the catheter can be washed out with a bladder syringe. If this fails to restore flow, the catheter should be changed. Continuous irrigation avoids the need to change the catheter and cuts down the infection rate (10.31).

Post-operative pain is minimal, unless the trigone has been trespassed upon. There is an urge to void, and some soreness in the urethra around the catheter, perhaps related to the balloon on the trigone. Elderly patients worry about an occasional involuntary escape of urine around the catheter, and need to be reassured.

If the drainage is reasonably clear, the catheter is removed after forty-eight hours. If removed sooner than this, local extravasation of urine gives rise to discomfort. The catheter may of course be left in longer if there is some special reason for doing so, for example chronic retention with a big atonic bladder, or men confined to bed on some other account, but the longer the catheter remains in the bladder the greater the risk of infection.

Hazards of transurethral resection

Perforation of the capsule is inevitable if an adenoma is to be completely resected. Tell-tale glistening of extravesical fat is often to be seen in the capsule at 3 and 9 o'clock, but may usually be safely disregarded, and gives rise to no harm. Very rarely one makes a big perforation, usually because the patient has suddenly coughed, or the obturator nerve has been stimulated. It is evident that something has gone wrong very quickly: the irrigating fluid does not run back properly when the resectoscope is removed from the sheath; the character of the patient's respirations changes; there may be an obvious suprapubic swelling.

When these signs appear, do not hesitate. Make a Pfannenstiel incision as soon as things can be made ready. There will be considerable fluid in the retropubic space, but the actual perforation is seldom seen. If there is any reason to suspect that the peritoneal cavity has been entered, make a formal opening in it, look for free fluid, and if there is any, carefully inspect the adjacent loops of bowel to see that none have been burnt or perforated. If the bowel has been injured, oversew it in the transverse axis, and protect the sutures with a plug of omentum. Usually it is only necessary to drain the retropubic space. In practice such perforation during transurethral resection of the prostate is exceedingly rare: it is far more common during resection of tumours of the bladder.

There is one even more rare, but very frightening combination of events, which I hope that my readers will never encounter. Rarely, when resecting the prostate of a frail and atheromatous patient, the prostatic arteries stand out like pipe-stems, and do not close despite patient application of the diathermy. Sometimes this bleeding occurs in association with a perforation. In either event, if it is impossible to control with the diathermy, it must be suture-ligated. In such a case, you must be prepared to go straight on to expose the prostatic cavity just as you would in an ordinary retropubic prostatectomy, seek out and underrun the offending vessel, and get perfect haemostasis.

Obturator nerve stimulation has been mentioned. If it occurs during the operation, have the cutting current turned down to the minimum power that will allow the loop to cut the tissue. If the adductors still jump, stop the resection, and insist that your anaesthetist paralyses the patient and effects a complete block at the motor end-plates. This may be impossible if the operation is being performed under spinal or epidural anaesthesia. The alternative is to infiltrate the obturator nerve with local anaesthetic.

The landmarks of the obturator nerve are the pubic tubercle, the femoral artery, and

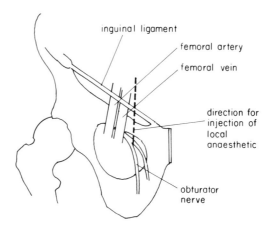

inguinal ligament
femoral artery
femoral vein
direction for injection of local anaesthetic
obturator nerve

10.32. Landmarks for the obturator nerve.

the symphysis pubis (10.32). Using a spinal needle, aim for the obturator foramen, letting the needle enter half way between the mid-inguinal point (where the pulsation of the femoral artery is felt) and the pubic tubercle. It passes downwards and medially, infiltrating and aspirating alternately, until the resistance of the medial edge of the obturator foramen is felt. About 10 ml of 1% lignocaine are needed, and you should wait five minutes for the block to take effect.

The TUR syndrome

This term is applied to two complications, each caused by loss of irrigating fluid into the venous circulation (Bird *et al.* 1982). Nowadays most resectionists use 4% glucose, 2% glycine, sorbitol, mannitol, or some similar non-ionizing fluid that will not cause haemolysis if it enters the blood-stream. Haemolysis is therefore very rare, but if distilled water is used for transurethral resection then haemolysis is an ever present risk. The obdurate old-fashioned resectionist who insists on distilled water in the face of all the evidence which shows it to be dangerous is asking for a lawsuit.

Even if one avoids haemolysis by using an isotonic solution, electrolytic complications may still follow infusion of a large volume of glycine or any of the other compounds. Dilution of the extracellular fluid lessens the differential concentration of extra- and intra-cellular sodium and potassium, which preserves the cell membrane potential, and the function of nerves and muscles. The consequences may be widespread and serious. First is a transient period when the circulatory volume is expanded and there is hypertension. Then, as the water overload diffuses into the tissue space, nerve and muscle complications follow, with the development of bizarre paralyses that mimic hemiparesis, cerebrovascular accident, or epileptiform fits. I have even seen transient blindness occur.

Fortunately the kidneys usually get rid of the excess water, and the glycine or glucose is metabolized without complication. This diuresis may be encouraged by giving frusemide, but it is seldom necessary. Hypertonic saline is not necessary—it merely frustrates the efforts of the body to get rid of the surplus water and threatens heart failure.

Although the diagnosis is made on clinical grounds, it is easily confirmed by having the plasma sodium concentration measured: it will be very low. Be on guard for this complication after a prolonged and difficult TUR in which large venous sinuses have been entered.

The one-hour rule

Forty years ago, when the great pioneers were establishing the technique of transurethral resection, most of the operations were performed under spinal anaesthesia, and after about an hour the patient would recover sensation. In this same period, when these same pioneers recognized the risks of haemolysis and the dilutional TUR syndrome, they appreciated that it was only encountered when the operation had gone on for more than an hour. This is hardly surprising, for these were the same patients in whom the glands were very large and where venous sinuses were most likely to be breached. Hence arose the notion of the 'one-hour rule', that is all transurethral resections must be discontinued after one hour. This is a curiously silly rule because it implies that there is some mysterious physiological clock, that 59.9 minutes is all right but 60.1 minutes is dangerous. I take no account of the time of the resection, but I do take very great care to avoid delay when large veins have been breached, and I do take the precaution of having the plasma sodium measured in those patients in whom the resection has been unduly prolonged.

Blood loss during the operation

Unless special precautions are taken, it is difficult to assess blood loss at operation. One may take an aliquot of the collected irrigation fluid, convert the haemoglobin to acid haematin using Drabkin's solution, and measure the colour with a colorimeter. An optimistic glance at the effluent in the collecting reservoir is a very unreliable way of estimating blood loss. On the whole, remember that it is the larger glands in which there is likely to be significant blood loss, and that if you guess the patient has lost one unit, he has usually lost two (Mackenzie et al. 1979).

In the past there have been innumerable suggestions for reducing loss of blood. They include administration of oestrogens, carbazochrome-salicylate, kutapressin, premarin, arotinin, and many others. Aminocaproic acid and its successors may reduce the loss of blood, but at the expense of forming stiff, tenacious blood clots which are very troublesome to remove. Dicynine minimizes capillary oozing, and may reduce bleeding by an insignificant amount, when the bleeding is insignificant, but does not, and cannot be expected to, stop bleeding from a cut artery or open vein. Ice-cold irrigating solution runs the risk of producing total body hypothermia.

Secondary haemorrhage

There is nearly always a little secondary haemorrhage, for the prostatic cavity is lined by slough, especially where the coagulating current has been used. In due course the slough must separate: as elsewhere in surgery, it does not always choose the tenth post-operative day to come away, but the patient should be warned of the occurrence of some discomfort and some pink staining of the urine about ten to fourteen days after the TUR. Only in 1% of patients is there enough bleeding to give rise to clot retention but for this reason the patient must be within easy distance of a hospital where his bladder may be washed out. Very rarely, once the bladder has been washed out and clots gently syringed away, bleeding may continue and if so, then the patient is returned to the operating theatre and the inner surface of the capsule inspected for the source of the bleeding.

Late post-TUR bleeding

This is a well-recognized late sequel of transurethral resection. Years after an apparently successful resection, the patient may return with haematuria, raising the suspicion of a bladder cancer. A routine pyelogram and cystoscopy shows no sinister cause for the bleeding, and the only abnormality seems to be a frill of tender pink granulations around the site of the otherwise well-resected prostate. I have never been able to refrain from taking a biopsy of this tissue which invariably shows mild chronic inflammatory change in residual adenoma (10.33).

Stricture

It is now clear that urethral stricture can be largely, if not entirely avoided, if the Otis urethrotome is used to slit the urethra whenever the sheath is gripped, even ever so slightly. Stricture formation takes place at three sites: the usual site is just inside the external urinary meatus; but it also forms at the penoscrotal angle, perhaps by pressure of the catheter on the angulated penis; and also just downstream of the external sphincter. The first two are easily dealt with by the passage of a bougie on three or four occasions. The stricture that forms near the external sphincter is far more sinister, since it is often accompanied by a degree of incontinence. Dilatation of the first two varieties may be assisted by internal urethrotomy, but there is a risk of making incontinence worse if the urethrotome is used near the external sphincter. For the same reason, if either of these strictures becomes so intractable that urethroplasty is contemplated, one should be reluctant to offer it when the stricture is adjacent to the sphincter.

Incontinence

Incontinence is the most feared of all complications of transurethral resection. The danger of cutting deeply distal to the verumontanum has been stressed since the beginnings of this type of surgery, but it cannot be the whole explanation of this complication. In some patients with post-TUR incontinence the verumontanum has been intact and the ring of sphincter not breached, but the tissues look shiny and smooth, losing their normal frilly softness. Mauermayer (1983) has shown that in some of these patients the external sphincter no longer

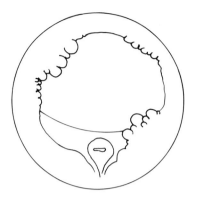

10.33. Granulations in prostate bed, causing late post-TUR bleeding.

contracts when stimulated. But there is more to post-TUR incontinence than mere damage to 'the sphincter'. In some patients a small nubble of apical tissue seems to keep the lumen half-open (10.34) and continence is restored only when the residual tissue is resected. In others the cause of the incontinence is that the patient started off with a very irritable or unstable bladder, and should not have undergone prostatectomy in the first place.

Retrograde ejaculation

Although retrograde ejaculation is less common after transurethral than after other forms of prostatectomy, it is still an important sequel. Some patients are very concerned about the dry ejaculate, and it is essential that the surgeon explains to the patient that this may occur. It is however unpredictable. Many patients with thorough resections are able to ejaculate perfectly well afterwards, even though cystography shows that the bladder neck is patent and the prostatic cavity wide open. Just as it is important to explain to the patient that retrograde ejaculation may take place after prostatectomy, and hence he is likely to be rendered infertile, so it must also be pointed out that it is not inevitable, and no guarantee of sterility. If the patient needs to be assured of perfect contraception, then vasectomy should be added to the operation.

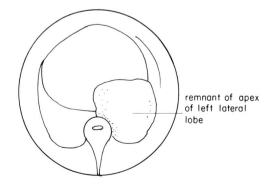

remnant of apex of left lateral lobe

10.34. Incontinence may be caused by a nubble of apical tissue left behind in the vicinity of the verumontanum.

Impotence

Sadly, a number of men complain that not only is there no ejaculate after transurethral surgery, but no erection either. I have never been able to discern a clear pattern in these patients. In some there seems to be an element of depression, in others it would seem that the TUR was the symbol, the last straw, of a diminishing sexual activity. What is important is that the surgeon should protect himself from possible litigation by making sure that the matter has been fully discussed with the patient (Blandy 1976; Madorsky 1976; Zohar *et al.* 1976).

Infection

Bacteraemia (page 41) may strike out of the blue after any endoscopic surgical operation and TUR is no exception. If the urine is known to be infected, then of course appropriate antimicrobial cover will be given to protect the patient throughout the time of the operation and for the first few days afterwards. But one must be equally aware that resection may stir up unsuspected microbes in the prostatic tissue, and force them into the blood-stream with the irrigating fluid (Robinson *et al.* 1982).

Epididymitis is so rare after transurethral surgery that it is no longer justified to perform vasectomy as a routine, but in patients who have had an indwelling catheter for a long time, or whose urine is grossly infected, it is still seen.

Post-operative urinary infection is almost inevitable if the catheter has to remain in position for more than a week (Symes *et al.* 1972). Our policy is to refrain from treating the infection, so long as the patient is well, until after the catheter has been taken out. A urine specimen is then cultured, and residual infection treated accordingly.

Modifications of standard transurethral resection

Small fibrous and bilharzial prostates

In small fibrous prostates, and in particular those due to scarring from schistosomal infection, there is a very short distance between the bladder neck, verumontanum, and sphincter, so that one must take extra care not to transgress the landmarks. Since there is no lump of lateral lobe adenoma to be enucleated, or spooned out of its capsule, there is no purpose in making a trench at 1 o'clock and 11 o'clock: it is more easy to find the veru in the usual way, resect down to the bladder neck at 6 o'clock, feeling with a finger in the rectum the thickness of the tissue, and then work out laterally on either side from 6 to 3 o'clock and 9 o'clock until a complete ring of the obstructing tissue has been removed all around (10.35).

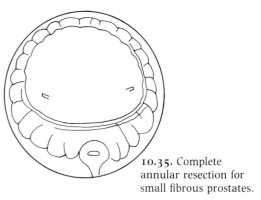

10.35. Complete annular resection for small fibrous prostates.

Bladder neck incision

This very ancient operation has been revived in recent years and has become very fashionable as an alternative to TUR. It claims to be followed by less retrograde ejaculation (though no alternative prospective series has ever been performed to support this claim). It is claimed to be safer, and to be followed by fewer complications (Moisey *et al.* 1982).

It may be indicated when the cause of the obstructed outflow is a failure of the bladder neck to relax in coordination with the contraction of the detrusor. Patients may be tested by being given phenoxybenzamine prior to the operation. Using a Collings knife, an incision is made through the ring of bladder neck tissue until it gapes (10.36). Some surgeons make only one incision; others make two. Since the cut has to be made right through the bladder neck muscle and any adjacent prostatic adenoma, it enters the capsule, and is often followed by alarming bleeding.

10.36. Bladder neck incision.

line of insision with Collings knife

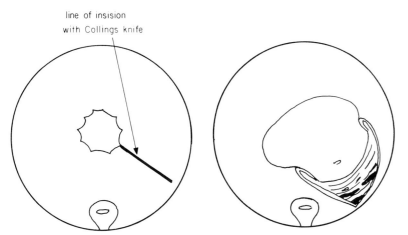

Despite vociferous claims for the advantages of this procedure, I have been repeatedly disappointed by its long term results in practice, and have again and again had to bring the patient back within months for a formal endoscopic resection of the offending tissue. The scanty published results do not impress one as being superior to those of transurethral resection for small glands. Its advantage however is that it is easy, needing no particular skill or training.

TUR for very large prostates

With a very large gland it may be difficult to see over the adenoma into the bladder. In such a case TUR is best avoided except when the patient is too ill for any open procedure. In such very rare cases TUR can be done through a midline perineal urethrostomy.

With less enormous glands, over whose middle lobe the ordinary resectoscope reaches comfortably, the stages of the TUR are just the same, but it is necessary to take extra care never to allow yourself to get disorientated.

The first stage, finding the landmarks, may be more difficult because the veru is pushed backwards, and it is necessary to lift up the resectoscope to see it. Similarly, a big bulky middle lobe must be removed to show the transverse fibres of the bladder neck. Instead of digging a channel to identify the bladder neck, it is better to cut away the dome of the middle lobe in a series of furrows and ridges, keeping it even, until the bladder neck fibres are exposed along the entire width of the middle lobe (10.37). To do this properly may mean that it is necessary to take out 20–30 g of tissue. The advantage is that at the end of formal resection of the middle lobe, the 5 o'clock and 7 o'clock vessels will have been uncovered and definitely closed with diathermy. Having obtained haemostasis, continue to remove the rest of the bulk of the middle lobe down to the upper edge of the verumontanum (10.38).

In the second stage of the resection of a large gland, sink a trench immediately adjacent to the anterior commissure, and work round the bladder neck, just as if a finger were enucleating a large adenoma from the capsule (10.39). To enable the mass of lateral lobe to fall medially in the desired way, this trench must be carried down to the level of the verumontanum, and in a long prostate this may call for two or three furrows, two or three complete travels of the loop (10.40). Freeing up the lateral lobe,

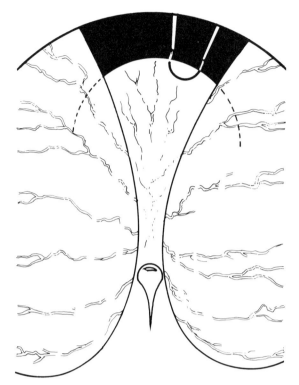

10.37. When the middle lobe is very big, make sure that it is trimmed away evenly across the top.

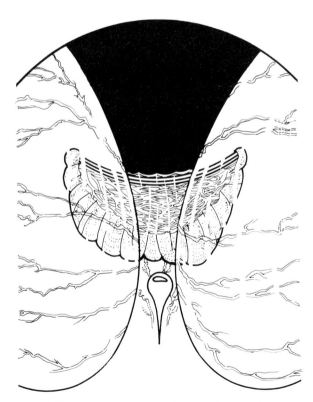

10.38. When the middle lobe has been resected right down to the bladder neck, make sure the 5 and 7 o'clock arteries are well coagulated.

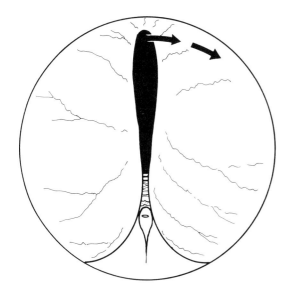

10.39. TUR for the big gland: start to free the lateral lobe beside the commissure.

10.40. Resect the freed-up quadrant of prostate down to the capsule before going on to the next part.

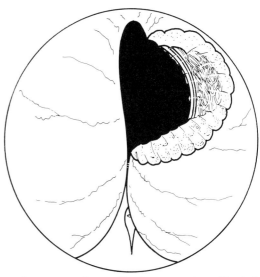

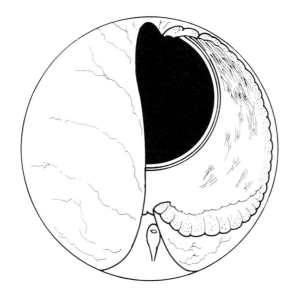

10.41. Main part of the large lateral lobe removed: leave the apical portion until the other side is done.

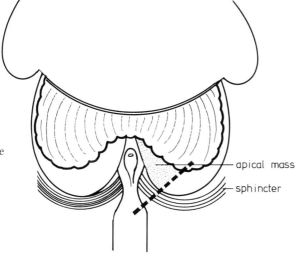

10.42. The hazard of resecting the apical mass in the very large adenoma. Note how far distal to the verumontanum the lateral lobe can extend, and how it deforms the external sphincter.

apical mass

sphincter

make sure that all the anterior Flocks' arteries have been well diathermized, and then set to remove the bulk of the lateral lobe as rapidly as is consistent with safety. Make each loopful as long and as deep as possible, and keep the pyramidal lump of lateral lobe trimmed off evenly, taking ridges and furrows from the inner as well as the upper surface of the lump. Avoid hollowing out the lateral lobe, so that a tiresome flap of mucosa does not flop down to hide the veru-montanum. As the work proceeds, remember that the prostatic cavity is barrel-shaped and it is necessary to swing the loop deeply into its hollow to spoon out the bread from the capsule.

Once the first side has been done, leaving only the apical tissue to be dealt with (10.41), spend time getting good haemostasis, for if bleeding is not controlled now, it is difficult to see the capsule clearly later on, since it becomes lined with a layer of blood clot. Once good haemostasis has been obtained, repeat the process on the other side. From time to time there may be concern about the patient's general condition after one lobe has been removed. It is sometimes safer to stop. Many a patient can void even when only one lateral lobe has been removed.

The third, tidying-up stage of TUR is especially difficult in large glands. A museum specimen of a large adenoma will show that each lateral lobe bulges right down beyond the veru and deforms the external sphincter (10.42). Remember this when trimming away the tissue on either side of the verumontanum. A finger in the rectum will help to bring up the adenoma from the periphery into the lumen of the urethra, and one should repeatedly check not only the position of the veru but also that of the external sphincter.

Remember that, in addition to the visible part of the external sphincter, there is also the invisible 'supramembranous' sphincter, and that the purpose of prostatectomy is not to clean out every shred of adenoma, but to get the old boy out of hospital, passing his water comfortably, and with perfect control. There is no prize for astonishing your residents with a gigantic pile of chips.

Carcinoma

In an obvious carcinoma of the prostate the intention is to carve a funnel from veru to bladder neck, both to remove obstruction and to obtain tissue for diagnosis. The cancer often invades the adjacent tissues so there is no clear distinction between 'bread' and 'capsule' (10.43). Occasionally one meets a Müllerian duct cancer, which is curiously glairy and once cut into, continues to spill into the lumen of the prostatic cavity like a breaking-down abscess.

Most carcinomas are relatively bloodless, and present easy technical operations for the beginner. Occasionally one may be caught out by fibrinolysins liberated by a large carcinoma or its metastases, which cause uncontrollable bleeding. The remedy is cyclocapron or its derivatives but one should whenever possible obtain laboratory confirmation of the need for it before operation. The tell-tale features are petechiae and ecchymoses in an old patient with suspected cancer of the prostate.

Since cancer of the prostate often invades the sphincter and renders the tissue stiff and rigid, it is small wonder that many of these men become incontinent. Warn the patient of this hazard, and be specially careful to spare the tissue adjacent to the verumontanum.

Prostatic calculi

Most prostatic calculi lurk in the plane between capsule and adenoma. They are easily wriggled out with the loop when the adenoma has been partially resected, and indeed offer a useful warning that you have approached the capsule, especially in the vicinity of the apex (10.44). Large stones may replace one or both lobes, but are trapped under the mucosa of the prostatic urethra, which must be deliberately cut away to allow the stones to be dislodged back up into the bladder, where they are crushed and removed by lithotrite and Ellik.

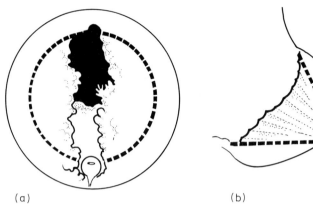

(a)   (b)

TUR after previous abdomino-perineal excision of rectum

Here the bladder and prostate have fallen back into the cavity formerly occupied by the rectum. It is difficult to see the verumontanum because it also falls backwards. The trick is to follow down the midline of the urethra, tilting up the resectoscope as you go. The steps of the resection are otherwise the same, though more difficult owing to the tilt of the prostate gland, and the inability to work with a finger in the rectum. Post-operative incontinence is more common after TUR when there has previously been an excision of the rectum, and one must be extra careful not to resect too much tissue in the vicinity of the verumontanum.

References

Barnes R.W. (1943) *Endoscopic Prostatic Resection.* Kimpton, London.

Bird D., Slade N. & Feneley R.C.L. (1982) Intravascular complications of transurethral resection. *Brit. J. Urol.* **54**, 564.

Blandy J.P. (1976) Benign enlargement of the prostate gland. In *Urology* (ed. by Blandy J.P.), p. 859. Blackwell Scientific Publications, Oxford.

10.43. TUR for carcinoma of the prostate. (a) The irregular appearance of the carcinoma may deform and obscure the verumontanum. Your intention (b) is to resect a generous cone from veru up to bladder neck.

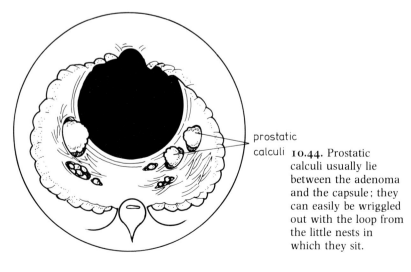

prostatic calculi

10.44. Prostatic calculi usually lie between the adenoma and the capsule; they can easily be wriggled out with the loop from the little nests in which they sit.

Blandy J.P. (1977) Surgery of the Benign Prostate. *J. Irish Med. Ass.* **70**, 517.

Blandy J.P. (1978) *Transurethral Resection*, 2nd edn. Pitman Medical, London.

Mackenzie A.R., Levine N. & Scheinman H.Z. (1979) Operative blood loss in transurethral prostatectomy. *J. Urol.* **122**, 47.

Madorsky M.L., Ashamalla M.G., Schussler I., Lyons H.R. & Miller G.H. (1976) Post-prostatectomy impotence. *J. Urol.* **115**, 401.

Mauermayer W. (1983) *Transurethral Surgery*. Springer, Berlin.

Moisey C.U., Stephenson T.P. & Evans C. (1982) A subjective and urodynamic assessment of unilateral bladder neck incision for bladder neck obstruction. *Brit. J. Urol.* **54**, 114.

Nesbit R.M. (1943) *Transurethral Prostatectomy*. Thomas, Springfield.

Robinson M.R.G., Arudpragasam S.T., Sahgal S.M., Cross R.J., Akdas A., Fittal B. & Sibbald R. (1982) Bacteraemia resulting from prostatic surgery: the source of bacteria. *Brit. J. Urol.* **54**, 542.

Symes J.M., Hardy D.G., Sutherns K. & Blandy J.P. (1972) Factors reducing the rate of infection after transurethral surgery. *Brit. J. Urol.* **44**, 582.

Zohar J., Meiraz D., Maoz B. & Durst N. (1976) Factors influencing sexual activity after prostatectomy: a prospective study. *J. Urol.* **116**, 332.

Chapter 11
Open prostatectomy

There are many variations on the theme of transvesical prostatectomy, which is the oldest of all methods of removing the adenoma, but they are virtually superseded in modern units by Millin's retropubic method (Blandy 1976, 1977).

Retropubic prostatectomy

Indications

Each surgeon must decide for himself when it is better to desist from an attempt at a TUR: each will have his own individual rules, dictated by experience, aptitude, the equipment that is available, and the general condition of the patient.

Small fibrous glands and cancers have no plane of cleavage, and should not be operated on by any open method if possible. Calculi in the prostate are better removed endoscopically. There are some patients in whom one must open the bladder in order to remove a stone or deal with a diverticulum, where it might be better to perform an open prostatectomy at the same time. Finally, every urologist must learn the retropubic approach, for it is the escape route from serious trouble. For the average prostate it has a significantly worse mortality and morbidity than the transurethral operation (Blandy 1978).

Special preparations

The preparations for all forms of prostatectomy are the same: find out the sensitivity of micro-organisms in the urine; have at least two units of blood cross-matched; above all, secure the services of an experienced anaesthetist.

Anaesthesia

Take the greatest care in selecting your colleague, but do not tell him what to do. If happy about the cardiovascular state of the patient, ask for a measure of controlled hypotension. There are many ways to provide this: some prefer an epidural anaesthetic, others a ganglion-blocking agent; many prefer the hypotensive effect of fluothane. It is not the technique but the doctor that matters: if your colleague provides controlled hypotension, then in turn you must keep your side of the bargain, and treat every capillary as if it was a major vessel. Haemostasis must be perfect or there will be a serious danger of reactionary haemorrhage. When ganglion-blockers are used, make sure that all lost blood is replaced—hypovolaemia in a paralysed symphathetic system can be lethal.

Position on the table

In our unit open prostatectomy is so rare that the decision is never made until cystoscopy has been performed. We leave the patient in stirrups: clean, shave and prepare the skin, and towel up again in the same position. If for some reason it has been obvious that an open procedure is going to be needed, the patient may be left supine.

Cystoscopy

It should go without saying that every patient must have the inside of the bladder carefully examined with the cystoscope before any prostatectomy is performed, to exclude cancer, stones, and other vesical pathology.

Incision

The Pfannenstiel incision is better than the midline one.

Steps of the operation

Having parted the bellies of the rectus muscle, wipe the peritoneum superiorly with a gauze-covered finger and insert Millin's self-retaining retractor, and put in the back-blade.

In the fat in front of the prostate there are several large veins, which must be sutured and divided. It helps to make a little pedicle of these veins by dissection with a Lahey swab

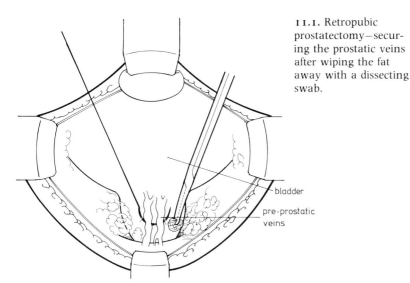

11.1. Retropubic prostatectomy—securing the prostatic veins after wiping the fat away with a dissecting swab.

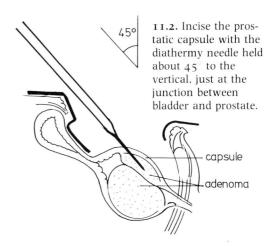

11.2. Incise the prostatic capsule with the diathermy needle held about 45° to the vertical, just at the junction between bladder and prostate.

capsule

adenoma

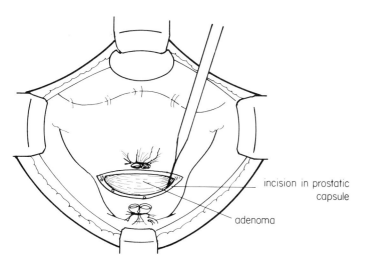

incision in prostatic capsule

adenoma

11.3. The capsule incised to expose the outer surface of the adenoma.

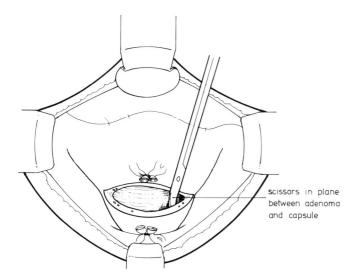

scissors in plane between adenoma and capsule

11.4. Define the plane of cleavage between capsule and adenoma with dissecting scissors, over the anterior and lateral aspects of the adenoma.

first (11.1). The incision in the prostatic capsule is made nearer to the neck of the bladder than is often supposed and illustrated. It is made obliquely, using a diathermy needle held 45° from the vertical and directed towards the anus (11.2). Make the incision little by little, to give ample time to seal off the little arteries by coagulation. Deepen this incision in the capsule to expose the shining white outer part of the adenoma (11.3). If the diathermy needle cuts into the adenoma, one may recognize the bread-like appearance so different from the woven texture of the capsule.

Open the plane between adenoma and capsule with scissors (11.4) and then enlarge-it with finger-tip and scissors. It is all too easy to enucleate the entire lateral lobe at this stage; indeed this was the classical technique, but Fergusson's modification is safer, as it preserves the veru and sphincter. After freeing up the front and sides of each lateral lobe, the finger is forced down in the midline into the cleft between each lateral lobe until it breaks into the prostatic urethra, (11.5); one can feel the pimple of the verumontanum

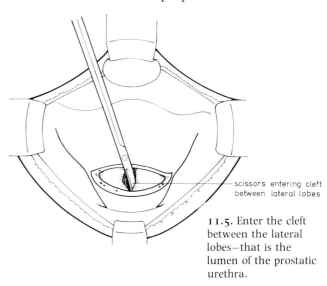

scissors entering cleft between lateral lobes

11.5. Enter the cleft between the lateral lobes—that is the lumen of the prostatic urethra.

on the posterior floor of the cavity. Now force
the finger-tip downwards and sideways until
the mucosa just to one side of the verumontanum cracks, allowing the finger to
slip into the plane between adenoma and
capsule. The same process is performed on the
other side of the verumontanum, leaving a
strip of intact urethral mucosa running up the
floor of the prostatic cavity (11.6). Each
lateral lobe is now enucleated completely and
delivered up into the wound with the
assistance of a vulsellum forceps (11.7).

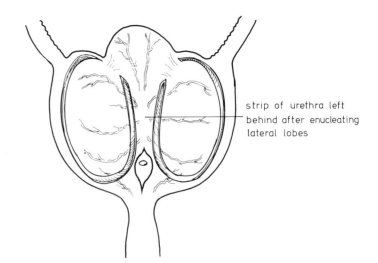

11.6. With your index finger cleave into
the plane between adenoma and capsule
just lateral to the verumontanum on
either side of the midline–in this way you
cannot damage the veru or the sphincter
distal to it.

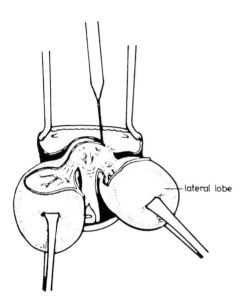

11.7. The lateral lobes are delivered, held
up and out of the prostatic cavity, and
the dissection of the middle lobe begun
with the diathermy needle.

Use a bladder neck spreader to stretch wide
the bladder neck and upper leaf of the capsule.
Identify the ureteric orifices. Pick up the
middle lobe along with the lateral lobes, and
cut along the line where middle lobe and
trigone join, lifting it up and away from the
posterior capsule and the seminal vesicles.
The two lateral lobes and the middle lobe now
form a single clump, attached only by the
strip of urethra which is cut off well above
the verumontanum (11.8).

Haemostasis

As in transurethral resection, the main
sources of haemorrhage are the arteries at 11,
1, 5, and 7 o'clock. The 11 and 1 o'clock
vessels (Flocks' arteries) were sealed off when
the capsule was incised with the diathermy.
The 5 and 7 o'clock vessels are seen in each
corner of the incision in the bladder neck, and

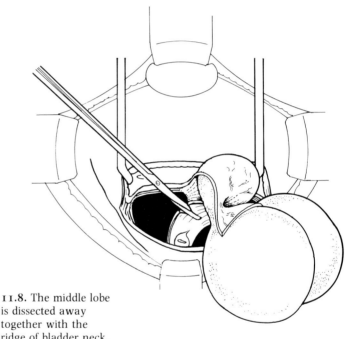

11.8. The middle lobe
is dissected away
together with the
ridge of bladder neck,
and the thin ribbon
of prostatic urethra is
cut across.

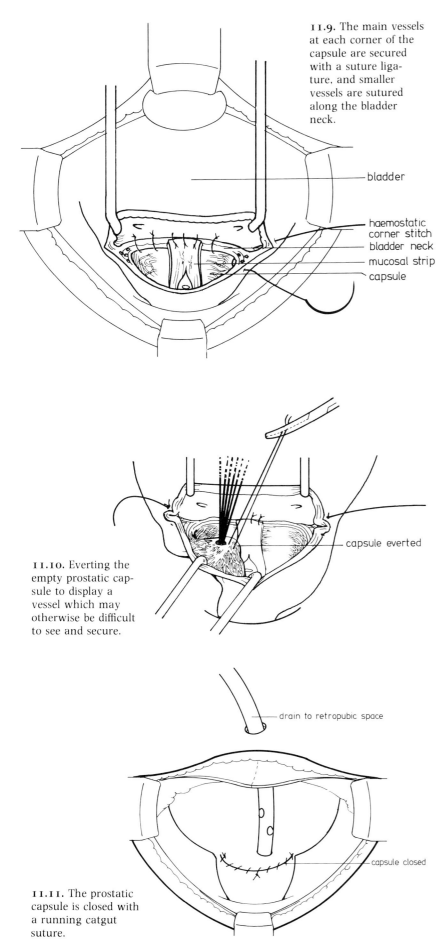

11.9. The main vessels at each corner of the capsule are secured with a suture ligature, and smaller vessels are sutured along the bladder neck.

— bladder

— haemostatic corner stitch
— bladder neck
— mucosal strip
— capsule

11.10. Everting the empty prostatic capsule to display a vessel which may otherwise be difficult to see and secure.

— capsule everted

— drain to retropubic space

11.11. The prostatic capsule is closed with a running catgut suture.

— capsule closed

are now suture-ligated with 2-0 chromic catgut leaving the needle long on the catgut at each corner, as this makes it easy to close the capsule in a few moments (11.9).

Now irrigate, identify, and suture-ligature each little artery along the edge of the bladder neck. If there is difficulty because of a continual ooze of blood welling up from the prostatic cavity, pack it firmly while the bladder neck vessels are sutured. Some of this is venous bleeding, which will stop within a few minutes. More often there is an artery or two that enters the prostatic capsule just where it cannot be seen. To bring it into view, a useful trick is to insert a strong suture into the inner aspect of the capsule, and pull the thin capsule inside out—deprived of its adenoma, the capsule is surprisingly pliable. A bleeding artery can now be seen, sutured or diathermized with ease (11.10).

The free strip of urethra is sutured to the neck of the bladder. Any untidy tags of tissue are trimmed away, and a final careful look is taken to make sure that haemostasis is perfect. There is no need to reconstruct the mucosal covering for the raw surface of the prostatic fossa.

A three-way irrigating Foley catheter is left in the bladder. Using the two sutures that were placed in each corner, the capsule is sutured (11.11) and the wound is closed with catgut leaving a tube drain down to the prevesical space.

Vasectomy is no longer indicated in prostatectomy since the post-operative incidence of epididymitis is now so low.

Post-operative care

Continue the irrigation with physiological saline until the effluent is clear, usually after twelve to twenty-four hours. The suprapubic drain is removed after twenty-four hours and the urethral catheter on the fifth post-operative day. The patient may go home on the seventh or eighth day (if all is well) and the sutures are removed on the tenth.

Hazards of open prostatectomy

The main danger of any prostatectomy is primary haemorrhage on the table. The enormous advantage of Millin's approach (Millin 1947) is the free access to the principal source of this bleeding, the vessels at each corner of the capsule. Because of this excellent access, the surgeon should make the best use of it, and make sure that the prostatic cavity is really dry before closing the wound. If the haemostasis is imperfect there will be bloody effluent, clot retention, and maybe the need to return the patient to the theatre to irrigate the clot away with an Ellik evacuator. If this is needed, a general anaesthetic will be required, and one should take the opportunity to examine the inside of the prostatic fossa with the resectoscope to identify and coagulate the offending vessel.

Deep venous thrombosis and pulmonary embolism are important complications after all forms of open prostatectomy but are almost unknown after transurethral resection. The reason for this discrepancy is not obvious (Mayo & Browse 1971; Hedlund 1976). To treat the thrombosis with anticoagulants courts the risk of provoking a major secondary haemorrhage. Low-dose heparin prophylaxis has its advocates, but seems to be followed by an unwonted incidence of wound haematoma and sepsis.

Persistent suprapubic fistulae occur only when there is an uncorrected outflow obstruction. It demands reintroduction of the catheter for two to three days.

Rectal fistula has been reported from time to time when an attempt has been made to enucleate a small fibrous, calculous, or malignant prostate in which there is no plane of cleavage, or, when there has been considerable bleeding, attempts have been made to control it with diathermy or suture ligatures that injure the rectum.

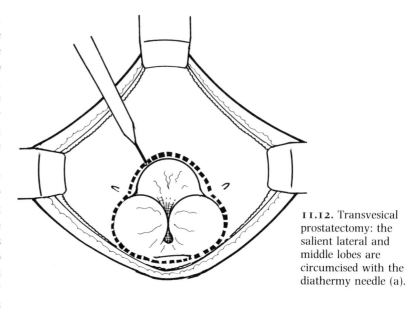

11.12. Transvesical prostatectomy: the salient lateral and middle lobes are circumcised with the diathermy needle (a).

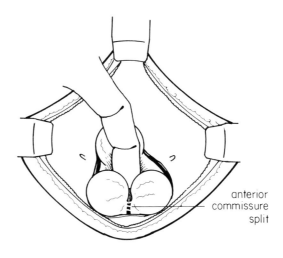

anterior commissure split

11.13. The index is thrust into the lumen via the internal meatus, and used to enucleate the lateral and middle lobes.

Transvesical prostatectomy

Historically the first type of prostatectomy (Blandy 1977) this method has a very limited place nowadays. It offers poor access to the prostate, and limited, rather blind control of bleeding. The access to the bladder obtained by adding a vertical limb to the Millin's capsular incision is better than through the conventional suprapubic cystostomy. Nevertheless the method ought, I suppose, to be mentioned somewhere.

Open the bladder through a Pfannenstiel incision. Incise the mucosa around the projecting prostatic lobes with the diathermy (11.12). Thrust the index finger into the internal meatus until it cracks open (11.13). It splits down the anterior commissure. Follow the crack into the plane between adenoma and capsule, first on one side and then on the other, wriggling the finger-tip now this way and now that until the lateral lobes can be plucked out. Pack the cavity with gauze for

four or five minutes, and suture-ligate the bleeding vessels in each corner as best you can (11.14).

Because haemostasis is so inexact, many surgeons put a purse-string suture around the neck of the bladder and a Foley balloon in the prostatic fossa. The purse-string is tied and the balloon inflated to effect a kind of primitive tamponade (Parton 1977).

Y-V plasty of the bladder neck

Y-V plasty has been replaced by TUR for the fibrous bladder neck contracture of adult males for which it was once used. If there is some other exceptional reason for open operation on the bladder or to attempt to reduce the size of the bladder, then partial cystectomy may be combined with a Y-V plasty.

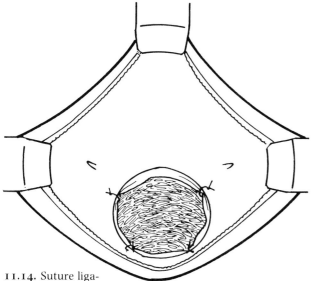

11.14. Suture ligatures are used to control haemorrhage at each of the four quadrants. A Foley balloon on traction may be left in afterwards to assist in haemostasis.

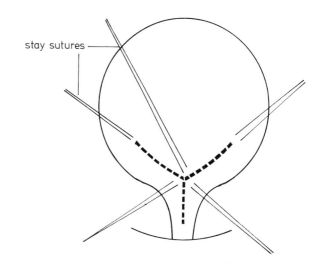

11.15. Stay sutures mark out the Y for the Y-V plasty of the bladder neck.

Preparations

The most important preparation is to ensure that the diagnosis is correct, and today one will demand clear urodynamic evidence of bladder neck obstruction before offering a Y-V plasty.

Anaesthesia

Controlled hypotension may be a special advantage in this procedure especially when the patient is obese.

Position

Supine.

Incision

Pfannenstiel.

Steps of the operation

The prevesical space is opened. The fat and peritoneum are swept upwards. Millin's self-retaining retractor is put in. Unless there is an indication for partial cystectomy, the bladder neck is opened between stay sutures in a long V (11.15). After opening the bladder, identify the ureters, and if necessary, mark them with catheters. Place a soft rubber catheter in the urethra, and incise the bladder neck in the midline to make a vertical limb to the Y (11.16). Stop this incision just proximal to the upper leaf of the levator ani, or when you have cut through a noticeable ridge of hypertrophied bladder neck (11.17). Leave enough of the distal urethra to allow a suture to be

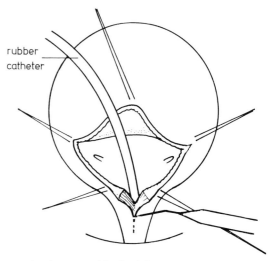

rubber catheter

11.16. The vertical limb of the Y is made by cutting down on to a rubber Jaques catheter in the internal meatus.

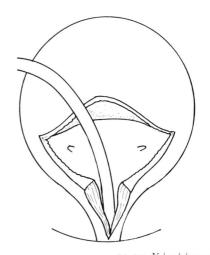

11.17. Y-incision completed.

placed. Five 3-0 sutures are placed and held in forceps (11.18), taking care to seize a good bite of urethra. After placing the stitches (11.19), remove the catheter and tie them. The wound is closed with drainage, and a small 14 Ch catheter is left indwelling for the first ten days.

Total prostatectomy

Indications

This is a subject of intense debate. Many urologists are still unconvinced that early radical prostatectomy for cancer offers the patient any better chance of survival than merely observing him and treating his symptoms as they occur. Others cite uncontrolled but persuasive statistics in favour of early and radical surgery (Chisholm 1985). I am frankly muddled and confused, and to date resist performing the operation for prostatic cancer.

Bitter experience has also taught me that the results of radical total prostatectomy for prostatitis are disappointing. In every one of the patients in whom I have performed this operation I have regretted it, and the patients have developed other, even more distressing symptoms.

Special preparations

One must have absolute histological evidence of the tumour from transurethral resection or a Trucut needle biopsy. The patient must be fully informed that the operation will make him impotent, and possibly may make him incontinent.

Position

Supine.

Incision

Pfannenstiel.

Steps of the operation

Leave a catheter in the bladder. Enter the prevesical space as in Millin's operation, and secure the great veins in front of the prostate and urethra by careful suture-ligature. Then incise the superior layer of the pelvic fascia for 2–3 cm on either side of the urethra. Dissect round the urethra to free it from its lateral and posterior attachments (11.20).

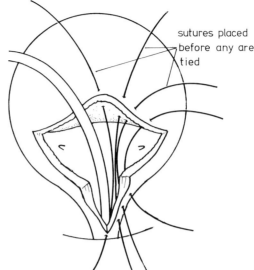

sutures placed before any are tied

11.18. The sutures are placed before they are tied.

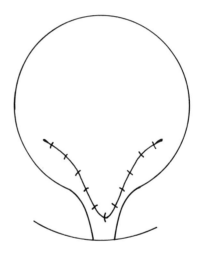

11.19. Completed Y-V plasty.

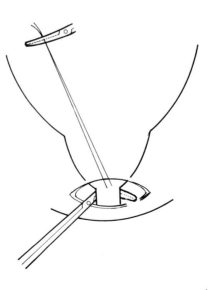

11.20. Total prostatectomy—after incising the pelvic fascia, mark the urethra with a stay suture and divide it just distal to the lower edge of the prostate.

11.21. Dissect behind the prostate as its lower cut edge is lifted upwards.

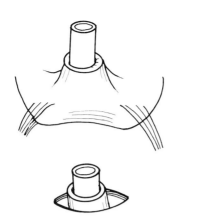

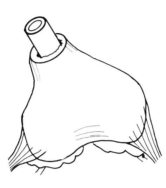

11.22. The prostate is retracted upwards to reveal the seminal vesicles and ampullae of the vasa.

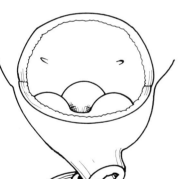

11.23. The bladder neck is cut across just above the prostate.

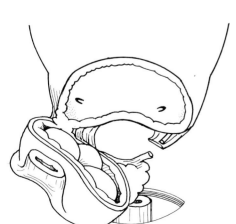

11.25. Division of the vas deferens on the left side.

Mark the urethra just distal to the prostate with a stay suture and the lower end of the prostate with another. Cut through the urethra between them, and lift up the distal cut edge of the prostate (11.21). Now keeping the scissors close to the prostate, dissect the plane between the layers of Denonvilliers' fascia, which may be opened to leave the posterior layer as a white sheet protecting the rectum. Continue to pull up the prostate and open up the plane until you feel and see the seminal vesicles marking the upper edge of the prostate (11.22).

Replacing the mobilized prostate, open the bladder along the border between bladder and prostate, catching each vessel with suture ligature (11.23). Insert a bladder neck spreader to open it out. Find and catheterize the ureteric orifices, and continue the incision around the bladder neck (11.24), little by little, taking each vessel with suture ligatures. A particularly large group of vessels will be found at each corner of the wound accompanying the ampulla of the vas (11.25). The prostate and vesicles are now removed.

A gap is now left which must be closed (11.26). Sometimes the bladder is easily

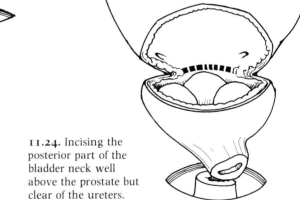

11.24. Incising the posterior part of the bladder neck well above the prostate but clear of the ureters.

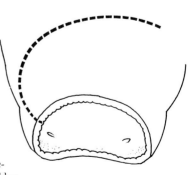

11.26. Prostate removed. If the bladder will not come down easily and without tension, the gap is bridged with a tubed flap (dotted line).

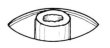

brought down to the urethra without any tension. In other instances it is fixed by fibrosis and cannot be brought down without strain. To bridge the gap, it is easy to make a ∩-shaped flap of detrusor, rather like a Boari flap (11.27), which is then closed over an indwelling catheter. The wound is closed with an indwelling catheter and a suprapubic drain (11.28).

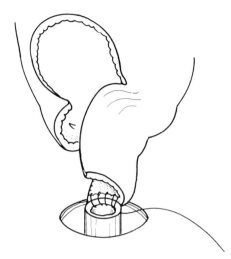

11.27. The bladder flap is swung down and sewn over a catheter to which it is closely tailored.

Hazards of the operation

Haemorrhage may be severe when the bladder neck is divided, and for this reason it is best to make the incision piecemeal and control the bleeding bit by bit as you go. If the prostate is very stuck and adherent, there is a risk of injuring the rectum. This is a good reason for keeping the scissors close to the prostate, and for attempting to enter the plane between the layers of Denonvilliers' fascia early in this part of the dissection.

References

Blandy J.P. (1976) Benign enlargement of the prostate gland. In *Urology* (ed. by Blandy J.P.), p. 859. Blackwell Scientific Publications, Oxford.

Blandy J.P. (1977) Surgery of the Benign Prostate. *J. Irish Med Ass.* **70**, 517.

Blandy J.P. (1978) *Transurethral Resection*, 2nd edn. Pitman Medical, London.

Chisholm G.D. (1985) *Carcinoma of the Prostate*. In *Textbook of Genitourinary Surgery* (ed. Whitfield H.N. & Hendry W.F.), p. 1001–1018. Churchill-Livingstone Edinburgh.

Hedlund P.O. (1976) Post-operative venous thrombosis in benign prostatic disease—a study of 316 patients using the I 125 fibrinogen uptake test. *Scand. J. Urol. Nephrol.* Supp **27**.

Mayo M.E., Halil T. & Browse N.L. (1971) The incidence of deep vein thrombosis after prostatectomy. *Brit. J. Urol.* **43**, 738.

Millin T. (1947) *Retropubic Urinary Surgery*. Livingstone, Edinburgh.

Parton L.I. (1977) Hryntschak prostatectomy: a review of 900 patients. *New Zealand Medical Journal*, **85**, 329.

Shuttleworth K.E.D. & Blandy J.P. (1976) Carinoma of the Prostate. In *Urology* (ed. by Blandy J.P.), p. 926. Blackwell Scientific Publications, Oxford.

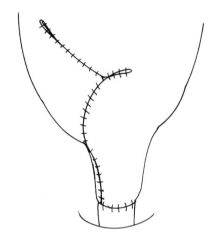

11.28. Completed tubed flap closes the gap without tension.

Chapter 12
Incontinence and fistulae in women

Stress incontinence

Indications

Advances in urodynamics and radiodiagnosis of recent years have made possible much more precise diagnoses of incontinence. No longer is it acceptable to rely on clinical tests or a patient's history. Urodynamic investigations will detect gross instability and bring to light neuropathic bladder lesions that escaped clinical observation. The investigation of these patients is beyond the scope of this book (McGuire *et al.* 1980; Abrams *et al.* 1983; Raz *et al.* 1979).

Marshall–Marchetti–Krantz operation

Precautions

After full radiological and urodynamic assessment, make sure of the sensitivity of the organisms in the urine, and have blood in reserve.

Position on the table

The patient is placed in the cystoscopy position with the legs supported on Lloyd-Davies stirrups allowing a second assistant to stand between the legs.

Incision

Pfannenstiel.

Steps of the operation

Pass a catheter. Dissect the prevesical space and clean the fat from the back of the symphysis and the front of the urethra and vagina (12.1). When this operation is done after previous suprapubic surgery, take great care in separating the peritoneum from the dome of the bladder, and the bladder from the symphysis pubis.

The sutures take hold of the vaginal wall on either side of the urethra. To help place them, a finger is placed in the vagina either side of the catheter by the second assistant, who stands between the patient's legs. Lifting his fingers tents up the paraurethral tissue of the vaginal wall in which the sutures are placed (12.2).

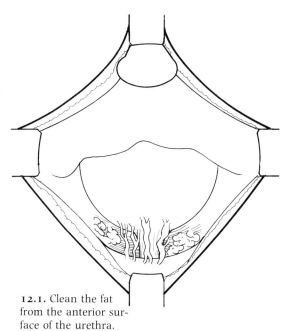

12.1. Clean the fat from the anterior surface of the urethra.

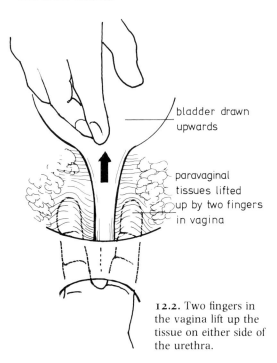

bladder drawn upwards

paravaginal tissues lifted up by two fingers in vagina

12.2. Two fingers in the vagina lift up the tissue on either side of the urethra.

Using o-chromic catgut on a curved atraumatic needle, place a row of sutures through the paravaginal tissue, and then through the periosteum and the extension of Gimbernat's ligament on the back of the symphysis. Have each suture held in forceps until three or four sutures have been placed on each side of the urethra (12.3).

Now ask the second assistant to lift the bladder up to take tension off the sutures, and tie them one after the other (12.4). Complete

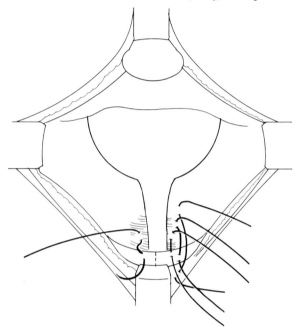

12.3. Place sutures between the vaginal wall on either side of the urethra and the periosteum behind the symphysis or Gimbernat's ligament.

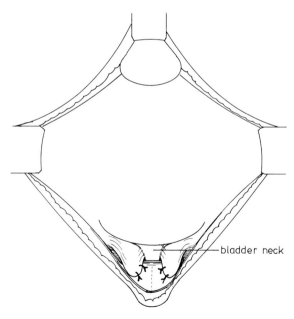

12.4. As the sutures are tied, the urethra and front of the bladder are brought up against the back of the symphysis.

the lifting up process by suturing the paravaginal tissues to the inferior fibres of the rectus sheath.

The wound is closed in layers with catgut. The catheter is left indwelling for ten days.

Hazards of the operation

Infection in a retropubic haematoma is a tiresome complication of this operation which should be prevented by meticulous haemostasis throughout. Difficulty in voiding is common for the first few weeks after an otherwise successful procedure, and should not give rise to alarm. Teach the patient to catheterize herself. Within two to three weeks all will be well.

Never promise complete success with any of these operations; always advise your patient to get thin and stay thin. Nothing makes for failure so much as adiposity.

Millin's sling operation

Indications

When the Marshall operation has failed, it may be done again with equally good success, but when it fails a second time, consider Millin's sling operation (Millin 1939).

Position and incision

These are the same as for the Marshall operation, and it is equally helpful to have a second assistant standing between the patient's legs.

Steps of the operation

Dissect the bladder and urethra away from the symphysis. This is often the most difficult part of the operation. The secret is to follow the back of the rectus abdominis right on to the bone of the symphysis, and then follow the periosteum of the symphysis using the diathermy needle to cut through the dense fibrous tissue so often present from previous surgery.

Once the urethra has been clearly defined, a right-angled forceps is passed around it to seize a tape (12.5). A ribbon of fascia about 2 cm wide is taken from the inferior edge of the aponeurosis of the rectus sheath (12.6). Leave one end attached, and sew the other to the tape. Use the tape to draw the ribbon underneath the urethra (12.7). Let the assistant lift the bladder with two fingers in

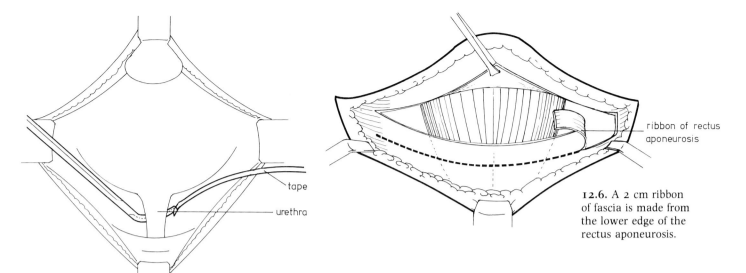

12.6. A 2 cm ribbon of fascia is made from the lower edge of the rectus aponeurosis.

ribbon of rectus aponeurosis

12.5. Sling operation: pass a right-angled forceps behind the urethra and seize a tape.

tape

urethra

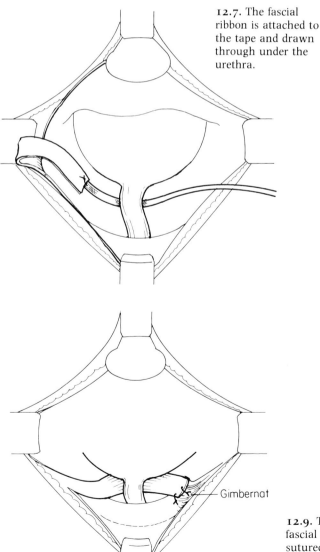

12.7. The fascial ribbon is attached to the tape and drawn through under the urethra.

12.9. The end of the fascial ribbon is sutured to Gimbernat's ligament.

Gimbernat

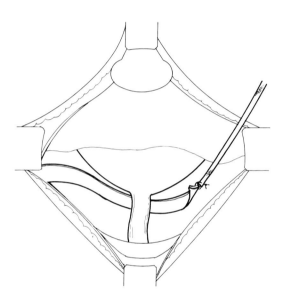

12.8. The ribbon should lie under the urethra and lower part of the trigone.

the vagina. Secure the free end of the fascial ribbon to Gimbernat's ligament or to the lower fibres of the rectus aponeurosis (12.8, 12.9). Non-absorbable sutures may be used for these last important stitches.

Hazards of the operation

In all these operations there is a risk of making a hole in the urethra, or between the urethra and the vagina, so when there is difficulty in getting around the urethra, it is better to make a deliberate incision in the anterior vaginal wall, identify the urethra, and guide the tape and the fascial ribbon beneath the urethra under direct vision.

Retention of urine is common after this operation as with the Marshall–Marchetti, and is dealt with by means of intermittent catheterization for a few weeks until the patient can void naturally without a residual urine.

Vesicovaginal fistula

Most vesicovaginal fistulae in this country follow hysterectomy, and result from injury to the trigone when there has been difficulty in dissecting the cervix from the back of the bladder (12.10).

In other countries a more difficult type of vesicovaginal fistula is seen, which follows neglected and obstructed labour. When the foetal head has been impacted in the pelvis for many hours, ischaemic necrosis destroys the trigone, the upper part of the urethra and the ends of the ureters (12.11). If the mother survives, she is left with a huge slough, always secondarily infected, which takes many weeks to heal. The end result is a kind of cloaca into which the bladder may bulge backwards, and into which both ureters may issue. Often the cervix is scarred and the products of menstruation retained in a haematocolpos. Traditional experience with this type of vesicovaginal fistula gave rise to the widespread notion that one must refrain from closing all vesicovaginal fistulae until forty days after the original injury. However true this may be of post-partum fistulae, it is certainly not true of the common fistulae seen after hysterectomy.

Special preparations

As soon as one suspects that fluid leaking per vaginam may be urine, it should be aspirated in a syringe and sent for blood urea estimation: if the fluid is urine, its urea concentration will be higher than that of the blood and the diagnosis is made.

The next investigation is an IVU. At this stage it is never certain whether the ureter is breached or whether there is a hole in the bladder (or both). If one or other ureter is obstructed, it usually signifies a ureterovaginal fistula.

The diagnosis is confirmed by cystoscopy and vaginal examination. Nowadays the fistula is always visible on cystoscopy, thanks to the brilliant light and irrigating systems of today, and there is no need for the traditional antics with methylene blue or milk. Even when a hole is seen, it is wise to exclude a coincidental ureteric lesion by making a bulb-ureterogram on the table at the same time.

Cystograms are a waste of time.

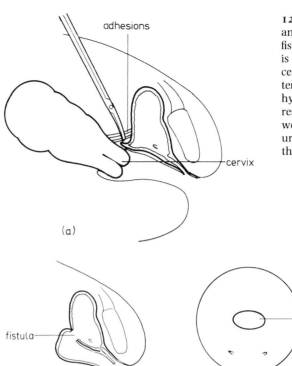

(a)

12.10. Formation of an 'easy' vesicovaginal fistula: (a) the bladder is tented up against the cervix and inadvertently cut during hysterectomy. The resulting fistula (b) is well away from the ureters and above (c) the trigone.

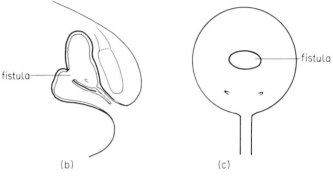

(b)   (c)

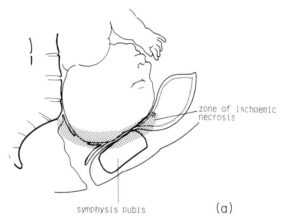

(a)

12.11. (a) Mechanisms of the formation of a large vesicovaginal fistula: prolonged pressure leads to ischaemic necrosis of the bladder, urethra, and cervix which slough away. (b) Post-partum vesico-vaginal fistula. There is a kind of cloaca into which enter the ureters, the scarred cervix, and the back of the bladder and trigone. The sphincter may be completely destroyed.

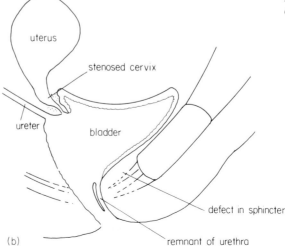

(b)

Position on the table

The cystoscopy position allows access to the vagina when an abdominal closure is performed; if the closure is to be attempted from below, then the patient is put into an exaggerated lithotomy position.

Closure of a small fistula per vaginam

Very small, easily accessible fistulae can be closed per vaginam. Place a suitable speculum in the vagina. A small balloon catheter is passed through the fistula, inflated, and pulled down (12.12). This brings the fistula into view. Its edge is circumcised (12.13) and the full thickness of vaginal wall mobilized all around, making sure that the plane between

vagina and bladder has been well opened up (12.14). Traction on the balloon makes this manoeuvre much easier. Now remove the balloon catheter and close the hole in the bladder with a series of 3-o chromic catgut sutures, all tied gently to avoid causing ischaemia to the tissues of the bladder. This suture line is closed in the sagittal plane (12.15). The defect in the vagina is closed with a second layer of interrupted 2-o chromic catgut sutures in the coronal plane so that the two suture lines cross, if at all, at

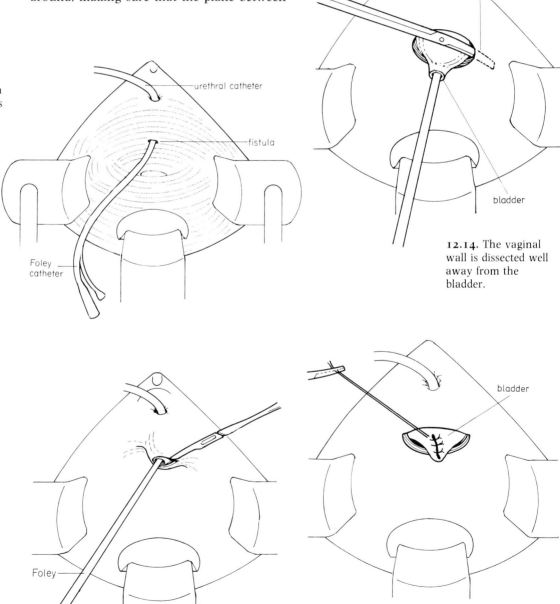

12.12. Closure of a small vesicovaginal fistula per vaginam: a small Foley catheter is put into the opening of the fistula to serve as a tractor.

urethral catheter

fistula

Foley catheter

vaginal wall

bladder

12.14. The vaginal wall is dissected well away from the bladder.

Foley

12.13. The margin of the fistula is excised.

bladder

12.15. The hole in the bladder is closed in the sagittal plane.

right angles (12.16). A small catheter, for
example 18 Ch, is left in the bladder on
continuous drainage.

Closure of large fistulae with omental plug

Incision

Unless the hysterectomy was a vaginal one,
reopen the incision used by the gynaecologist:
both the Pfannenstiel and the vertical incision
give adequate access for this operation.

Steps of the operation

Open the peritoneum and dissect away
adherent loops of small bowel, and the knots
of fallopian tube that are often left tethered to
the back of the bladder and vaginal stump.
Mobilize the sigmoid up and out of the pelvis.

Now open the bladder in the midline
between stay sutures (12.17) and as soon as

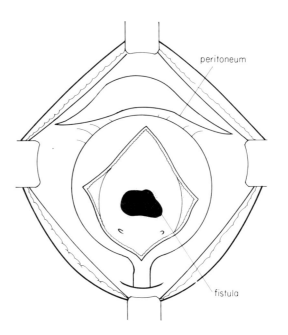

12.17. Closure of a larger vesicovaginal fistula—the bladder is opened and the ureters catheterized.

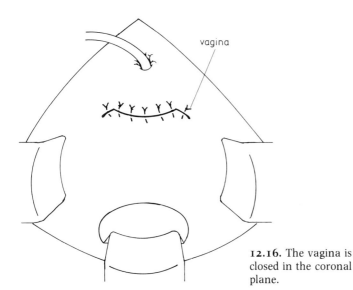

12.16. The vagina is closed in the coronal plane.

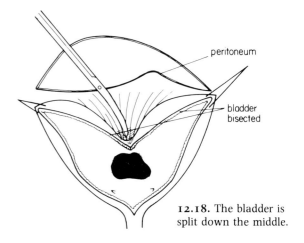

12.18. The bladder is split down the middle.

you can, pass a ureteric catheter up each
ureter and fix it to the skin.

Strip the peritoneum off the back of the
bladder, and split the bladder down in the
midline (12.18), carefully picking up all the
little arteries with 4-0 chromic catgut suture
ligatures to prevent continual and tiresome
bleeding. Continue in the midline until you
come to the fistula.

Place a stay suture near the edge of the
fistula on either side to lift it up. This makes it
easier to cut round the hole, using a long-
handled fine knife. Use dissecting scissors to
work between the trigone and the vagina
(12.19) until some 2–3 cm of healthy

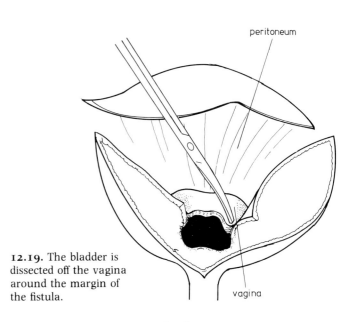

12.19. The bladder is dissected off the vagina around the margin of the fistula.

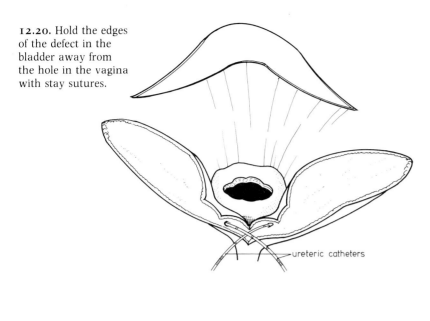

12.20. Hold the edges of the defect in the bladder away from the hole in the vagina with stay sutures.

ureteric catheters

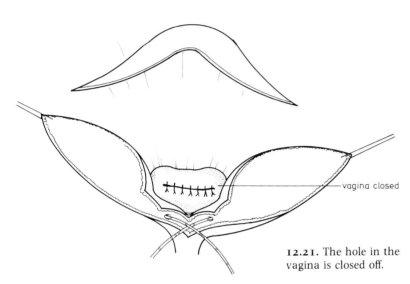

vagina closed

12.21. The hole in the vagina is closed off.

bladder has been lifted up from the vagina (12.20). During this dissection, it is comforting to be able to feel catheters in the ureters and to know that they are out of harm's way.

The hole in the vagina is closed with 2-0 chromic catgut, taking a generous bite of the vaginal wall and rolling the tissues at the upper end of the vagina forwards into the defect. These sutures are tied, but not so tightly as to cause ischaemic necrosis (12.21).

Before closing the bladder, the vagina is to be covered up with a plug of omentum (Walters 1937). Frequently it is easy to find a long loose lump of omentum hanging down from the transverse colon and simply lay it into the sutured vault of the vagina. In other cases it is more difficult, and one must detach the omentum from the transverse colon by dissecting along the bloodless line of embryological attachment between omentum and bowel, taking care not to injure the vessels of the mesocolon. Very occasionally it may even be necessary to detach the omentum from the greater curvature of the stomach by dividing the short gastric vessels (12.22).

With 3-0 chromic catgut sutures, stitch the omentum to the bottom of the gap between vagina and bladder, spreading it out so that

12.22 The great omentum is detached from the transverse colon and led through a hole in the mesocolon.

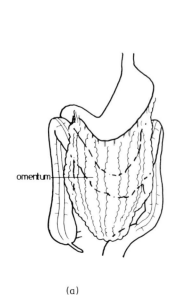

omentum

(a)

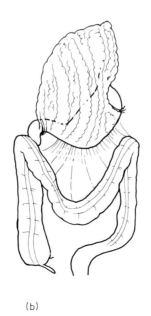

(b)

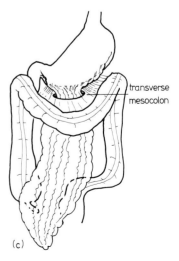

transverse mesocolon

(c)

the whole of the vault of the vagina is covered with the omentum (12.23).

Close the incision in the bladder with two layers of continuous or interrupted 3-0 chromic catgut (12.24). Usually the bladder comes together easily, but when the gap has been particularly big and it seems as if there may be some tension on the wall of the bladder, it is better to rotate one of the halves of the bladder (12.25) to fill the gap, even if this means mobilizing one-half of the bladder by dividing the superior vesical pedicle on that side.

It is my practice to attempt to keep the suture line dry for the first few days by catheterizing the ureters and for this purpose, a Gibbon catheter is placed in each ureter. The Gibbon catheter passes through the abdominal wall and up the opposite ureter, its plastic flanges being very apt for being sutured to the skin (12.26). The bladder is drained with a Foley catheter and the retropubic space with a tube drain.

Post-operative care

Catheter, splints, and drain are each connected to closed sterile collecting systems. Although some surgeons use suction on the urethral catheter to keep the system dry, it has not been necessary in my own series. The retropubic drain is removed after forty-eight hours; the ureteric catheters continue to drain urine for five or six days but then serve only as a splint and when they cease to drain should be removed. The urethral catheter remains for two weeks.

Difficult fistulae with trigonal injury

Here the anatomy varies so much that it is impossible to lay down rules for a condition which, in this country, is seen only in patients referred from overseas. Use a generous midline incision because it may be necessary to mobilize the omentum or form an ileocaecal segment.

Great care may be needed in order to clear the pelvis of adhesions. When the peritoneum is separated from the back of the bladder, it is opened between stay sutures.

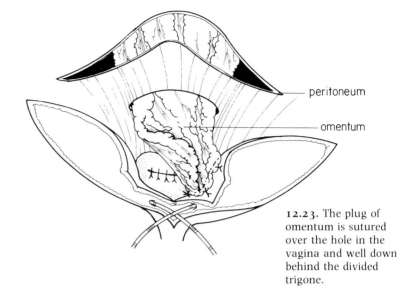

12.23. The plug of omentum is sutured over the hole in the vagina and well down behind the divided trigone.

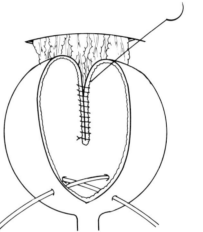

12.24. The divided bladder is closed up the middle.

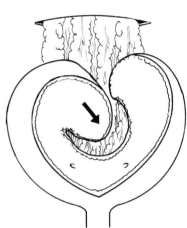

12.25. When the bladder defect is very large, rotate one half of the bladder wall round to fill the hole.

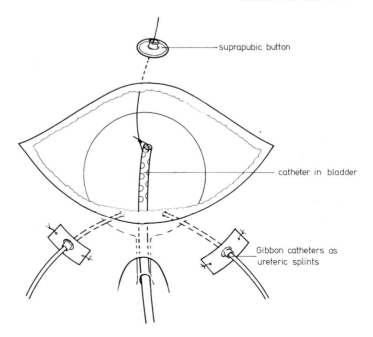

12.26. Gibbon catheters are left in as ureteric splints, and a suprapubic button and nylon stitch helps retain the catheter in the bladder.

12.27. Closure of a difficult urethro-trigono-vaginal fistula. Split the front of the bladder down the middle, having identified and taped the ureters.

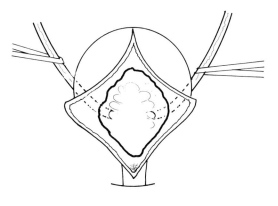

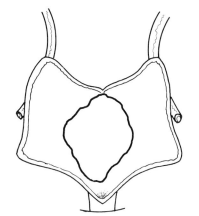

12.28. The bladder is divided down to the edge of the defect.

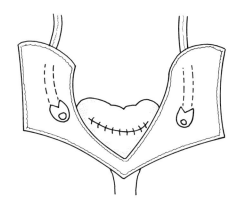

12.29. Each ureter is reimplanted into the half-bladder after closing the vaginal hole.

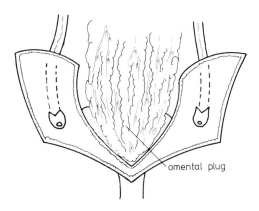

12.30. Omentum is packed down over the suture line in the vagina.

omental plug

12.31. The ureters are protected with Gibbon catheter splints; the bladder is closed over the omental plug.

In these giant fistulae preliminary cystoscopy is unhelpful because there is neither urethra nor trigone, and it is impossible to identify either of the ureters from below. The first step is to find the ureters in the pelvis, as they cross the bifurcation of the common iliac arteries. Each ureter is traced down to the scarred area, and identified with a silicone sling (12.27).

The next task is to find the urethra. If only a short length of urethra is left behind (12.28), an edge of the internal sphincter may still be discovered, with a little searching, and in such a case it may be possible to reconstruct the bladder around this margin. Here the operation is much as was outlined above, except that the remnant of the bladder is so small, oedematous and stiff. However, if the bladder can be reconstructed around a catheter—however small it seems—it will regenerate in an astonishing way and return to a normal volume within a few weeks.

One practical difficulty to be faced is that the ureters may no longer be opening onto the trigone. If they are still present, it may be possible to incorporate them into the re-fashioned bladder, closing the fistula with the assistance of a plug of omentum as described above.

More often the ureters have been destroyed in the sloughing process that led to the destruction of the trigone, and they now open into the common cloaca that is formed by the upper vagina and the remnant of the front wall of the bladder. When the cervix has also been injured and has stenosed, then hysterectomy is usually necessary.

Once or twice it has been possible to close the bladder and reimplant the ureters into its wall with a tunnel-and-cuff technique protected by a pair of splints (12.29–12.31) but

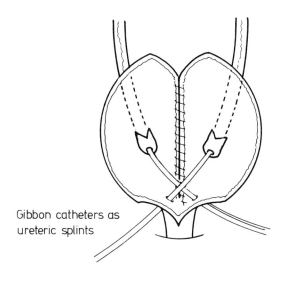

Gibbon catheters as ureteric splints

this demands a certain minimum amount of bladder. When even this minimum has been destroyed by ischaemia or fibrosis, then it may still be possible to restore continence and a semblance of normality by forming a new bladder out of the caecum (see page 125). Since it is impossible to foretell whether the patient will be continent or not, it is safer to put the ureters into the ileum, reserving the option of an ileal conduit if, after all this effort, the patient remains hopelessly wet and miserable.

In such a case it may be possible to make good use of the bits of bladder that are left, useless though they may be for forming a new one. Having closed off the hole in the vagina, and covered it with a lump of omentum, strip off the mucosa from the remnants of the halves of the bladder, and use these thick muscular leaves to cover over the defect in the vagina and to support the remnant of the internal sphincter. Finally, join the caecum to the stump of the urethra (12.32–12.34).

Use of the gracilis muscle graft

Indications

Some surgeons with the most experience of post-partum vesicovaginal fistulae (Hamlin & Nicholson 1969) would use the gracilis muscle where I, with less experience, prefer to attempt to close the hole with omentum. Nevertheless the gracilis muscle is so easy to use, so easy to fix into a fistula, and so successful for cases where other methods have failed, that perhaps it should be used as the technique of first choice. I have found it of particular benefit in recurrent vesicovaginal fistulae that have followed radiotherapy, where other techniques, such as the use of the omental plug, have failed, no doubt because there has been so much radiation damage to the tissues with which one was trying to deal in the first place.

Position on the table

The cystoscopy position is ideal. The thigh should be prepared down to the knee and suitably towelled off (12.35).

Steps of the operation

First the vagina is approached, after making an episiotomy incision if its entrance is tight. A suitable self-retaining catheter is inserted

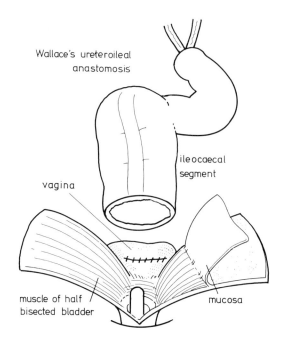

12.32. Ileocaeco-cystoplasty reconstruction of gross urethrotrigonal fistulae: the ileocaecal segment is mobilized after splitting the bladder and closing off the vaginal hole. The mucosa is stripped off each half of the bladder. Ureters are anastomosed to the tail of ileum.

Wallace's ureteroileal anastomosis

ileocaecal segment

vagina

muscle of half bisected bladder

mucosa

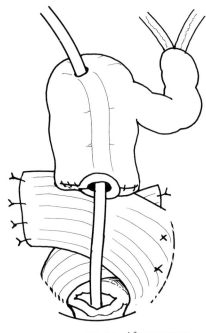

12.33. After narrowing the caecal lumen, it is anastomosed to the urethra in front of the omentum and the crossed bladder muscle flaps.

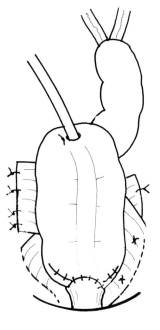

12.34. Completed reconstruction: the uretero-ileal anastomosis is protected with indwelling splints and a catheter left in the caecum via the appendix stump.

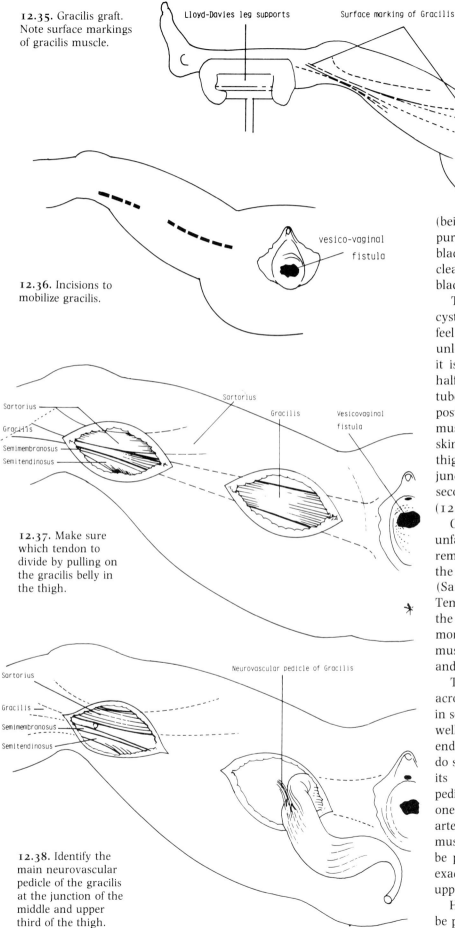

12.35. Gracilis graft. Note surface markings of gracilis muscle.

Lloyd-Davies leg supports

Surface marking of Gracilis

12.36. Incisions to mobilize gracilis.

vesico-vaginal fistula

Sartorius
Gracilis
Semimembranosus
Semitendinosus

Sartorius

Gracilis

Vesicovaginal fistula

12.37. Make sure which tendon to divide by pulling on the gracilis belly in the thigh.

Neurovascular pedicle of Gracilis

Sartorius
Gracilis
Semimembranosus
Semitendinosus

12.38. Identify the main neurovascular pedicle of the gracilis at the junction of the middle and upper third of the thigh.

(being a urologist, I use Millin's for this purpose). The fistula is dissected out, the bladder closed, and a generous plane of cleavage developed around the hole between bladder and vaginal wall.

Then the gracilis muscle is prepared. In the cystoscopy position it is usually very easy to feel the gracilis muscle belly in the thigh, unless the patient is particularly obese, when it is found by incising along a line starting half-way between pubic tubercle and ischial tuberosity and extending down to the medial posterior tendons near the knee joint. The muscle belly is often distinctly seen under the skin. After identifying the gracilis in the thigh through a short incision over the junctions of the middle and upper third, a second short incision is made near the knee (12.36).

Obviously, to the urological surgeon, this is unfamiliar territory. He may desperately try to remember the mnemonic he was taught for the primary FRCS, 'Say Grace before MeaT' (Sartorius–Gracilis–semiMembranosus–semi Tendinosus), to remind himself of the order of the rows of tendons in this situation. But a more sure way to get it right is to pull on the muscle belly of the gracilis in the midthigh, and see which tendon moves (12.37).

There is no point in cutting the tendon across too near down, for tendon is no good in sealing off a fistula—what is needed is good well-vascularized muscle. Divide the lower end of gracilis where it seems convenient to do so. Pull up the upper end, and free it from its adjacent structures: there are three pedicles, two very fine and unimportant ones, and one large one, containing nerve artery and vein, on which the viability of the muscle depends. This big upper pedicle must be preserved at all costs. It is found almost exactly at the junction of the middle and upper third of the gracilis (12.38).

Having mobilized the muscle, it now has to be provided with a tunnel, under the fat and the stiff fascial line that marks the fold of the groin, up and into the vagina. This tunnel is made with scissors, assisted with a finger, and emerges into the raw area at the apex of the vagina where the bladder has been sutured and there is a defect to be covered up (12.39). Pass a forceps along this tunnel, grasp the tendon of gracilis and so draw the gracilis up along the tunnel. It is always most gratifying and surprising to see how easily it lies in its new position. A generous amount of good, well-vascularized tissue is now available with which to cover up the suture line in the bladder (12.40). In these patients it is seldom possible to find enough vaginal wall to close over the muscle belly, but as long as it is attached firmly to the tissues around the vault of the vagina, covering up the fistula, the naked muscle will soon become epithelized. The bladder should be drained with a catheter for two weeks (12.41).

Hazards of these operations

The chief danger of any of these operations to close vesico-vaginal fistulae is ischaemia and tension on the suture lines. For this reason adequate mobilization of the bladder and vagina must be carried out before trying to close even the most easy and supple of them. The effects of radiotherapy are usually more widespread than the appearance of the tissues might lead one to suspect, and the surrounding soft tissues are on the brink of ischaemic necrosis, so that whenever possible, additional blood supply should be brought to the site—hence the advantage of the gracilis or the omentum. The siting, choice of calibre, and material from which catheters and drains are made, are of crucial importance to success and need great care: vesicovaginal fistulae have already caused so much misery to the patient that everything must be done to make certain that the first operation to cure it is the last.

Urethral diverticula in females

Indications

Urethral diverticula may be complicated by infection, stones, and carcinoma. In the first two of these, all that is required is excision of the diverticulum.

Position on the table

Lithotomy.

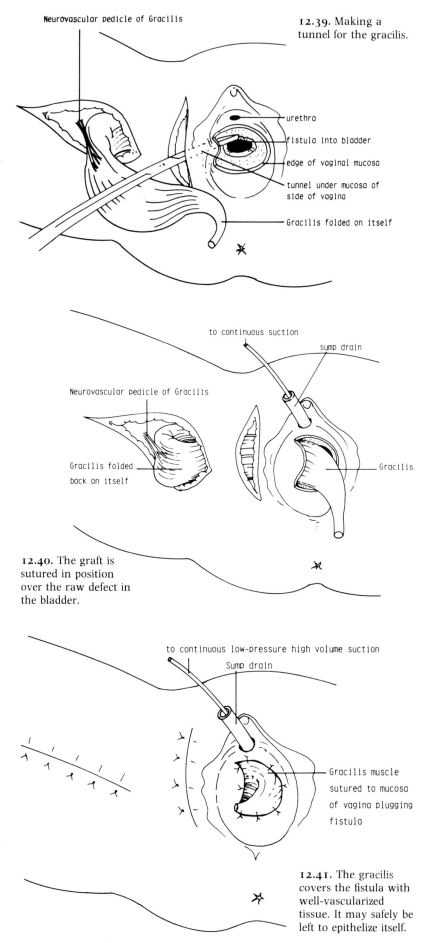

12.39. Making a tunnel for the gracilis.

Neurovascular pedicle of Gracilis

urethra
fistula into bladder
edge of vaginal mucosa
tunnel under mucosa of side of vagina
Gracilis folded on itself

to continuous suction
sump drain

Neurovascular pedicle of Gracilis

Gracilis folded back on itself

Gracilis

12.40. The graft is sutured in position over the raw defect in the bladder.

to continuous low-pressure high volume suction
Sump drain

Gracilis muscle sutured to mucosa of vagina plugging fistula

12.41. The gracilis covers the fistula with well-vascularized tissue. It may safely be left to epithelize itself.

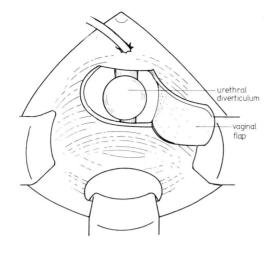

12.42. Approach to a urethral diverticulum through a laterally based vaginal flap.

urethral diverticulum

vaginal flap

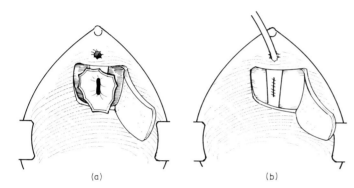

(a)　　　　　(b)

12.43. (a) The diverticulum is trimmed away and (b) closed off, and (c) the laterally based flap sutured back in position.

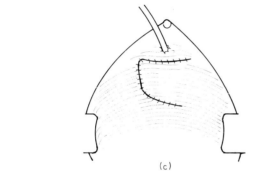

(c)

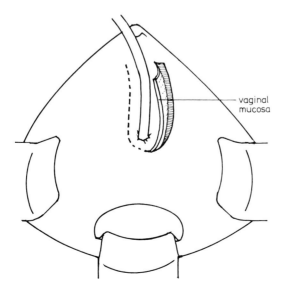

vaginal mucosa

12.44. Urethroplasty in the female: using a 22 Ch catheter as a mould, raise a tube of vaginal mucosa which is wider on one side than the other.

Steps of the operation

A catheter is passed and left in the bladder. A suitable self-retaining retractor is placed in the vagina (Millin's is very suitable). Cut a C-shaped flap with its base to one side. When this trapdoor is lifted, the diverticulum is exposed (12.42). The flap is retracted to one side, and the diverticulum dissected down to its opening into the urethra. In some diverticula the wall is made up of spongy tissue like the female urethra, suggesting a congenital origin. In others it is formed of scar tissue, suggesting an origin in an abscess in a paraurethral gland. Open the diverticulum and remove the surplus wall, but allow a little margin for sutures when closing it over the catheter. The urethra is closed and the vaginal flap sutured back into place with 3-0 chromic catgut (12.43). To avoid a haematoma in the vaginal wall, use a tampon made of sterilized Reston foam, doubled on itself and trimmed to size, which may be removed after forty-eight hours (Woodhouse *et al.* 1980).

Reconstruction of the female urethra

The distal few centimetres of the urethra may have been destroyed by injury, especially the disrupting fracture of the pelvis that results in a sagittal tear in the anterior wall of the vagina. It may also be needed when the urethra has had to be taken away because of carcinoma. There are two problems to be solved: first, the formation of a new tube; and second, the restoration of urinary continence.

Simple urethroplasty

Often it is enough to make a new urethra by rolling up a tube as in the second stage of a male urethroplasty. On two occasions I have found that this simple manoeuvre was enough not only to produce a satisfactory new urethral tube, but also resulted in a return of continence. When there is too little spare lining in the adjacent vagina to provide an adequate width of tissue for a new urethra, it may be necessary to borrow skin from the labia.

Steps of the operation

With a suitable speculum in the vagina and a catheter in the proximal stump of the urethra or the neck of the bladder, a skin strip is raised first on one side of the catheter (12.44) and then on the other so as to embrace a 22 Ch catheter comfortably. The vaginal wall is then thoroughly mobilized on each side of the urethra until it can be easily brought together without tension. The 22 Ch catheter is now taken out and replaced with a narrow 10 Ch catheter and the skin tube is closed with 3-0 chromic catgut (12.45). The vaginal tissue is brought together over the new urethra with interrupted everting mattress sutures that bring together all the subjacent tissue as well. The two suture lines do not overlap if the first incision is made eccentrically (12.46).

Use of a labial patch

First measure the length of urethra which has to be replaced and mark out on one or other of the labia minora the size of the skin patch that is needed, using a 22 Ch sound as a guide (12.47). Raise an isolated skin island and provide it with a thick pedicle of labial fat and the subcutaneous muscle that is similar to the dartos in the male (12.48). Burrow between the labium and the urethra

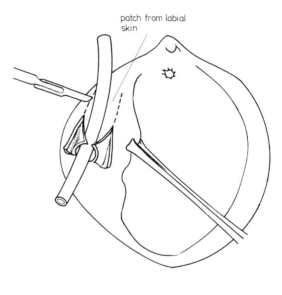

12.47. Labial patch: mark out width and length of the patch you will need, using a 22 Ch catheter as a guide.

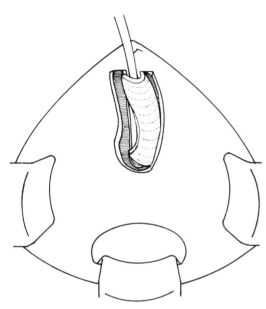

12.45. Sew the tube to make a complete urethra. Mobilize the vaginal wall thoroughly on either side.

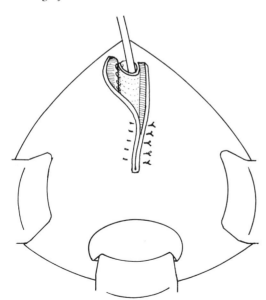

12.46. The closure of the vaginal wall leaves a suture line which is not directly over the suture line of the new urethra.

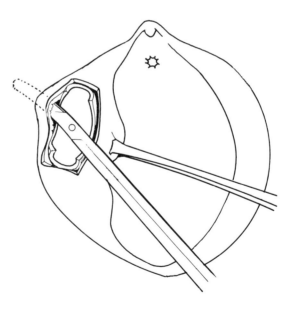

12.48. The patch is dissected from the labium in the plane between dartos and skin so that the patch is provided with a laterally based pedicle.

12.49. A tunnel is made from the labium under the vaginal wall towards the defect in the urethra which is to be repaired.

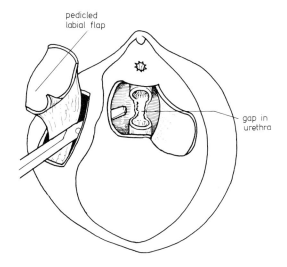

12.50. The patch is sutured over the gap in the urethra.

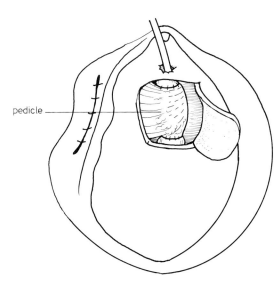

with scissors to make a tunnel (12.49) and draw the skin flap on its pedicle through the tunnel so that it occupies the defect in the urethra (12.50). If the defect is in the middle of the urethra, a laterally based trapdoor flap in the vaginal wall gives good access.

In some patients this reconstruction of the urethra is enough to restore continence. In others it is not enough, and one may have to perform a Young–Dees type of narrowing at the neck of the bladder.

References

Abrams P., Feneley R. & Torrens M. (1983) *Urodynamics*. Springer, Berlin.

Hamlin R.H.J. & Nicholson E.C. (1969) Reconstruction of urethra totally destroyed in labour. *Brit. Med. J.* **2**, 147.

Marshall V.F., Marchetti A.A. & Krantz K.E. (1949) The correction of stress incontinence by simple vesico-urethral suspension. *Surg. Gynec. Obstet.* **88**, 509.

McGuire E.J., Lytton B., Kohorn E.I. & Pepe V. (1980) The value of urodynamic testing in stress urinary incontinence. *J. Urol.* **124**, 256.

Millin T. (1939) Some observations on the surgical treatment of urinary incontinence. *Proc. Royal Soc. Med.* **32**, 777.

Raz S., Maggio A.J. & Kaufman J.J. (1979) Why Marshall–Marchetti operation works, or does not. *Urology*, **14**, 154.

Walters W. (1937) Omental flap in the transperitoneal repair of recurring vesicovaginal fistulas. *Surg. Gynec. Obstet.* **64**, 74.

Woodhouse C.R.J., Flynn J.T. & Blandy J.P. (1980) Urethral diverticulum in females. *Brit. J. Urol.* **52**, 305.

Chapter 13
Penis and scrotum

The surgery of the penis and scrotum ante-dates recorded history, for the earliest cave paintings record this and other ritual mutilations. In the Australian aboriginal practices of Arintha and Tokalosi, following circumcision at initiation to the totem, subincision of the urethra, again and again, marks a man's advancement in the hierarchy of his tribe. Not all mutilations were ritual: amputation was practised on prisoners of war, particularly captives destined to guard the harem. Even in England the ancient penalty for treason included excision of the 'privy parts' as part of the package of hanging, drawing, and quartering. Surgeons came late upon the scene (Remondino 1891; Ghalioungui 1963; Blandy 1977).

Circumcision

Indications

The normal prepuce may be fully retracted to allow the glans penis to be washed by the age of two or three years. If it cannot be retracted by the third year, then circumcision is advisable (Gairdner 1949). Where soap and water are scarce, circumcision may be a useful prophylactic measure against penile cancer. In this country there is no surgical indication for it before the age of two or three, when the need is limited to 1 or 2% of children, and the hazards of the operation are far less than they are when it is done in infancy (King 1982). Circumcision should be neat and careful, for it is no less important to the patient than plastic surgery to his nose. It is not to be delegated to the least experienced and most clumsy member of the surgical team.

Ritual circumcision of the newborn, though still widely practised, is not a surgical procedure: it is of great interest to the anthropologist as a persistent echo of a stone-age practice. True meatal stenosis, calling for meatotomy, is exceedingly rare. The normal infant prepuce does not slide back and should not be meddled with (Johnston 1976).

Preparations

Older children and adults requiring circumcision are admitted on the day of operation with the precautions normal for a general anaesthetic.

Anaesthesia

Too light an anaesthetic may occasion an erection which may be tiresome and call for extra care in securing haemostasis. As so often with so-called 'minor surgery' it calls for the most experienced anaesthetist, not the beginner.

Steps of the operation

With the penis in its normal relaxed position, feel for the bulge formed by the corona of the glans and make a clean incision along the convexity of this bulge just through the skin (13.1). A knife makes a cleaner incision and leaves a neater scar than do scissors. Incise the prepuce in the dorsal midline, taking care not to injure the glans, which should be pro-

13.1. Circumcision: an incision is made along the bulge of the corona glandis through the skin only. The prepuce is split in the midline and retracted, and a second incision made through the reflected 'mucosa'. The separated foreskin is detached and the clean-cut edges sutured with interrupted 5-0 catgut sutures.

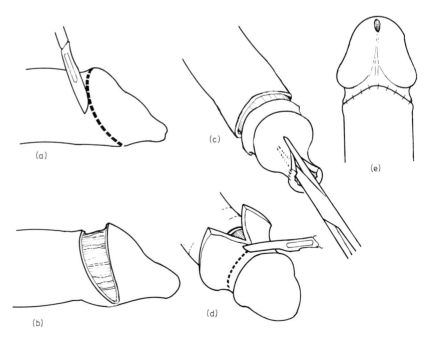

tected with a probe or forceps. The prepuce can then be pulled right back to expose the sulcus behind the corona glandis. This sulcus must be carefully cleaned of adherent smegma, and all the adhesions between prepuce and glands must be fully released.

Again using knife rather than scissors, cut cleanly round the edge of the sulcus 3 mm proximal to the glans. The foreskin is now removed by dividing the subcutaneous tissue, taking care to pick up and tie every small vessel that is cut across, using 4-0 catgut.

Diathermy is dangerous in circumcision but only because it is so often used without common sense precautions (Mitchell & Dobbie 1976). If the penis is surrounded with a saline-soaked swab to ensure good conduction of current, diathermy can be used safely. Never lift up a small penis away from the body when using diathermy, for this means that the current must return through the shaft of the penis and may lead to coagulation of its main arteries and be followed by the gangrene so feared by our medical protection societies.

Suture the skin with 4-0 or 5-0 catgut using neat, closely spaced sutures. A dressing is unnecessary. The suture line is smeared with sterile vaseline and covered with gauze until the child returns to the ward. Afterwards it may be washed and dried gently in the usual way.

In adults the cleft between the skin of the glans and the prepuce may be obliterated and it may be necessary to carve the glans penis from its thick adherent prepuce, leaving the glans quite raw at the end of this procedure. If this is left to granulate on its own, it will return to an appearance far more normal than after any attempt to resurface it with split skin. This re-epithelization may take two to three weeks.

Paraphimosis

Indications

When confronted by an adult with para-phimosis, attempt to reduce it as soon as possible. While preparations are being made to get the patient to the operating room, ice-cold saline may be applied to the penis in a pack.

Anaesthesia

When the paraphimosis has been established for several days a general anaesthetic is needed.

Technique

Whitaker's method is the best: grasp the tip of the glans and pull the penis out as far as possible, squeezing the glans firmly to reduce oedema (13.2). Then slide the roll of prepuce

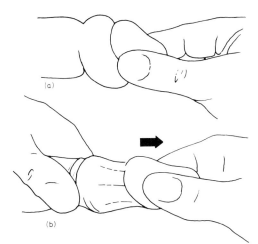

13.2. Paraphimosis: to reduce the swelling, pull the glans firmly forwards and then slide the ring of the paraphimosis forwards over it.

forwards over the glans. Exceptionally, it may be necessary to incise the tight white band proximal to the oedematous roll.

Priapism

Priapism is a surgical emergency. Irrigation of the distended spongy tissue with heparinized saline, nerve blocks, hypotensive drugs, and similar manoeuvres are in general useless, although the recent suggestion of using 1:200,000 adrenaline (Brindley 1984) is worth trying. To prevent the delicate structure of the corpora cavernosa from being ruined by a deposit of fibrin, decompression is needed at once (Forsberg et al. 1981).

Winter's procedure

The most simple procedure is to make a hole between the fascia that separates the distended corpora cavernosa and the flaccid corpus spongiosum and bulb, for in a priapism the glans and spongiosum are never distended.

This may be easily performed using a sharp pointed knife, inserted through the flaccid glans, just deeply enough to cut through the projecting dome of the part of the corpus cavernosum that protrudes into the glans penis (13.3). An alternative is to use the Trucut biopsy needle to remove a few cores of tissue, including the fascial septum separating the distended from the flaccid tissue (13.4). Either of these methods may be effective: they only take a second or two, and should always be tried first. Unfortunately they are not always successful.

Corpus–corpus anastomosis

The next progressively invasive procedure is to cut a window out of the septum between distended and flaccid tissues, and anastomose them together. The anastomosis may be made anywhere along the shaft of the penis: I prefer to incise near the bulb.

Position

The patient is put in the cystoscopy position.

Anaesthesia

The patient is anaesthetized, but not necessarily fully relaxed.

Incision

A short midline incision near the base of the penile urethra is held open with a self-retaining retractor (13.5). The plane between corpus spongiosum and corpus cavernosum on one side is easily dissected with the aid of a bougie in the urethra. Cut an elliptical window 1.5 cm in length from the side of the corpus spongiosum adjacent to the corpus cavernosum, and cut an identical window in the latter opposite the first. Using heparinized saline, irrigate the stiff 'redcurrant jelly' material from the corpora cavernosa until the blood flows freely. Anastomose the two windows together using 5-0 arterial suture material (13.6).

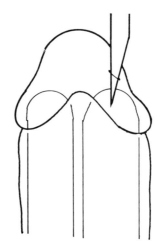

13.3. The corpora cavernosa protrude well up into the flaccid glans penis. A fine knife may be used to create an opening between the two systems.

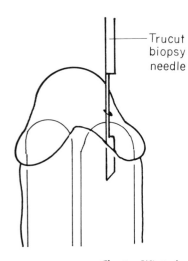

13.4. Chester Winter's procedure: a Trucut biopsy needle is used to take out a core from the septum between the corpus cavernosum and the glans.

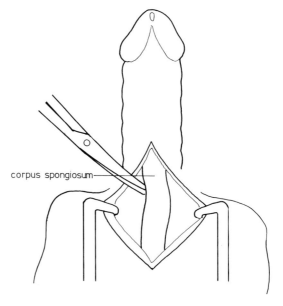

corpus spongiosum

13.5. Priapism: corpus–corpus anastomosis: through a midline incision over the penoscrotal junction dissect into the plane between corpus spongiosum and corpus cavernosum on one side.

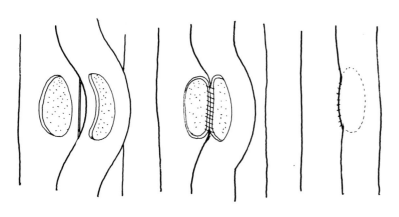

13.6. Cut out elliptical windows in the firm fascia covering the adjacent corpora and anastomose them together with fine vascular suture material.

13.7. Sapheno-corporal anastomosis: the long saphenous vein is exposed in the thigh and its tributaries divided between ligatures.

long saphenous vein

13.8. The distal end of the saphenous vein is brought through a subcutaneous tunnel to a window cut in the side of one of the corpora cavernosa.

saphenous vein

13.9. Degloving injury of the penis: as an emergency measure the shaft of the penis may be buried under the scrotal skin.

avulsed skin

scrotal tunnel

(a)

(b)

Sapheno-corporal anastomosis

When the corpus–corpus anastomosis does not control the priapism (and it is by no means always successful), the third step is to anastomose the saphenous vein to the corpus cavernosum on one side or the other.

Steps of the operation

Make an incision along the long saphenous vein in the thigh (13.7) for about 10 cm, securing and ligating all its tributaries with fine catgut. Irrigate the vein firmly with heparinized saline and make sure that shreds of adventitia do not indent its wall. Make a tunnel under the fat from groin to penis on that side. Make a second incision over the root of the penis. The free end of the saphenous vein is now anastomosed to an elliptical window in the corpus cavernosum (13.8).

Hazards of these operations

The results of these operations are good if done within forty-eight hours of the onset of priapism, but there is no guarantee that any or either of these procedures will (a) prevent the priapism returning within a period of twelve hours or (b) assure restoration of potency. Since the outcome is so uncertain, make sure that the patient clearly understands that one cannot be certain of the result, for be sure of one thing—the patient who becomes impotent after all your efforts will assuredly blame you, never himself for leaving things too late. These patients are notoriously ungrateful, resentful, and litigious (Hinman 1960).

Penile degloving injuries

Partial or complete avulsion of the skin of the penis is seen in a variety of domestic or industrial accidents. It is seen from time to time as a result of inept ritual operations. Always attempt to conserve as much skin as possible, for even when it has been avulsed completely, it will serve as a useful skin graft if carefully cleansed and laid bare of all the subcutaneous fat.

Alternatively, when most of the penile skin has been avulsed, the shaft of the penis is buried under the scrotum as a first-aid manoeuvre (13.9). The surplus scrotal skin is used to clothe the penis at a second-stage operation (13.10).

Closed fracture of the penis

The corpora cavernosa have been fractured from time to time, usually by a woman scorned, who in her fury breaks the erect penis, splitting the corpus cavernosum and rupturing Buck's fascia. The history is typical and the swelling characteristic. Although cases have been reported of spontaneous recovery with return to normal function by simply waiting for the haematoma to resolve, the more usual procedure (13.11) is to sleeve back the penis to expose the tear, repair it, and restore the skin to its former position (Laubscher 1972).

Accidental amputation of the penis

Little boys suffer this injury at the hands of a particularly inept circumcision attempt. Here the amputated distal glans should be saved, kept in ice, and sutured back into position. I have seen one such successful case.

In adults the injury is occasionally seen in severely deranged schizophrenics. If the amputated member can be saved, it should be cooled. Using microvascular techniques, reanastomose as many of the penile arteries and nerves as can be found (13.12). The cavernous system is relied upon for venous return. Cases are on record where not only has the penis survived, but erection has returned.

Impotence

Amost every year sees a new prosthesis for splinting the flaccid penis (Finney 1982). Before accepting a patient for this type of surgery a most careful preliminary investigation must be carried out (Montague 1982; Marshall et al. 1982). One must have objective evidence that there are no true erections taking place during deep REM sleep. Any operation to insert an artificial prosthesis must necessarily destroy the delicate structure of the erectile system.

Recent advances in microvascular surgery give promise of a more rational approach to well-selected cases, using the inferior epigastric artery to restore blood flow to the penis (McDougal & Jeffery 1983).

13.10. Degloving injury: at a second stage, skin from the scrotum is borrowed to furnish a complete covering for the penis.

13.11. Fracture of the penis: (a) the history and the swelling make the diagnosis; (b) the penile skin is pulled back after making a circumferential incision to expose the tear in the corpora; (c) the corpus cavernosum is repaired; and (d) the skin sleeve is restored.

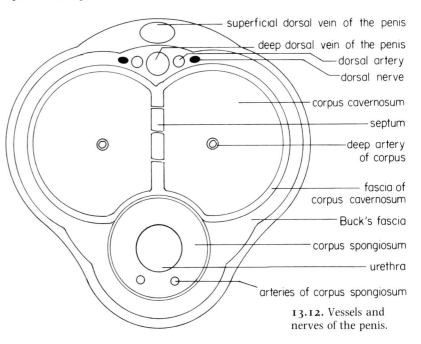

13.12. Vessels and nerves of the penis.

Anaesthesia

General.

Position on the table

Cystoscopy.

Steps of the operation

Through a short, vertical, midline, perineal incision each corpus cavernosum is exposed first on one side and then on the other. A short incision is made into Buck's fascia to enter the spongy tissue of the corpus. Hegar's dilators of increasing size are used to make a tunnel inside the corpus cavernosum from the bulb of the glans. Measure off the Hegar's dilator the length of prosthesis that is needed, and also the calibre. There are many different types of prosthesis available, and surgeons doing many of these operations will have a complete set from which to choose (Bennett 1982). The most simple is the semi-rigid Small–Carrion prosthesis (13.13). The Jonas flexible model contains a bendable silver wire which allows the stiffened penis to be placed in a dependent or an erect position at will. The long-term aftermath of these prostheses has perhaps yet to be fully evaluated, but it seems that if patients are carefully selected, and well motivated, this type of implant can be most successful.

I have no experience of the more sophisticated inflatable-deflatable Brantley–Scott device for which it is necessary to prepare oneself by proper training, if good results are to be obtained (Bennett 1982).

Peyronie's disease

Be cautious to avoid operating on men with Peyronie's disease unless you are absolutely forced to: they will blame you for impotence afterwards, and the end-result is nearly always less satisfactory than the patient hopes for.

Today the excision of the plaque and its replacement by a graft of skin has been replaced by more simple operations that take a reef on the longer side to correct the deformity of the penis. These procedures do not correct the defective filling of the corpus cavernosum distal to the plaque, however, and it is important to warn the patient that all the operation can do is to straighten out the penis.

Anaesthesia

General

Position on the table

Cystoscopy.

Steps of the operation

Jonas' modification of Nesbit's reefing operation is simple to do and avoids the need to cut out any of Buck's fascia (Jonas 1983). The penile skin is sleeved down after making

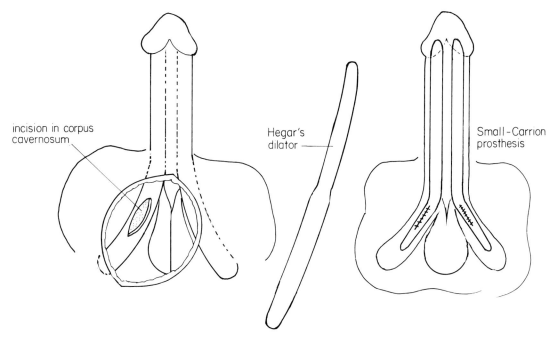

13.13. Insertion of the Small–Carrion prosthesis for impotence: (a) one corpus cavernosum is approached through a midline scrotal incision, opened and (b) a track made with Hegar's dilators through which the prosthesis may be inserted; (c) the corpus is closed.

incision in corpus cavernosum

Hegar's dilator

Small-Carrion prosthesis

a circumferential incision behind the glans (13.14). With a tourniquet around the base of the penis, saline is injected into the corpus on one side to produce an erection. This makes it possible to mark out the site, on the convexity of the penis, that must be reefed (13.15). If the angulation is upwards, then it is necessary to dissect the corpus spongiosum away from the corpora cavernosa, and insert the reefing sutures on the underside of the cavernosa (13.16).

A series of 3-0 prolene sutures are placed to gather the fascia together over an ellipse judged to correct the deformity. The placing and the number of these sutures must be assessed from time to time by reapplying the tourniquet and inducing an artificial erection again. Additional sutures are added or taken away until the penis stands up straight. Then the skin is sleeved back and sutured to its original position.

Partial amputation of the penis

Indications

For Stage 1 and 2 cancer of the penis, where radiotherapy has been tried without success (Salverria *et al.* 1979; El-Demiry *et al.* 1984), then partial amputation is indicated. It also gives good results in early carcinoma of the penis and is a satisfactory alternative when facilities for radiation therapy are not available.

Special preparations

No special preparations are needed unless the penis is grossly infected, when circumcision should be performed and the glans cleaned up with local antiseptic irrigation and systemic chemotherapy.

Position on the table

Supine.

Steps of the operation

Place a Doyen's non-crushing clamp well proximal to the site of incision to keep the field bloodless. The amputation should be 3 cm proximal to the palpable edge of the tumour.

Make the ventral skin flap longer than the dorsal one so that the incision around the penis is elliptical. Retract the sleeve of skin. Divide the corpus spongiosum 1 cm distal to the division of the two corpora cavernosa (13.17). Close the thick cylinders of Buck's

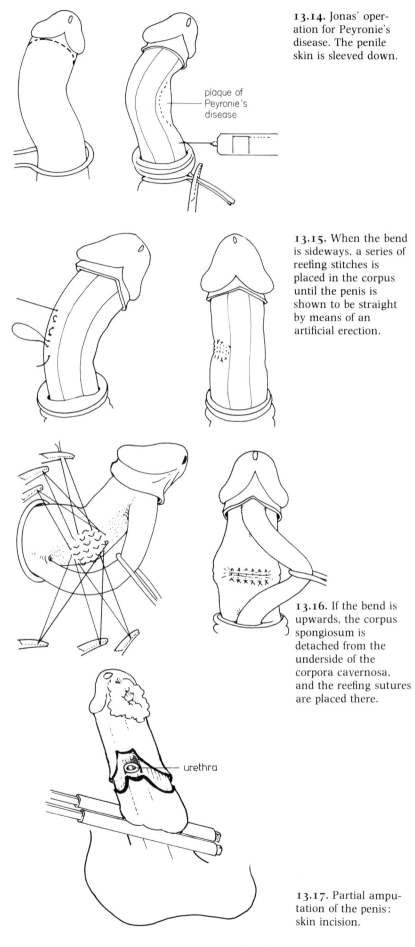

13.14. Jonas' operation for Peyronie's disease. The penile skin is sleeved down.

plaque of Peyronie's disease

13.15. When the bend is sideways, a series of reefing stitches is placed in the corpus until the penis is shown to be straight by means of an artificial erection.

13.16. If the bend is upwards, the corpus spongiosum is detached from the underside of the corpora cavernosa, and the reefing sutures are placed there.

— urethra

13.17. Partial amputation of the penis: skin incision.

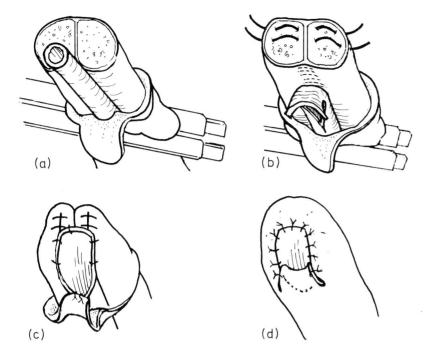

(a)

(b)

(c)

(d)

13.18. The skin is slid back and the corpora cut across. Interrupted 1-0 chromic catgut closes the corpora together. The urethra is spatulated and sewn

over the united cavernosa and the ∩-shaped flap of skin used to make an elliptical anastomosis between skin and urethra to prevent stricture.

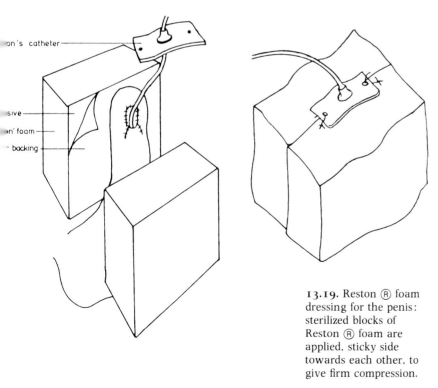

bon's catheter

sive

on' foam

backing

13.19. Reston ® foam dressing for the penis: sterilized blocks of Reston ® foam are applied, sticky side towards each other, to give firm compression.

fascia with o-chromic catgut. Spatulate the corpus spongiosum on its ventral aspect, and suture the splayed urethra to the end of the closed corpora cavernosa (13.18). The ventral tongue of skin is tucked into the slit in the urethra so that there is a long elliptical suture line which prevents subsequent stricture. A 12 Ch Gibbon's catheter is left indwelling.

Haematoma is prevented by applying a pressure dressing made of two blocks of sterile Reston foam, sticky sides facing each other: this prevents venous ooze and provides a comfortable dressing. The wings of the Gibbon's catheter may be sutured to the dressing. Dressing and catheter may be removed after two to three days (13.19).

Hazards of the operation

In former days stricture was almost inevitable at the end of the divided urethra. The method described here avoids this inconvenience. Secondary infection of the wound may be largely prevented by using metronidazole prophylactically (400 mg every eight hours).

Radical amputation of the penis

Indications

Radical amputation of the penis is the only way to cure the patient of cancer when the growth has reached the scrotum and has invaded the middle part of the shaft of the penis. For such patients irradiation is seldom feasible or effective. Radical amputation is also indicated when cancer recurs after failure of partial amputation to control the growth (Blandy 1976).

Using the method described here, I routinely remove not only the penis, but the testicles along with the majority of the scrotal skin. This reflects the pecularities of the age incidence of penile cancer in the locality served by the London Hospital, where it is a disease of very elderly men to whom the loss of the testes is of little consequence. The procedure leaves the patient with a clean perineum, resembling a vulva. Where it is obviously desirable (for example in a younger patient) to conserve the testicles, the operation may be appropriately modified.

Special precautions

Metronidazole and an antibiotic capable of dealing with spore-bearing Gram-positive infection should be given as prophylaxis against infection in this area, especially when so many of these patients have a growth that is already septic and stinking.

The psychological trauma of losing the penis needs to be considered: expert psychiatric help may be needed to reinforce tactful explanation and discussion by the surgeon and the nursing team.

Blood loss may be considerable and three units should be available.

Anaesthesia

Controlled hypotension may be particularly helpful in this operation.

Position

The patient is placed in the cystoscopy position giving access to the perineum and the inguinal regions.

Steps of the operation

When there is a large fungating mass, begin by thoroughly washing the penis and scrotum with Betadine and enclose the mass in a sterile rubber glove, tied tightly around the penile shaft. The skin is prepared again with iodine and the legs covered with leggings.

Make a ∩-shaped scrotal flap as for urethroplasty. Dissect down to the bulbospongiosus muscle and urethra (13.20). The incision of the scrotal flap is now carried anteriorly to divide the scrotum in the midline up to the base of the penis, which is circumcised well away from any induration that might suggest infiltration by cancer.

Retracting the lateral skin flap out to the external inguinal ring, to expose the spermatic cord, cross-clamp and divide the cord and secure its vessels by suture-ligature (13.21). Dissect all the tissues from the external inguinal ring medially and downwards to the pectineus fascia and the deep fascia of the thigh, sweeping everything towards the midline. Repeat this process on the other side, dividing the cord at the external ring, and cleaning everything medially.

Retract the upper edge of the skin to expose the prepubic fat and the suspensory ligament of the penis (13.22). Large veins need careful ligation between the root of the penis and the symphysis and it is easier to dissect the penis from the symphysis and rectus sheath if a diathermy needle is used.

Pull the entire mass firmly downwards while continuing to dissect against the front

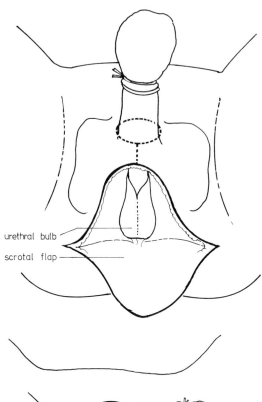

urethral bulb
scrotal flap

13.20. Radical amputation of the penis: start by raising the ∩-shaped scrotal flap and exposing the urethra and bulbospongiosus muscles.

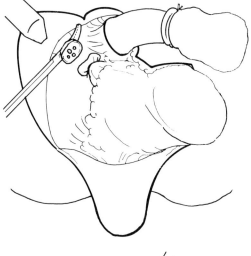

13.21. The right spermatic cord is clamped, doubly transfixed and ligated, at the external ring.

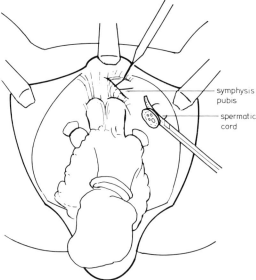

symphysis pubis
spermatic cord

13.22. The left cord has been cut, and the suspensory ligament of the penis is divided with the diathermy needle, clearing the tissues away from the front of the symphysis.

of the symphysis, until its inferior margin is exposed, and the triangular space that is bounded by the diverging corpora cavernosa and the inferior margin of the symphysis is entered. Here the dorsal vein of the penis and, on either side, the two deep arteries of the penis should be suture-ligated before they are accidentally torn (13.23).

Lift up the mass of penis and scrotum, and free up the corpus spongiosum from the inferior surface of the corpora by dissecting in the plane between them for 5–6 cm. Hold the free length of corpus spongiosum in an atraumatic Potts' clamp and cut it across (13.24).

It is not necessary to erase the corpora cavernosa from their tough attachment to the ischial rami, but they should be dissected sufficiently far back until a crushing clamp can be placed across each one to allow it to be divided safely (13.25). Oversew each corpus using o-chromic catgut to occlude the tough sleeve of Buck's fascia. Repeat this on the other side. The specimen is now free, and leaves a cleanly dissected perineum in which the urethra hangs down from the bulb. The urethra is now slit along its inferior midline, and the strip spread out and sutured to the front of the symphysis with fine 3-0 catgut sutures (13.26). Into the apex of the slit

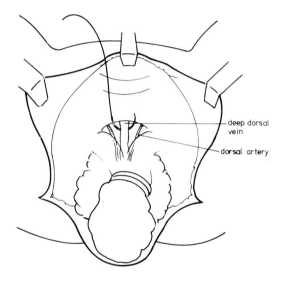

13.23. The deep vein of the penis and the deep arteries of the penis are suture-ligated and divided.

deep dorsal vein

dorsal artery

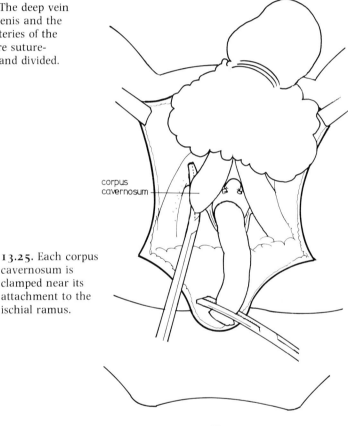

corpus cavernosum

13.25. Each corpus cavernosum is clamped near its attachment to the ischial ramus.

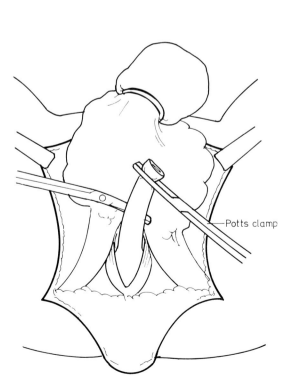

Potts clamp

13.26. Both corpora cavernosa are over-sewn, and the spatu-lated urethra attached to the front of the symphysis.

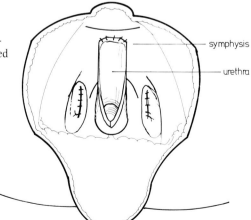

symphysis

urethra

13.24. The corpus spongiosum and urethra are separated from the corpora cavernosa, clamped, and cut across.

urethra is sutured the tip of the ∩-shaped
scrotal flap, and the edges of scrotal skin are
brought to the edges of the urethra (13.27).
This forms a stricture-proof anastomosis. A
catheter is left indwelling for four to five days.

Hazards of the operation

A little cellulitis of the edges of the scrotal skin
is commonly seen in these infected patients.
Sometimes a little of the edge of the skin will
undergo necrosis, but healing always takes
place without the need for a skin graft, and
with minimal scarring.

Inguinal node dissection

Inguinal node dissection for cancer of the penis
is deferred for three months after amputation
or radiotherapy to the primary lesion. It should
only be performed (a) when a lymphangio-
gram has excluded metastases in the pelvis,
when block dissection of the groin nodes
would not be worth-while and (b) when fine-
needle aspiration has given cytological proof
of cancer in the node. These criteria are rarely
present. It is not worth putting the patient to
all the discomfort and inconvenience of a
block dissection, to say nothing of the persistent lymphoedema of the lower limb that inevitably follows, when the nodes prove to be
negative, or, worse, when massive recurrence
of tumour occurs in the pelvis within a few
weeks of the operation. The technique of node
dissection used in my practice is a simple one,
even though most of the patients so treated
have been given pre-operative radiotherapy
to the nodes in the groin, and the skin is
affected.

An oblique incision is made parallel with
the skin crease (13.28). The skin edges are
retracted, exposing all the tissue within the
triangle bounded by the inguinal ligament,
the sartorius and the gracilis muscles. The
saphenous vein is divided between ligatures
at the inferior apex of the triangle; fat and
fibrous tissue at each border of the triangle
are progressively divided until the deep
fasciae are found, then the whole mass removed
en bloc (13.29, 13.30). Laid bare in the floor
of the femoral triangle are the femoral artery
and vein. In most of my cases I have simply
sutured the skin edges together without
tension, using a suitable soft drain, and a
Reston foam pressure dressing. However,
when the inguinal region has been heavily
irradiated, it is a wise precaution to protect
the femoral vessels with the thickness of the

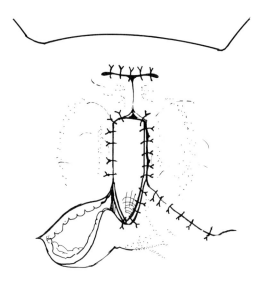

13.27. The scrotal
skin is folded in and
sewn to the edges of
the spatulated urethra
on each side, while
the ∩-shaped scrotal
flap is let in to the
apex of the urethra to
make a stricture-proof
anastomosis.

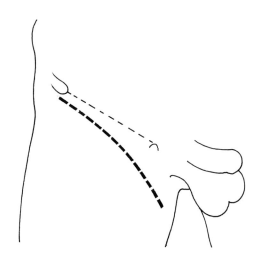

13.28. Incision for
inguinal node dis-
section.

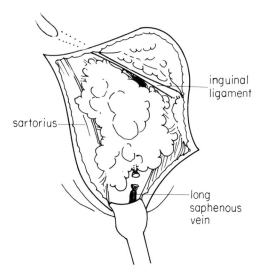

sartorius

inguinal
ligament

long
saphenous
vein

13.29. All the tissue
within the femoral
triangle is removed *en
bloc*.

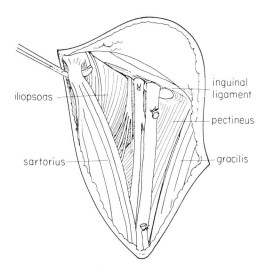

13.30. Structures displayed after inguinal node dissection.

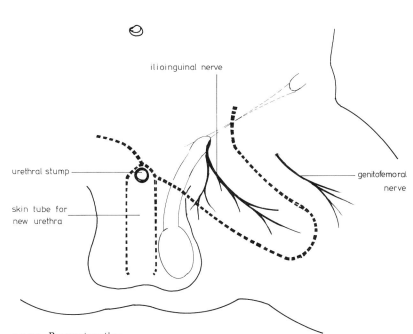

13.32. Reconstruction of the penis. The urethra is formed from the skin of the front of the scrotum using a 24 Ch catheter as a guide. A full thickness dermofat graft is cut to include the cutaneous distribution of the ilio-inguinal nerve from the medial upper part of the thigh.

sartorius muscle: this is easily detached from its upper origin (13.31) and swung across to be sutured in front of the femoral canal. Should there be necrosis of the overlying skin, infection will be prevented from reaching the vessels, so avoiding the risk of massive secondary haemorrhage.

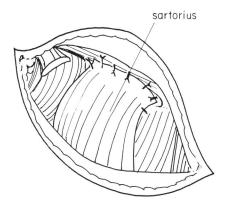

13.31. To cover and protect the femoral vessels, the sartorius is detached and sutured to the inguinal ligament.

Reconstruction of the penis

Indications

The penis may be lost after Fournier's gangrene, or removed by accident or for cancer. Each case calls for an individualized approach, in which the help of a plastic surgeon should, whenever possible, be sought. One method is as follows (Kaplan & Wesser 1971).

Steps of the operation

First reconstruct the urethra using a full-thickness skin tube from the front of the scrotum, rolling it up over a 24 Ch catheter as a stent (13.32). This leaves a 24 mm wide raw defect along the front of the scrotum.

A full thickness pedicled skin flap is constructed for the new penis. If it is taken from the medial aspect of the thigh (13.33, 13.34) it incorporates the cutaneous branches of the ilioinguinal nerve as they emerge from the external inguinal ring, and care is taken to preserve these fine nerves in the subsequent dissection. The raw surface on the upper thigh is covered with split skin.

At a second stage, six to eight weeks later, the new penis is formed by turning in the full thickness graft from the thigh, including the new urethra (13.35). There are, it should be mentioned, many other techniques for reconstructing the penis, one useful modification

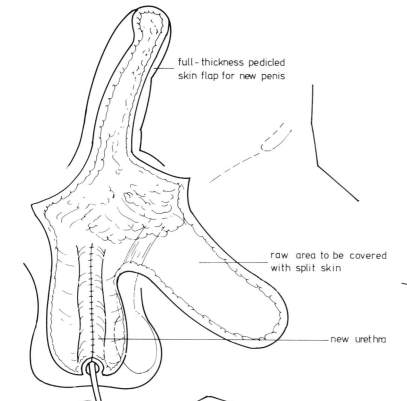

full-thickness pedicled skin flap for new penis

raw area to be covered with split skin

new urethra

13.33. The urethral skin tube has been completed, leaving a broad defect in the front of the scrotum, to be covered with the skin flap from the thigh which, in turn, is covered with split skin taken from the other thigh.

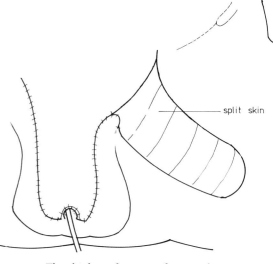

split skin

13.34. The thigh graft is sewn to the scrotum, covering the new urethra; the raw surface on the inner aspect of the thigh is covered with split skin.

being the incorporation of the gracilis muscle within the pedicled tube of thigh skin, to give it extra bulk and blood supply (Persky *et al.* 1983). But like all such reconstructed penises, the end result is always a disappointment: it looks unlike the real thing; its sensation is not that of the glans penis; and the patient cannot have a normal erection. Unless all these points are very carefully explained to the patient before beginning this long and difficult series of staged operations, he will be bitterly disappointed.

References

Bennett A.H. (1982) The inflatable and malleable penile prosthesis. In *Management of Male Impotence*, (ed. by Bennett A.H.), p. 210. Williams & Wilkins, Baltimore.

Blandy J.P. (1976) Penis and Scrotum. In *Urology*, (ed. by Blandy J.P.), p. 1049. Blackwell Scientific Publications, Oxford.

Blandy J.P. (1977) Circumcision. In *Contemporary Obstetrics and Gynaecology*, (ed. by Chamberlain G.V.P.), p.240. Northwood, London.

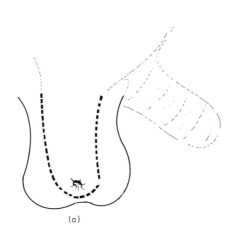

(a)　　　(b)

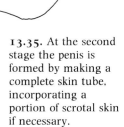

13.35. At the second stage the penis is formed by making a complete skin tube, incorporating a portion of scrotal skin if necessary.

Brindley G.S. (1984) New treatment for priapism. *Lancet*, **ii**, 220.

El-Demiry M.I.M., Oliver R.T.D., Hope-Stone H.F., & Blandy J.P. (1984) Reappraisal of the role of Radiotherapy and Surgery in the Management of carcinoma of the Penis. *Brit. J. Urol.* **56**, 724.

Finney R.P. (1982) Rigid and Semirigid penile prostheses. In *Management of Male Impotence* (ed. by Bennett A.H.), p. 198. Williams & Wilkins, Baltimore.

Forsberg L., Mattiason A. & Olsson A.M. (1981) Priapism—conservative treatment versus surgical procedures. *Brit. J. Urol.* **53**, 374.

Gairdner D. (1949) The fate of the foreskin. *Brit. Med. J.* **2**, 1433.

Ghalioungui P. (1963) *Magic and Medical Science in Ancient Egypt*. Hodder & Stoughton, London.

Hinman F. (1960) Priapism: reasons for failure of therapy. *J. Urol.* **83**, 420.

Johnston J.H. (1976) Congenital abnormalities of the bladder and urethra. In *Urology*, (ed. by Blandy J.P.), p. 619. Blackwell Scientific Publications, Oxford.

Jonas U. (1983) *Demonstration of modification of Nesbit's operation*. Boerhaave Symposium, Leyden.

Kaplan I. & Wesser D. (1971) A rapid method for constructing a functional sensitive penis. *Brit. J. Plastic Surg.* **24**, 342.

King L.R. (1982) Commentary: neonatal circumcision in the United States in 1982. *J. Urol.* **128**, 1135.

Laubscher W.M. (1972) Fraktur van die penis. *S. Afr. Med. J.* **46**, 1044.

Marshall P., Morales A. & Surridge D. (1982) Diagnostic significance of penile erections during sleep. *Urology*, **20**, 1.

McDougal W.S. & Jeffery (1983) Microscopic penile revascularization. *J. Urol.* **129**, 517.

Mitchell J.P. & Dobbie A.K. (1976) Surgical Diathermy in urological practice. In *Scientific Foundations of Urology*, **2**, (ed. by Williams D.I. & Chisholm G.D.), p. 432. Livingstone, Edinburgh.

Montague D.K. (1982) The evaluation of the Impotent Male. In *Management of Male Impotence*, (ed. by Bennett A.H.), p. 52. Williams & Wilkins, Baltimore.

Persky L., Resnick M. & Desprez J. (1983) Penile reconstruction with Gracilis pedicle grafts. *J. Urol.* **129**, 603.

Remondino P.C. (1891) *History of Circumcision*. Davis, Philadelphia.

Salaverria J.C., Hope-Stone H.F., Paris A.M.I., Molland E.A. & Blandy J.P. (1979) Conservative treatment of carcinoma of the penis. *Brit. J. Urol.* **51**, 32.

Chapter 14
Operations on the male urethra

Hypospadias

Indications

'Every man-child has the natural right to write his name in the snow.' The most trying disadvantage of a trivial hypospadias is the difficulty the little boy experiences in directing the jet of urine. It is not necessary to operate on boys with a urethra that opens near the base of the glans, when there is no chordee, but it is sometimes necessary to divide a little web of skin that arches across the meatus and makes the jet spray out.

Some parents are particularly anxious about this very minor deformity. If so, then it can be readily put right by the 'meatus advancement glanuloplasty' or MAGPI operation of Duckett (1981) (14.1). The web is slit in the midline: the incision is carried deeply into the glans, extended to its tip, and then closed transversely (a).

The skin is then circumcised just proximal to the meatus, taking great care not to make a hole into the urethra (b).

Drawing the meatus towards the tip of the glans with a fine skin hook, approximated the edges of the skin with 2 or 3 sutures. This will bring the meatus to the tip of the penis (c).

After trimming away surplus foreskin the edge of the circumcision is closed, if necessary sliding skin down from the surplus prepuce (d). The child need only stay in hospital for the day, or possibly overnight.

Having said this, there are many boys with severe hypospadias, a marked chordee, and a deformity that unquestionably calls for correction. Such children should, where possible, be referred to a surgeon who has experience of many of these cases, for in his hands the operation can frequently be done in a single stage. In few other surgical operation does practice matter so much. For the average urologist who may be called upon to deal with hypospadias only two or three times a year, the two-stage operation of Byars is reliable and easy to perform (Byars 1955).

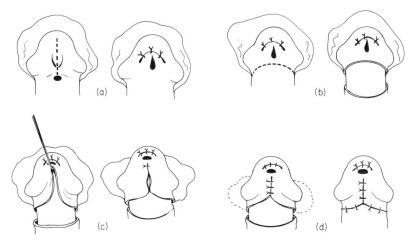

14.1. Meatus advancement glanuloplasty or MAGPI operation of Duckett. (a) The glans is split across the web and closed transversely (b). The penis is circumcised just proximal to the urethra, the meatus is drawn towards the tip of the glans and the skin closed in the midline, if necessary bringing down surplus foreskin (c). After trimming away any redundant foreskin the circumcision is closed (d).

First stage

A stay suture in the glans holds it straight. The skin on the ventral aspect of the penis is incised in a complete circle around the sulcus behind the glans, distal to the opening of the urethra (14.2). The urethra is dissected away from the corpora cavernosa and allowed to drop back. Firm bands of fibrous tissue may tether the urethra to the underside of the corpora cavernosa, keeping the penis curved in an arc. The chordee is only corrected when all this fibrous tissue is removed. Continue the dissection down towards the bulb until the

14.2. Hypospadias, first stage: correction of the chordee. A circumferential incision is made (a, b) and the sleeve of skin allowed to drop back with the urethra (c) which is dissected away from the fibrous bands which tether it to the corpora cavernosa.

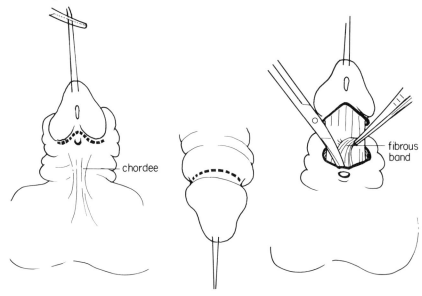

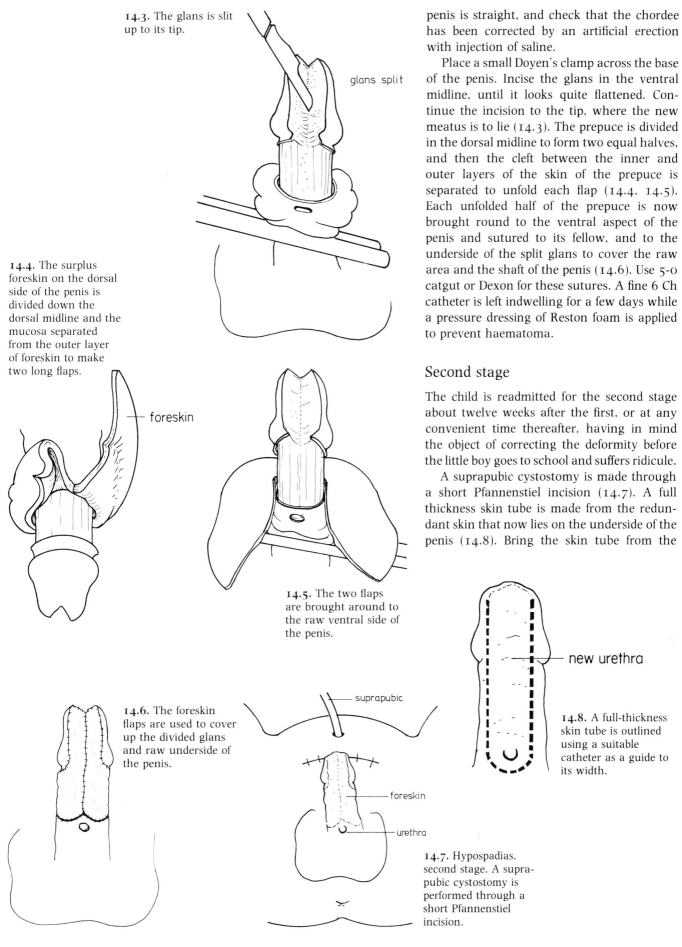

14.3. The glans is slit up to its tip.

glans split

14.4. The surplus foreskin on the dorsal side of the penis is divided down the dorsal midline and the mucosa separated from the outer layer of foreskin to make two long flaps.

— foreskin

14.5. The two flaps are brought around to the raw ventral side of the penis.

14.6. The foreskin flaps are used to cover up the divided glans and raw underside of the penis.

suprapubic

foreskin

urethra

14.7. Hypospadias, second stage. A suprapubic cystostomy is performed through a short Pfannenstiel incision.

— new urethra

14.8. A full-thickness skin tube is outlined using a suitable catheter as a guide to its width.

penis is straight, and check that the chordee has been corrected by an artificial erection with injection of saline.

Place a small Doyen's clamp across the base of the penis. Incise the glans in the ventral midline, until it looks quite flattened. Continue the incision to the tip, where the new meatus is to lie (14.3). The prepuce is divided in the dorsal midline to form two equal halves, and then the cleft between the inner and outer layers of the skin of the prepuce is separated to unfold each flap (14.4, 14.5). Each unfolded half of the prepuce is now brought round to the ventral aspect of the penis and sutured to its fellow, and to the underside of the split glans to cover the raw area and the shaft of the penis (14.6). Use 5-0 catgut or Dexon for these sutures. A fine 6 Ch catheter is left indwelling for a few days while a pressure dressing of Reston foam is applied to prevent haematoma.

Second stage

The child is readmitted for the second stage about twelve weeks after the first, or at any convenient time thereafter, having in mind the object of correcting the deformity before the little boy goes to school and suffers ridicule.

A suprapubic cystostomy is made through a short Pfannenstiel incision (14.7). A full thickness skin tube is made from the redundant skin that now lies on the underside of the penis (14.8). Bring the skin tube from the verge of the dropped-back normal urethra to the tip of the glans. The skin tube should be adjusted to equal the circumference of the urethra appropriate to the age of the boy. Form the tube around a bougie of appropriate size, that is one which fits the normal proximal urethra snugly (14.9). Suture the skin tube with very fine 5-0 catgut sutures. The skin of the underside of the penis is now approximated with fine everting sutures of the same material (14.10). At this stage, thanks to the generous amount of skin that has been brought round to the underside of the penis, there should be no tension on any of the suture lines, but the little organ will swell with oedema and erections in the next few days, and to guard against disruption of the suture line it is a wise precaution to make a dorsal relaxing incision (14.11). This heals with an insignificant scar within ten days.

The suprapubic tube is clamped and removed after ten days. Occasionally a small fistula develops along the line of the reconstructed urethra: if so, leave it alone for at least three months, and then close it in the following way.

Closure of penile urethral fistulae

Mark out a Y-shaped flap of skin, over the little hole (14.12). Mobilize the skin all round, well away from the fistula, and close the fistula with one or two 5-0 catgut sutures. Advance the tip of the V into the vertical limb of the Y so that the hole is covered up with full thickness skin. Close the skin with interrupted 5-0 catgut and protect the suture line with a very fine catheter (for example 6 Ch) for seven days.

The late harvest of hypospadias

Adults are occasionally referred with a typical combination of fistulae, chordee, and stricture, dating from efforts in childhood to close their hypospadias. These are difficult to deal with, and the golden rule is to avoid making use of the skin of the penile shaft, which is usually sadly scarred and deformed. The method I have found best is described under the section on one-stage island patch urethroplasty, of which it is a variant (page 222).

Extrophy and Epispadias

All errors in development of the lower abdominal wall present difficulties in management. They are all very rare, and they give rise to controversy amongst even the most exper-

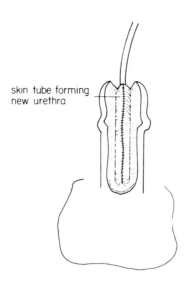

skin tube forming new urethra

14.9. The skin tube is sutured over the catheter.

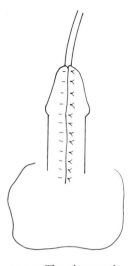

14.10. The glans and penile skin are closed over the skin tube.

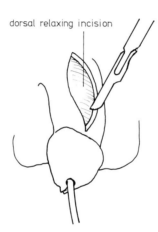

dorsal relaxing incision

14.11. A dorsal relaxing incision prevents any tension on the reformed skin tube.

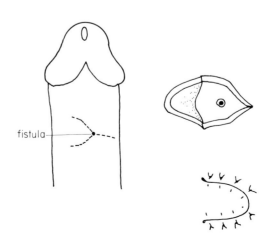

fistula

14.12. Closure of pinhole penile urethral fistula.

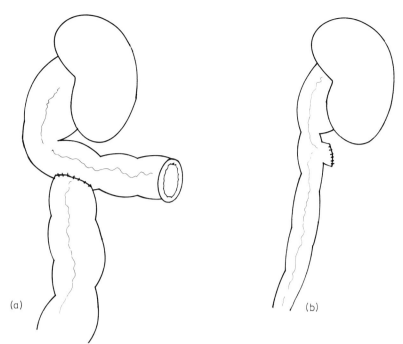

must be familiar with this entity. Treatment of the valve itself may not be enough when the child has grossly dilated ureters and an enormous bladder. Loop ureterostomy (14.13), nephrostomy, or suprapubic cystostomy may be urgently needed especially when obstructive uropathy is made worse by infection. The essential lesion is a spinnaker-shaped valve, set obliquely in the posterior urethra, whose two cusps allow only a trickle of urine to escape between them (14.14).

14.13. Diagram of Innes Williams' modified loop ureterostomy. (a) The ureter is brought out to the skin, which permits free drainage while at the second stage, when the time comes (b) to close the ureterostomy, the urine runs freely down the distal limb.

ienced paediatric urologists. The reader, faced with such a problem, should if possible refer the child to a specialist paediatric centre rather than try his hand at an operation which he may do only once or twice in his lifetime (Eckstein, Hohenfellner & Williams 1977).

Congenital posterior valves of the urethra

Congenital urethral valves are far from uncommon but, alas, often misdiagnosed. One in three of these boys present in the first three months of life, half of them in the first year, but a significant number escape detection until the lad is older, so that the 'adult' urologist

Special preparations

The diagnosis is made by a cystogram. This demonstrates a dilated posterior urethra, trabeculated and hypertrophied bladder and ureters. If renal function is impaired the child may need preliminary decompression, at first using percutaneous nephrostomy drainage (page 71) but later the modified loop nephrostomy of Innes Williams gives good drainage and less difficulty with later closure (Williams 1975). However, unless the child is severely uraemic, it is best to remove the cause of the obstruction by destroying the valves.

Endoscopic division of posterior urethral valves

In a tiny baby the small paediatric resectoscope may not pass without risk of injury to the narrow urethra, but through a small perineal incision a urethrostomy is made that allows insertion of the resectoscope. The valves are seen when the irrigating fluid is shut off and the cusps of the valve belly out

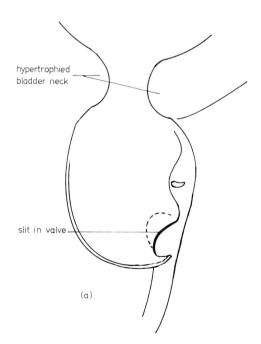

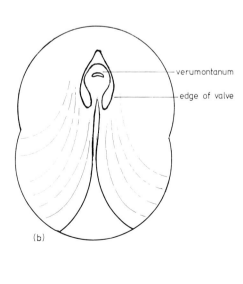

14.14. Congenital urethral valve in the male: there is a spinnaker-shaped valve set obliquely in the urethra, with a big anterior curtain and a narrow slit-shaped hole in the middle.

towards you. It is only necessary to slip the loop of the resectoscope under the anterior curtain of the valve and touch the cutting current for a second for the valve to disappear. On withdrawing the resectoscope the urine pours out. A tiny urethral catheter is left in position for three to four days to allow the perineal urethrostomy to seal off.

Not every urologist will have access to a paediatric resectoscope, but one can still deal with valves using an ordinary child's endoscope with a 0° or 30° telescope and a ureteric catheter with a wire stylet. Cut the tip off the ureteric catheter for about 5 mm, and bend the end of the wire into a slight hook-shape (14.15). Advance the wire to the edge of the valve, hold the diathermy cable to the other end of the stylet and touch the cutting current. (I have often had to use this simple trick when operating overseas.)

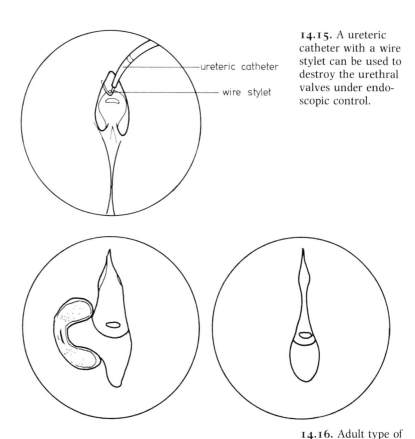

14.15. A ureteric catheter with a wire stylet can be used to destroy the urethral valves under endoscopic control.

14.16. Adult type of urethral valves.

Congenital urethral valves in adults

In young men and adults the congenital posterior urethral valve is more difficult to diagnose. It presents as a fleshy mound just to each side of the verumontanum. Above this the prostatic urethra is distended. Today, most of these young men have undergone extensive cineurography and urodynamic investigations, and one can identify the site of obstruction at the level of the verumontanum, but is anxious not to cause incontinence.

With the resectoscope, allow the irrigating fluid to run in and out: this shows the fleshy lumps meeting together (14.16). Take a tiny segment out of the lump on one or other side of the verumontanum. Unlike valves in children, these are quite thick and firm, and in section show prostatic glandular elements. There is often an immediate and gratifying return of a good urine flow, with decompression of the upper tracts, and no need to remove any tissue from the other side. So far, in my series, there has been no incontinence and no interference with ejaculation (Szemat-Nikolajenko & Cukier 1978).

Congenital anterior urethral valves— double urethra

This is a curious congenital deformity which may appear in several variations. During the embryological development of the male urethra, two urethrae are formed, one above the other. The second urethra may or may not open on the meatus and into the bladder: as a rule it is blind ending and rather narrower than the normal one. There is a septum between them which is not always perforated. In some patients symptoms only develop in adult life, when the septum between the two channels gives way; in others it seems to have been perforated since childhood (14.17).

The result of this is that on voiding, the second urethra fills up with urine, forcing the anterior part of the septum up against the lumen of the good urethra like a flap-valve— hence the name, congenital anterior urethral valve (14.18). The condition, though not

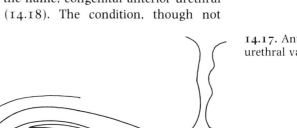

14.17. Anterior urethral valves.

14.18. Urethra occluded when child tries to void.

common, is not rare either, and alas, is often missed. I have recently been obliged to perform renal transplantation in such a child for whom repeated endoscopic assessments had been carried out without the diagnosis ever being considered. The simplest operation is to divide the anterior septum: this can be done endoscopically. If this leaves the patient with an ugly mega-urethra that causes symptoms, then a formal reconstruction of the urethra may be performed.

Endoscopic division of anterior urethral 'valves'

In children the paediatric resectoscope and a tiny Collings knife may be used. In adults it is easier to use the Storz–Sachse cold urethrotome, since it allows a clear view and gives rise to no bubbles.

The hole in the septum is easily recognized if one knows where to look for it, that is in the midline, in the middle part of the bulbar urethra. Sometimes there is more than one opening. It is simply slit open, the incision being taken the whole length of the septum (14.19), so that there is no residual flap valve

to give rise to obstruction. A catheter is left in for twenty-four hours.

Open reconstruction of the congenital anterior 'valve'

This is an easy operation as long as one understands that the second 'double' channel of the urethra is made like the normal one with a corpus spongiosum of its own. With the patient in the lithotomy position, make a midline incision (14.20). Retract the scrotal skin, and dissect down on the urethra, keeping in the midline with the assistance of a bougie in the normal urethral channel. Remove the bougie, and distend the urethra with a syringe and saline: this will fill out the second urethra (14.21). Open it between stay sutures. Trim away the surplus tissue of the sac of the urethra, and having removed the mucosa, approximate the walls of the second urethra

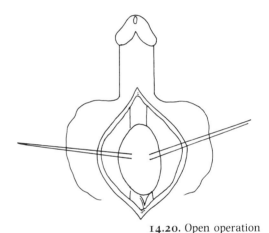

14.20. Open operation for anterior urethral valves.

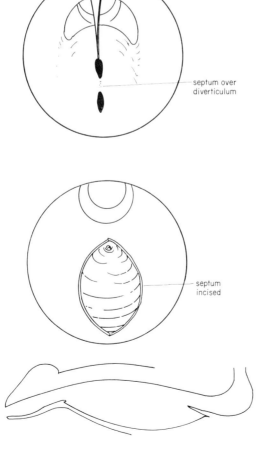

14.19. Endoscopic view of anterior urethral valves. The cold knife slits up the thin septum between the two barrels of the urethra.

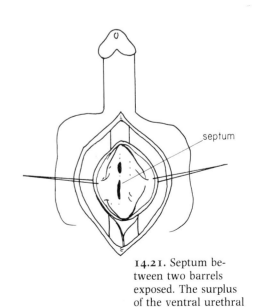

14.21. Septum between two barrels exposed. The surplus of the ventral urethral wall is trimmed away.

over the holes in the septum to close them off (14.22).

Occasionally previous infection and abscess formation has obliterated the tissue planes, and after making the dissection, one is left with a defect in the floor of the normal urethra which is easily dealt with using a pedicled island patch (see page 221) (14.23).

Urethral injury

Injury to the perineal urethra

The patient has fallen astride a rail, the handle-bar of his cycle, or has been kicked in the perineum. There is a clear history of the injury, a swelling in the perineum, and perhaps blood issuing from the urethra. Classically the main danger in the olden days was that infected urine would extravasate into the soft tissues of the perineum and give rise to necrosis of the overlying skin (14.24). This is still a risk today, and if the patient comes to the hospital after some delay, when there is considerable bruising and extravasation of fluid in the perineum, it should be evacuated and drained. There is, however, no need to attempt to join the ends of the urethra together. A suprapubic cystostomy should be made using a trochar and supracath, or a formal exposure. After about a week, when the local inflammation and bruising has settled down, the urethra may be examined with the urethroscope. If it looks well healed, the suprapubic tube is clamped and removed when the patient is voiding well. In the majority of these cases the urethra heals without a need for further surgery.

In a few, less fortunate patients, a stricture develops at the site of the injury, but it is always a short stricture in the mid-bulbar urethra which is the easiest site for a one-stage urethroplasty (see page 221).

Urethral injury associated with fractured pelvis

Nothing gives rise to such intense controversy as the topic of the management of the ruptured urethra that is associated with a fracture of the pelvis. The principles that should determine your approach to these cases are no different from the principles of good trauma surgery elsewhere (Glass *et al.* 1978).

Initial management

Many of these patients arrive shocked, with multiple injuries of which the fractured pelvis

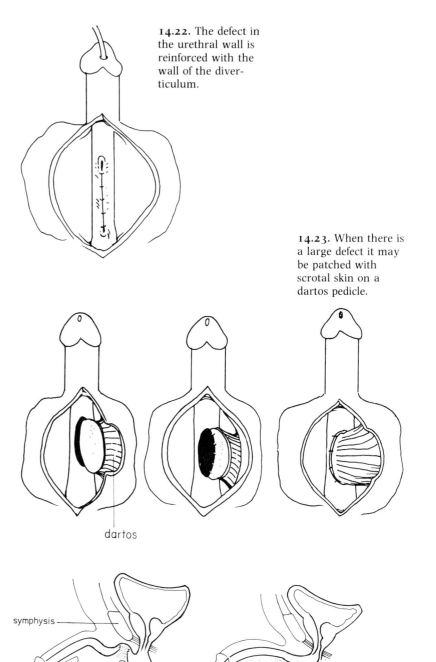

14.22. The defect in the urethral wall is reinforced with the wall of the diverticulum.

14.23. When there is a large defect it may be patched with scrotal skin on a dartos pedicle.

dartos

symphysis

extravasated urine

is sometimes the least important. Others are relatively fit and well, but have had a fractured pelvis, and one suspects that there may be an injury to the urethra because there is blood at the external meatus and the patient has been unable to pass urine.

In the first group, the overriding concern is to restore lost blood, close sucking wounds of the chest, and deal where appropriate with head injuries. Massive transfusion of blood may be needed, and the resuscitation team need to know that urine is being formed. The

14.24. Rupture of the perineal urethra: no attempt should be made to effect a primary repair; it is better to perform a suprapubic cystostomy and merely drain any extravasated blood and urine which has collected in the perineum.

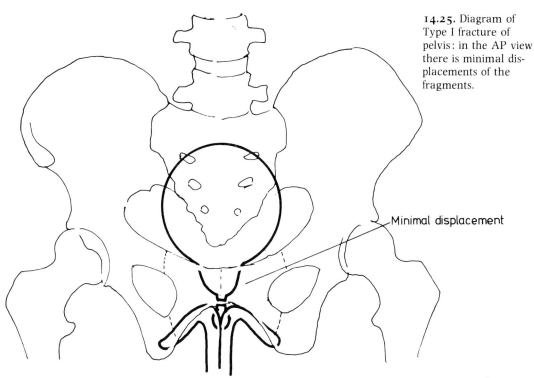

14.25. Diagram of Type I fracture of pelvis: in the AP view there is minimal displacements of the fragments.

Minimal displacement

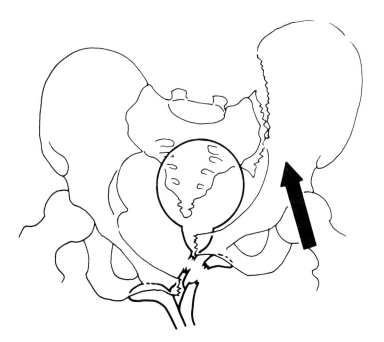

14.26. Diagram of Type II fracture of pelvis: one half-pelvis is displaced carrying with it the bladder and prostate.

question often arises, is it safe to pass a urethral catheter? The short answer is that if an experienced urologist is at hand, then a soft 12 Ch catheter may be slipped up the urethra: if it slides easily into the bladder and clear urine comes out, then the problem is (temporarily) solved.

Others prefer to obtain a urethrogram, using 25 ml of water-soluble contrast medium injected aseptically via a 12 Ch catheter placed in the anterior urethra, as soon as the X-rays of the pelvis have been taken. If the contrast goes easily into the bladder, a catheter will follow easily; if contrast extravasates, indicating a complete or partial rupture of the urethra, then it is prudent to insert a suprapubic cystostomy tube (page 117). To a large extent your choice of method at this stage will be determined by your radiographic facilities and expertise. When in doubt, a suprapubic catheter is the safest manoeuvre.

In the second group of patients, who are not shocked, and whose only injury is the fracture of the pelvis, the management is governed by the appearance of the X-ray. There are, broadly speaking, two types of fracture of the pelvis: (a) Type I, where there is minimal displacement in the anteroposterior view (14.25); and (b) Type II, where one half-pelvis has been displaced upwards, with a fracture in the region of the symphysis in front, and a fracture or dislocation of the sacro-iliac joint behind (14.26).

When there is minimal displacement in the

AP view, there can still be a backwards shift of the urethra in the lateral view, giving rise to an S-shaped bend in the urethral lumen (14.27).

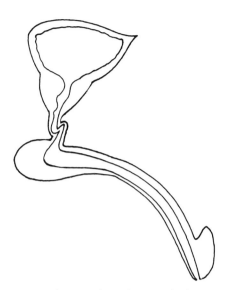

14.27. Type I fracture, lateral view. The bony segment has carried the prostate and the urethra backwards. If the urethra is in continuity there will be an S-shaped bend.

In the second group, where there is displacement of the half-pelvis, one can be reasonably sure that the bladder and prostate will be attached to one innominate bone, while the bulbar urethra remains tethered to the other: the urethra will have torn across at its most narrow part, that is the membranous urethra (14.28).

Although in the initial stages of the management of these patients it is perfectly safe and proper merely to insert a suprapubic catheter until expert help is available, the ultimate intention of the surgeon must be to restore continuity to the urethra with the minimum gap and displacement. A urethrogram, performed as described above, may show whether the urethra is torn or not, but gives less information than urethroscopy. If a 0° telescope is passed up the urethra under anaesthesia, and in the cystoscopy position, it is possible to identify the tear in the urethra, and to see whether or not there is much displacement. Curiously, the tear is always downstream of the 'external sphincter'.

If it is easy to see up into the bladder, a urethral catheter may be slid up and past the tear. It is left in for about two weeks, and then the patient is followed by endoscopy and urethrography in the usual way.

Often the pelvis heals after minimal dis-

placement fractures, with the upper part of the prostatic urethra coming to lie a little behind the bulbar urethra, so that a kind of S-shaped bend, with two septa, is formed. These are easily divided with the cold-knife urethrotome or a Collings knife, and the patient needs no urethroplasty at all (14.29).

This kind of internal urethrotomy is, of course, impossible if the lumen has been

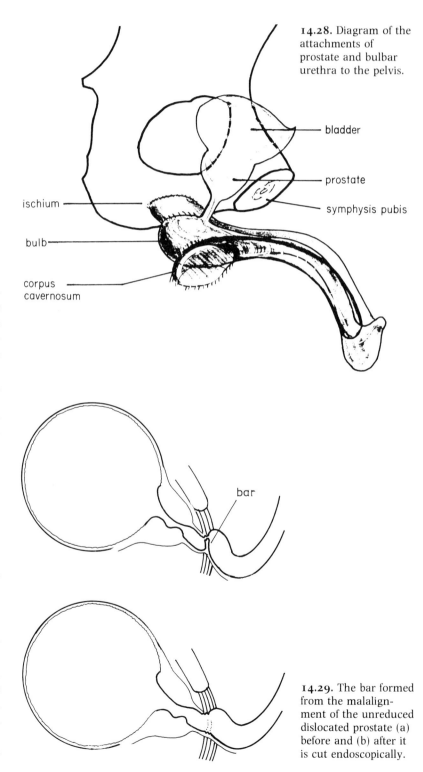

14.28. Diagram of the attachments of prostate and bulbar urethra to the pelvis.

bladder

prostate

symphysis pubis

ischium

bulb

corpus cavernosum

bar

14.29. The bar formed from the malalignment of the unreduced dislocated prostate (a) before and (b) after it is cut endoscopically.

allowed to become completely obliterated. In such a patient, in whom a suprapubic catheter has been left *in situ*, but nothing has been done to restore continuity to the lumen of the urethra, it is sometimes possible to pass one cystoscope down through the suprapubic into the prostatic urethra, and see its light shining across a narrow septum, with a second cystoscope passed up the urethra; and on occasion one can cut through the barrier and so allow the patient to escape without a urethroplasty (14.30).

Hence, if urethroscopy, urethrography, or the attempt to pass a soft 12 Ch rubber catheter demonstrates that the urethra has been torn right across, it is my firm conviction that an attempt should be made to re-establish continuity to the urethra, and this will need a formal open operation (Hayes *et al.* 1983; Patterson *et al.* 1983; Al-Ali & Husain 1983).

The same consideration applies to the second grossly displaced group of fractures, only here the forces which are keeping the ends of the ruptured urethra apart are the same forces that make it difficult for the orthopaedic team to reduce the fracture-dislocation of the pelvis. Clearly there is no urgency in reducing the gap, but it is necessary to reduce the dislocated pelvis and restore urethral continuity before the pelvis is fixed in scar tissue. The ideal time is when the patient is resuscitated, for example about five or six days after admission.

If possible, the displaced fracture should be reduced and held in position by means of external fixation. The external fixation device should be applied in such a way that access is still allowed to the pelvis through a Pfannenstiel incision.

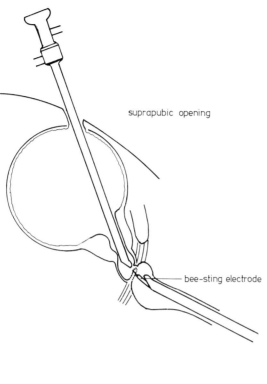

14.30. Cutting down upon the light of a cystoscope introduced through the suprapubic opening, or on to a bougie, may open the way through the bar formed after an old membranous rupture.

suprapubic opening

bee-sting electrode

Restoring continuity to the ruptured urethra

Through the Pfannenstiel incision, the retropubic space is opened and clot and debris are sucked out. A bougie is passed along the urethra, and its tip seen to emerge in the distorted tissue at the floor of the pelvis. The bladder is opened between stay sutures, and the prostate moved to and fro with a finger in the internal meatus. In some patients the prostate has become kinked upwards and sideways (14.31), and it needs to be turned in the right direction for its torn lower end to lie against the lower end of the membranous urethra.

In patients where for any reason the pelvis cannot be reduced (and not all pelvic fractures can be secured with external fixation) then the prostate and bladder must be got down to the membranous urethra by dividing their attachments to the side of the pelvis on the dislocated side. As a rule, only one or two bands of the puboprostatic ligament need to be divided, and one or two vessels secured with ligature or diathermy. Thus set free, the prostate lies against

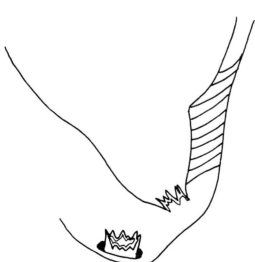

14.31. Ruptured membranous urethra in Type II facture.

the membranous urethra without any tension at all (14.32). How it is retained in position is of little consequence: a few catgut sutures between its capsule and the pelvic fascia are all that is needed, for there is no tension between the ends of the urethra (14.33). One should avoid putting traction on a Foley balloon, since this may give rise to ischaemic necrosis at the neck of the bladder and damage the internal sphincter upon which continence of urine may depend (14.34).

Having mobilized and replaced the dislocated prostate, the lumen is splinted with a suitable narrow silicone catheter and the wound closed with appropriate drainage. Where the ends heal together there is of course likely to be some shrinking of the scar, and a tendency for a stricture to form, but it seldom needs more than an occasional dilatation or internal urethrotomy, and urethroplasty can be avoided.

If urethroplasty is required, so long as pains have been taken to reduce the dislocated prostate and bring the urethral ends together, then the gap to be bridged is a short one, and the urethroplasty not only easy to do, but likely to give a successful result (Blandy 1980).

Dilatation of a stricture

Indications

Of all the operations in surgery, dilatation of a stricture may claim to be the most ancient, if not the most respectable. There is evidence that man inherited gonorrhoea from his simian ancestors. History records many martyrs to stricture: Epicurus committed suicide when he could no longer keep his own stricture dilated; Napoleon was obliged to seek help at the moment of his empty victory in Moscow. Even solemn Socrates thought strictures (in others) fit subject for a joke (Attwater 1943). Sadly, urethral dilatation over the years has come to be delegated to the novice in the urology clinic, yet no operation is more distressing to the patient or more apt to bring disaster. The records of any long standing stricture case will list the 'easy' passage of a 22/24 Ch bougie without incident for many years, until one day the handwriting changes. A new assistant inherits the clinic. He makes a false passage. He records pain, bleeding, possibly bacteraemia. The patient returns for dilatation at more frequent intervals until with time, the new assistant has learnt the need for a sensitive touch and a gentle one—qualities which, alas, cannot be learnt in books.

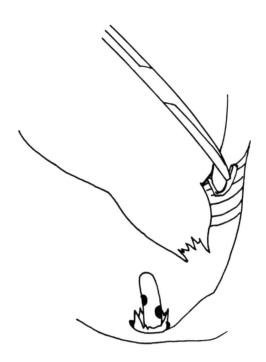

14.32. Re-establishing continuity of the urethra. The first task is to divide the pubo-prostatic ligaments on one side.

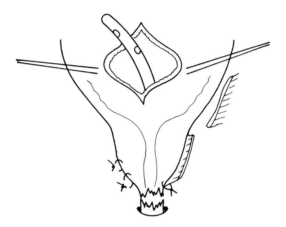

14.33. Once the prostate has been set free, there is no tension on the anastomosis.

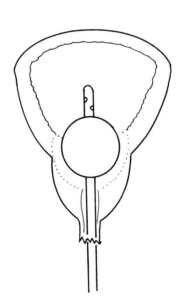 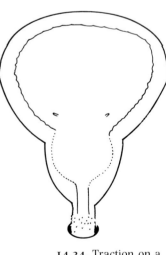

14.34. Traction on a Foley catheter may cause necrosis of the bladder neck.

Anterior urethral strictures

Fill the urethra with 15 ml of 1% lignocaine gel containing 0.25% chlorhexidine, and leave it, with a penile clamp to stop the gel running out, for four minutes.

For anterior strictures, use Wyndham-Powell's anterior straight bougies (14.35). Select the size recorded in the notes or, if

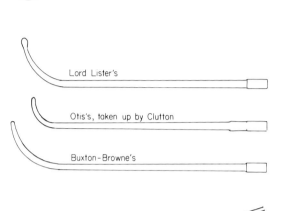

14.35. Wyndham-Powell's anterior urethral bougie.

14.36. Varieties of urethral sound.

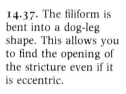

Lord Lister's

Otis's, taken up by Clutton

Buxton-Browne's

14.37. The filiform is bent into a dog-leg shape. This allows you to find the opening of the stricture even if it is eccentric.

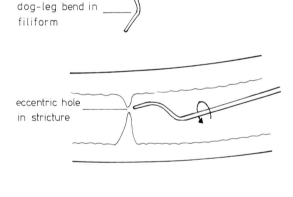

dog-leg bend in filiform

eccentric hole in stricture

14.38. Filiform bougie screwed on to flexible follower.

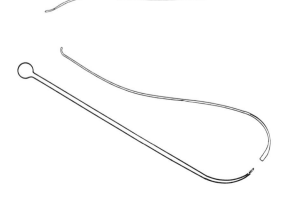

14.39. Filiform and steel follower.

starting with a new patient, try a 16 Ch bougie to begin with and select smaller or larger ones as needed. Dilatation of a stricture aims to stretch the scar tissue, not to disrupt it. It should not be painful, it should not bleed, and it should need no force at all. Stop when blood appears or when the patient suffers pain. Aim to enlarge the stricture little by little to start with. Double the interval between dilatations: for example after the first dilatation, bring the patient back in two weeks, after the second, in four, and so on, until your patient attends only once a year.

If dilatation is difficult, painful, or impossible, then the stricture should be examined under anaesthesia using the optical urethrotome, and an internal urethrotomy performed.

Posterior urethral strictures

The same rules apply to strictures of the posterior (bulbar and membranous) urethra, except that one needs a curved bougie. There are several different kinds of bougie (14.36): I prefer the polished steel bougie devised by Otis and copied by Clutton with a relatively short 'hockey-stick' curve. Again, gentleness and sensitivity are essential and it is important not to overdilate and make things worse. Far better bring the patient back in two or three weeks.

Filiforms and followers

Take a filiform bougie, and dip its tip into boiling water to soften it and allow it to be bent into a dog-leg (14.37). This allows the tip to be rotated to find its way into a stricture with an eccentric hole. Very gently rotating and wriggling the filiform allows it to go down the urethra and into the bladder. There is never any place for forcing it. There is a characteristic feel when the filiform knots itself into the urethra, which one must learn by experience. It is also necessary to learn the equally characteristic sensation of the filiform entering a false passage through a tear in the urethral mucosa.

Once safely in the bladder, a flexible follower (14.38) is screwed into the female end of the filiform and passed on through the stricture into the bladder, gently dilating the urethra *en route*. Flexible followers do not give the surgeon such a sensitive feel of the urethra as do steel ones, and once the filiform is definitely in the bladder, it is often more safe and sure to attach a steel screw-on bougie to the filiform (14.39).

Internal urethrotomy

Internal urethrotomy is a very ancient operation. It can be done blind, by attaching a urethrotome (for example Otis's urethrotome —14.40) to the filiform bougie, opening its jaws, and withdrawing the sharp blade of the knife. The sharp blade cuts about 3 mm into the lumen of the urethra, but this incision can be repeated as often as necessary until the required dilatation has been achieved. My own modification of Otis's urethrotome (14.41) has

the added advantage that it gives a more precise feeling of the length of the stricture but it is otherwise similar in principle.

Optical urethrotomy

Using Sachse's method, after filling the urethra with lubricating gel, the optical urethrotome (14.42) is advanced down the urethra until the stricture is seen. If the ring of stricture is obviously very short, the knife is advanced,

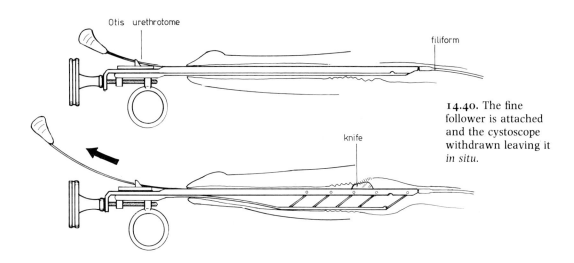

14.40. The fine follower is attached and the cystoscope withdrawn leaving it *in situ.*

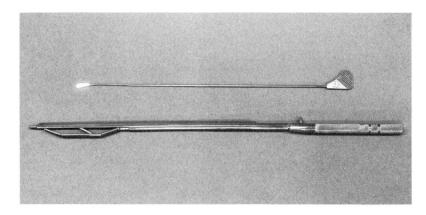

14.41. Author's urethrotome which gives a bougie-*à boule* calibration of the urethra (courtesy of Genitourinary Manufacturing Co.).

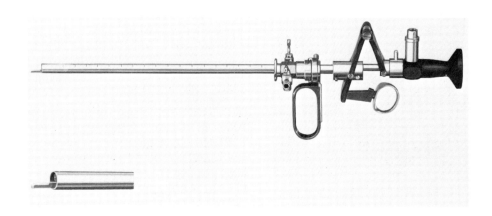

14.42. Storz cold-cutting urethrotome for internal urethrotomy under direct vision (courtesy of Karl Storz).

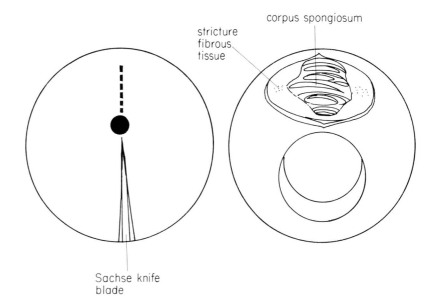

14.43. Endoscopic view of internal urethrotomy. All the fibrous tissue must be divided.

corpus spongiosum

stricture fibrous tissue

Sachse knife blade

and the stricture stroked through until all the fibrous bands of scar tissue under the mucosa have been divided (14.43).

If it is difficult to know which one of several holes is the right lumen to enlarge, or if the structure is long, and one cannot be sure where it ends, then a ureteric catheter should be passed under vision up through the stricture, and kept there as a guide during the subsequent internal urethrotomy.

After the urethral stricture has been laid open completely from one end to the other, opinions differ as to the need for, or the necessary duration of a catheter. Sachse uses no catheter in straightforward uninfected cases; I always leave a 16 Ch silicone catheter *in situ* for twenty-four hours.

Precautions

When performing optical urethrotomy remember that the irrigating fluid will run into the venous sinuses of the penis just as easily as it runs into veins during transurethral resection of the prostate. For the same reason, it should be saline or isotonic glycine, not distilled water, or there is a risk of haemolysis and the transurethral syndrome.

Infection is an important matter in internal urethrotomy since the bloodstream will receive the irrigating fluid and any organisms that happen to contaminate it. Every effort should be made, therefore, to cover the patient against known microbial infection, and if the urine is infected, a catheter should be left in position until the raw area in the urethra has sealed off.

Follow up

Strictures tend to recur, and every patient with a urethral stricture must be followed for ever. It is not enough to evaluate his urethra by means of a flow-rate alone, for the flow is proportional to the square of the diameter of the lumen, and may be compensated for by hypertrophy and increased pressure of the detrusor. It is not enough to evaluate the urethra by means of bougies *à boule*, for passage of a bougie must in some measure dilate the stricture. Increasing experience suggests that the only safe way to evaluate a stricture is to observe it by urethroscopy, and to document it by urethrography. However, when assessed by all available methods, it seems that internal urethrotomy alone gives adequate control (that is it avoids the need for further treatment) in about half the patients for at least a year. It has the supreme advantage that it is safe, it is quick, and it can easily be repeated. However, when it has been tried and has failed, then one should consider more permanent methods of curing a urethral stricture, that is urethroplasty. The method of urethroplasty is determined by the site and nature of the stricture.

Meatal stricture

A soft stricture often forms just inside the external meatus after instrumentation or transurethral surgery. As a rule, these strictures only need to be gently dilated on three or four occasions to remain open permanently. They probably can be prevented by the use of a prophylactic internal urethrotomy with the

Otis or similar urethrotome before starting a transurethral resection.

Others are seen associated with *balanitis xerotica obliterans (Lichen sclerosus et atrophicus)*: they return as soon as they are dilated, and should be treated by meatoplasty. Certain congenital strictures in very small boys may need incision *(meatotomy)*, and this can always be tried once.

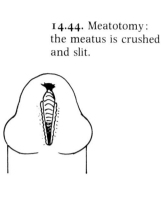

14.44. Meatotomy: the meatus is crushed and slit.

Meatotomy

Crush the meatus with mosquito forceps and incise it (14.44). Smear the incision with sterile vaseline, and instruct the mother to keep the end parted by gently manipulating it in the bath each day. An older child may be shown how to insert a suitable dilator (the plastic guard from a disposable intramuscular needle is about the right size) every day for a month.

Meatoplasty

In *balanitis xerotica obliterans*, and when meatotomy has failed, a ∩-shaped flap of skin is let into the slit urethra to keep it permanently open (Blandy & Tresidder 1967). If the patient has not been circumcised, begin by making a formal circumcision (page 192) but form the ∩-shaped flap in doing so. If the patient has been circumcised, begin by making the ∩-shaped flap (14.45, 14.46). Let it hang down, and open the terminal centimetre of the urethra: in *balanitis xerotica obliterans* the narrow zone may extend up the urethra for 2–3 cm. Sew the flap into the opened-up urethra using interrupted 4-0 or 5-0 catgut (14.47). By taking care in shaping the flap, one can end up with a very normal-looking meatus, but the patient must be warned that despite all your care, when he voids, he will spray (14.48).

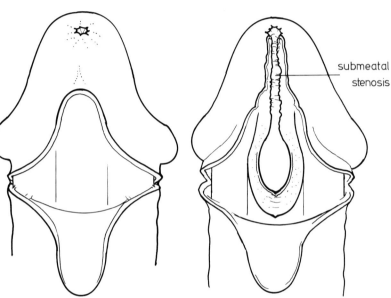

submeatal stenosis

14.45. Meatoplasty: a ∩-shaped flap is formed from the ventral penile skin and allowed to drop back.

14.46. The stenosed distal urethra is opened right down into healthy corpus spongiosum.

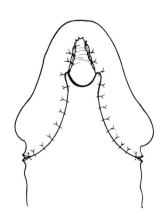

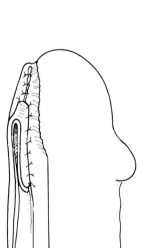

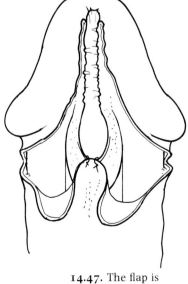

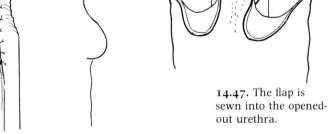

14.48. End-result of meatoplasty: the flap forms a permanent inlay with a long elliptical suture line which, even allowing for contracture, will not stenose again.

14.47. The flap is sewn into the opened-out urethra.

Short strictures of the anterior urethra

Today the one-stage island patch has become the standard method of urethroplasty, and needs no special preparations or equipment (Blandy & Singh 1975; Blandy 1980).

Position on the table

As for cystoscopy.

Anaesthetic

Profound general anaesthesia is needed, with every effort to avoid an erection.

Steps of the operation

Pass a 22/24 Ch bougie down to the stricture and have it held firmly in the midline. Cut down on to the stricture through the scrotal skin rather than the shaft of the penis (14.49). To obtain access to the anterior part of the urethra, it may be necessary to evaginate the shaft of the penis a little (14.50). This

manoeuvre adds a little to the difficulty of the operation, but avoids tension on the skin of the shaft of the penis and the risk of post-operative fistula.

Cut down on to the urethra and open it right along the full length of the stricture until healthy corpus spongiosum has been opened (14.51). Run a 4-0 haemostatic catgut suture along the bleeding edges of the corpus spongiosum to prevent bleeding (14.52).

Make a template for the patch, using tin foil from a catgut package, and mould it over a bougie about 24 Ch in calibre. Select a suitable part of scrotal skin from the edge of the incision and plan to provide it with a dartos pedicle that will stretch easily along the length of the stricture in the penile urethra. The skin is now separated from the pedicle with scissors

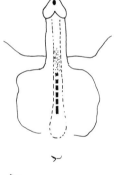

14.49. One-stage island patch urethroplasty for strictures in the penile urethra. To avoid making an incision in the skin of the penis itself, the shaft of the penis is everted through an incision in the scrotum.

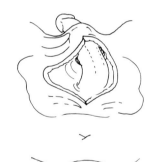

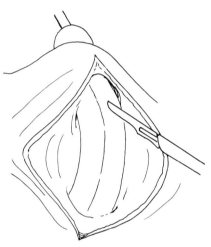

14.50. The whole length of the stricture is laid open.

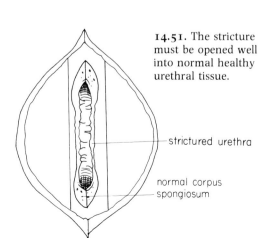

14.51. The stricture must be opened well into normal healthy urethral tissue.

strictured urethra

normal corpus spongiosum

14.52. Haemostasis with a running suture through the urethral mucosa and the outer layer of the corpus spongiosum.

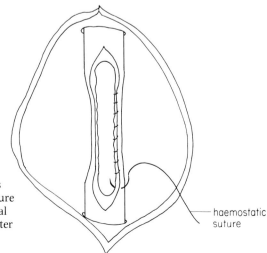

haemostatic suture

(14.53) that enter the plane between dartos and skin. It is important to take pains to ensure that the incision only goes through the skin and not the dartos as well.

The patch with its muscular blood supply can now be turned over and sewn into the defect in the urethra (14.54). Use 3-0 chromic catgut and attempt when possible to keep the knots on the outside of the new urethra. Before closing it, making sure that a 16 Ch silicone catheter sits comfortably along the urethra and in the bladder (14.55).

If it has been necessary to evert the penis, return it to its normal position and close the incision in the scrotum with everting fine nylon mattress sutures. A thin Penrose drain is left at the inferior edge of the incision and a compression dressing of Reston foam is kept in position with a T-bandage for the first twenty-four hours to prevent haematoma formation.

Replacing the anterior urethra after previous hypospadias repair

Adults are seen with severe chordee, fistulae, and stricture, in whom previous attempts, often multiple, have been made to repair a hypospadias. The penile skin is often very scarred and damaged, and there are often a number of fistulae. To attempt to make use of this skin is to invite disaster (Flynn *et al.* 1980).

Steps of the operation

Holding the penis up straight with a suture, a circumferential incision is made just proximal to the corona glandis, and the entire skin sleeve of the penis is dissected back to expose the shaft. In doing this dissection, the small fistulae are cut across, but at this stage, disregarded (14.56).

Often there is a very severe chordee, as if the original new urethra formed from a buried skin strip (the usual method employed in former times for hypospadias) has failed to keep up with the growth of the penis. The entire scarred and stenosed urethra is dissected away, down to healthy tissue. As this is done, so the penis is straightened out (14.57).

One may check that the chordee has been corrected by injecting saline into a corpus cavernosum after applying a tourniquet to the base.

Using tin foil from a catgut package as a template, moulded over a 24 Ch bougie, measure the length and width of skin patch

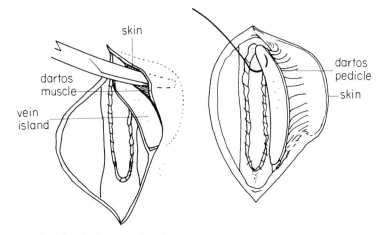

14.53. An island of scrotal skin is cut and provided with a pedicle of dartos.

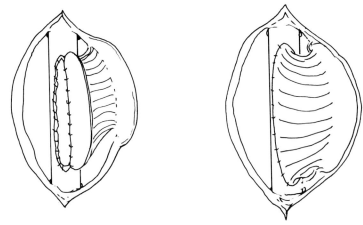

14.54. Skin island sewn into defect in urethra.

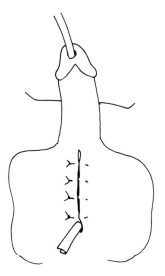

14.55. Scrotal incision closed. The shaft of the penis is not incised.

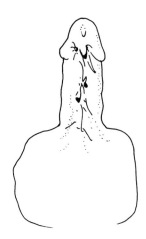

14.56. Late result of hypospadias operated on many times previously: there are multiple fistulae, scarring and chordee as well as a stricture.

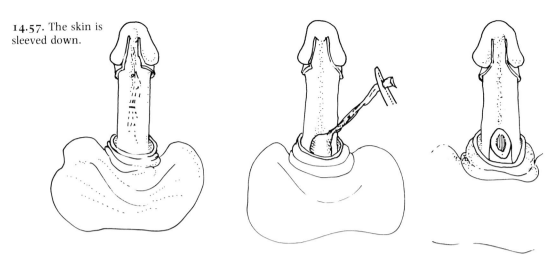

14.57. The skin is sleeved down.

that is needed to bridge the gap with a complete new skin tube formed from a dartos-pedicled island patch. The skin is most conveniently supplied from the scrotal skin, and given a pedicle that is based anteriorly and can be swung up to fill the gap (14.58). The skin patch and pedicle are formed as in the previous description, leaving a long elliptical defect in the scrotum. The skin patch is sewn into a tube over a 16 Ch silicone catheter (14.59), and drawn up inside the sleeve of

penile skin until it reaches the tip of the glans, where it is sutured, the seam of the skin tube being attached with a few interrupted 3-0 chromic sutures to the midline underneath the corpora cavernosa (14.60). The proximal end of the skin tube is similarly anastomosed to the opened out healthy part of the urethra. Finally the penile skin sleeve is drawn back over the new skin tube, and the defect in the scrotum is closed with a Penrose drain (14.61).

The silicone catheter is left in position for fourteen days.

14.58. Using tin foil as a template, a patch of skin large enough to replace the missing urethra is marked out on the skin.

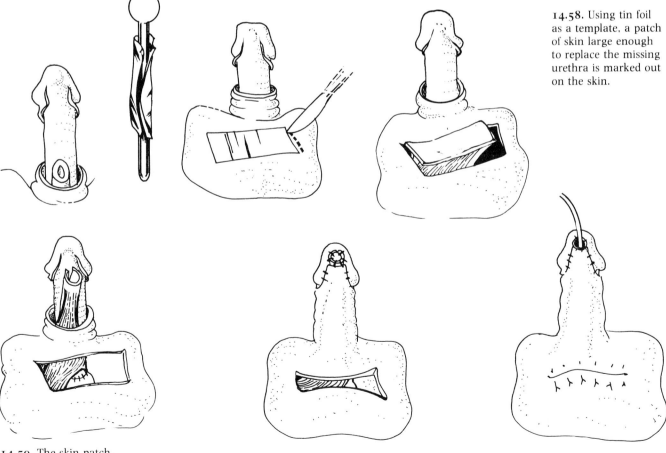

14.59. The skin patch, on a dartos pedicle, is formed into a tube.

14.60. New skin tube sewn in position.

14.61. Completion of restoration.

Follow-up

Although this operation gives a very satisfactory new urethra and the chordee correction provides a very serviceable penis, some patients find that the dartos pedicle stands out under the skin of the scrotum like a bowstring, especially when the penis is erect. Twice I have had to divide this pedicle at a second operation after three or four months when the skin tube has picked up a good secondary blood supply. Another minor problem has been the appearance of hairs at the end of the glans penis.

Complicated and infected strictures of the anterior urethra

Some old strictures are seen in which many para-urethral abscesses and fistulae as well as old scarring make it impossible to perform the operation in a single stage. Here it is more safe to revert to the old two-stage urethroplasty of Johanson & Swinney. In the first stage all the diseased tissue is cut out, leaving a long defect in the penile shaft (14.62). Since this may provide insufficient skin for an effective reconstruction, at the end of the first stage a flap of scrotal skin is rotated into the defect (14.63).

After three or four months, the urethra is reconstructed from this scrotal inlay, rolling a skin tube over a 24 Ch bougie, closing it with interrupted 4-0 sutures, and bringing the skin over it.

Short strictures in the bulbar urethra —one-stage island patch

Indications

Nearly any stricture in the bulbar or membranous urethra may be repaired in a single stage by using a modification of the island patch urethroplasty (Blandy & Singh 1975; Vijayan & Sundin 1983).

Steps of the operation

The patient is in the lithotomy position. Prophylactic antimicrobial cover is given with metronidazole and ampicillin, against Gram-negative infection and the spore bearing organisms so prevalent in the perineum.

Anaesthetic

A hypotensive anaesthetic is not essential, but one should avoid any technique that invites erection or congestion of the penis.

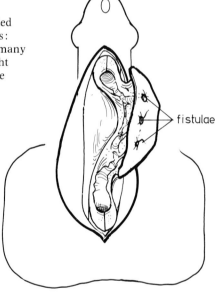

14.62. Complicated anterior strictures: where there are many fistulae and a tight chordee the entire diseased corpus spongiosum is removed.

fistulae

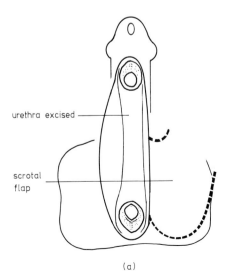

urethra excised

scrotal flap

(a)

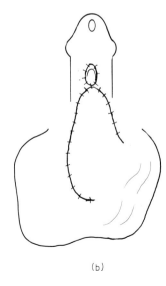

(b)

14.63. The gap left by removing the diseased urethra and straightening out the chordee is filled (a) by means of a skin flap taken from the adjacent scrotum which is rotated up (b) into the defect.

Steps of the operation

A ∩-shaped scrotal flap is formed, with a rather flat apex and each limb ending up just anterior to the ischial tuberosity (14.64). If the flap is not taken sufficiently far back there is insufficient access to the bulbar urethra and unnecessary difficulty in suturing the flap in position. The incision is carried through skin and dartos, sealing the small vessels carefully, step by step, but avoiding diathermy on the flap side for fear of coagulating vessels in its base. Keep a generous lining of fat on the flap and try not to disturb the vessels and nerves in the base of the flap. The flap is allowed to hang down (14.65).

Pass a 24 Ch bougie down to the face of the stricture and have it held steady in the midline to identify the urethra. Dissect down in the midline until the bulbospongiosus muscle is found (14.66). Separate the muscle from the bulb, divide it in the midline and reflect each half to either side like the pages of a book (14.67). Incise the urethra in the midline directly on to the bougie about 2 cm downstream of the obstruction. The normal corpus spongiosum will bleed smartly from the open spongy tissue, and this should be controlled with a running 4-0 chromic catgut suture bit by bit as the incision is extended, otherwise there is a continual ooze of blood that makes the subsequent operation more difficult (14.68).

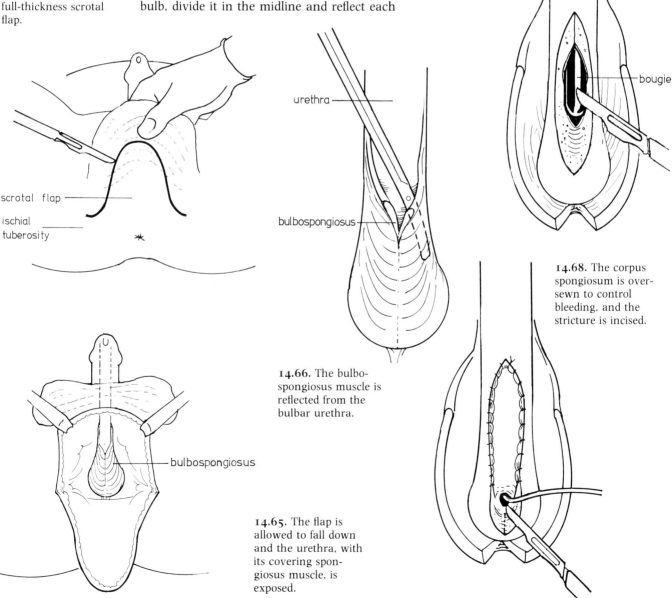

14.64. Short stricture in the bulb: the one-stage island patch operation. Outline a full-thickness scrotal flap.

scrotal flap

ischial tuberosity

14.65. The flap is allowed to fall down and the urethra, with its covering spongiosus muscle, is exposed.

bulbospongiosus

urethra

bulbospongiosus

14.66. The bulbo-spongiosus muscle is reflected from the bulbar urethra.

14.67. The urethra is opened on to a bougie, just distal to the stricture.

bougie

14.68. The corpus spongiosum is over-sewn to control bleeding, and the stricture is incised.

The stricture must be incised right up until healthy tissue is reached and in a bulbar stricture, this is often to within a few millimetres of the verumontanum. Make the incision a centimetre at a time and keep control of the bleeding by running the haemostatic suture along on each side. It is essential to carry the incision right past the stricture, and the only way to make sure is to put a finger in the urethra and feel that there are no strands of undivided scar tissue.

Insert a nasal speculum upside down to reveal the verumontanum and the edge of urethra at the lower end of the prostatic cavity (14.69).

Mark out the skin patch from the tip of the scrotal flap, measuring it with a tin foil template if necessary. The scrotal skin should be stretched with skin hooks, and the incision should just go through the dermis, not through the underlying dartos. Develop the plane between dartos and skin with dissecting scissors until the patch can be brought into the urethra without any tension at all (14.70).

Stitching the patch into the defect in the urethra is made easier if a 3-0 chromic catgut needle is first partially straightened out (14.71). Holding it in a needle-holder so that it almost points straight ahead, pass the needle up under the edge of the urethra, and as the tip of the needle emerges in the lumen of the urethra, grasp it with a long needle-catcher or artery forceps, and advance it up towards the bladder until the catgut emerges behind the shank of the needle (14.72). Needle and catgut can then be withdrawn. Five stitches are placed in this manner, and threaded through the tip of the skin patch

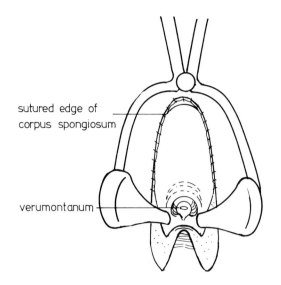

14.69. The incision of the stricture is continued until you emerge into healthy urethra and can see the verumontanum, using a nasal speculum.

sutured edge of corpus spongiosum

verumontanum

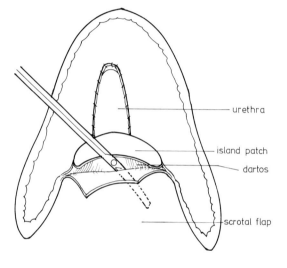

urethra

island patch

dartos

scrotal flap

14.70. An island patch is prepared from the skin at the tip of the scrotal flap, and is provided with its own dartos pedicle.

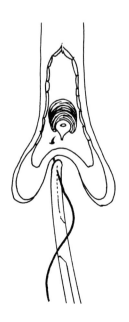

14.72. The modified needle is advanced under the edge of the urethra until its tip is seen, when it can be seized and taken up towards the bladder until the needle is free.

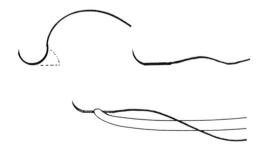

14.71. Preparing 3-0 catgut needle for urethroplasty. The curved shank is straightened out.

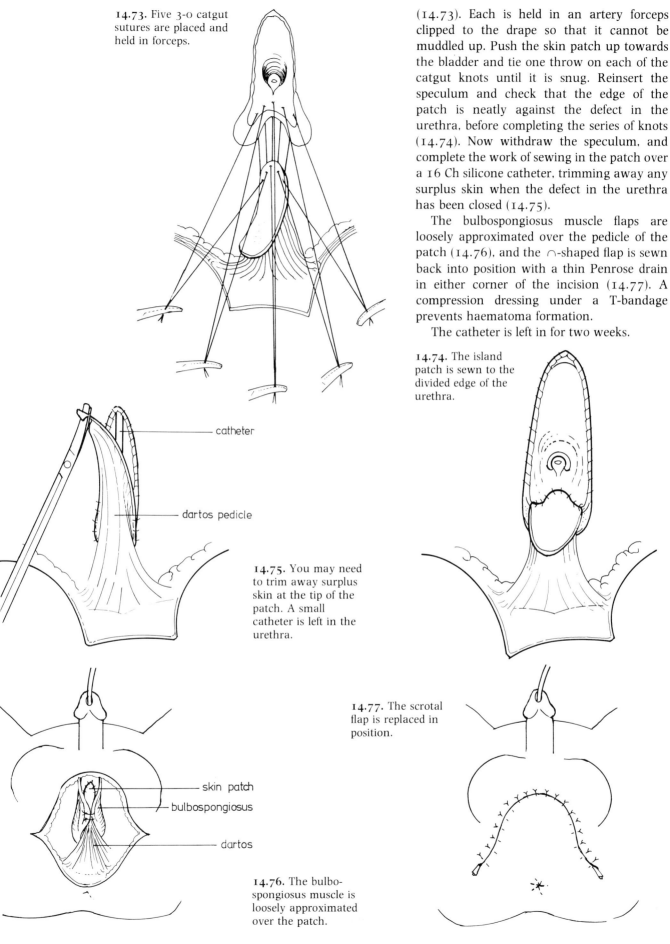

14.73. Five 3-0 catgut sutures are placed and held in forceps.

(14.73). Each is held in an artery forceps clipped to the drape so that it cannot be muddled up. Push the skin patch up towards the bladder and tie one throw on each of the catgut knots until it is snug. Reinsert the speculum and check that the edge of the patch is neatly against the defect in the urethra, before completing the series of knots (14.74). Now withdraw the speculum, and complete the work of sewing in the patch over a 16 Ch silicone catheter, trimming away any surplus skin when the defect in the urethra has been closed (14.75).

The bulbospongiosus muscle flaps are loosely approximated over the pedicle of the patch (14.76), and the ∩-shaped flap is sewn back into position with a thin Penrose drain in either corner of the incision (14.77). A compression dressing under a T-bandage prevents haematoma formation.

The catheter is left in for two weeks.

14.74. The island patch is sewn to the divided edge of the urethra.

catheter

dartos pedicle

14.75. You may need to trim away surplus skin at the tip of the patch. A small catheter is left in the urethra.

14.77. The scrotal flap is replaced in position.

skin patch

bulbospongiosus

dartos

14.76. The bulbospongiosus muscle is loosely approximated over the patch.

Infected or complicated strictures of the posterior urethra: two-stage scrotal flap urethroplasty

Indications

Today the two-stage scrotal flap urethroplasty is very seldom indicated, for there is hardly a case that cannot be dealt with using the dartos-pedicled one-stage method. However, it is still useful when there are many fistulae and much sepsis, as in the classical watering-can perineum of the neglected case (Kinn & Fritjofsson 1983).

Steps of the operation

The scrotal flap is raised with a broad posterior base as described above for the one-stage operation. In the type of patient for which one may consider a two-stage repair, it may not be possible to choose just which part of the scrotal skin to select, but begin by cutting out all the diseased tissue and making the best of what is left over. The principle of the ∩-shaped flap can easily be adapted to any part of the scrotum (14.78).

Having cut away all the diseased tissues, the urethra is slit open as far as may be needed to get right past the strictured tissue in each direction. A series of sutures using 3-0 catgut is now placed between the apex of the flap and the proximal limit of the incision in the urethra (14.79). Five sutures are placed first and the flap drawn into position (14.80). Then the scrotum is closed around the laid-open urethra with adequate drainage (14.81).

Today it is very rare to find a stricture that

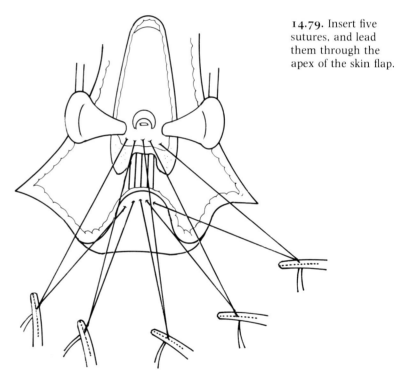

14.78. Modified scrotal flap for use in presence of old scarring or fistulae in the midline: base the flap on one or other side.

old scars and fistulae

14.79. Insert five sutures, and lead them through the apex of the skin flap.

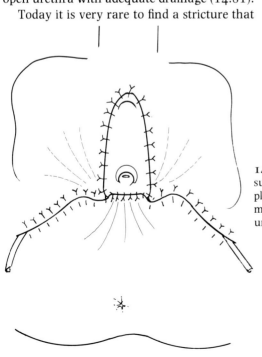

14.81. The other sutures are now placed so as to approximate scrotal skin to urethra all round.

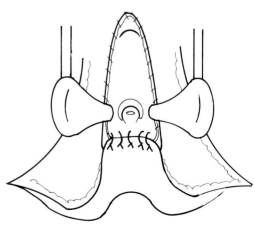

14.80. The top five sutures are tied, bringing the flap up into the opened-out urethra.

extends the whole length of the urethra, but when it is found, and when it cannot be dealt with by a pair of dartos-pedicled patches in a single stage, then the scrotum is cleft and the urethra slit up right to the end of the penis (14.82).

Second stage

After about six weeks (an interval which depends upon many individual circumstances) a new urethra is formed. A complete tube of skin is raised over a 24 Ch bougie that acts as a guide to the size of the urethra (14.83). The skin tube is closed over a 16 Ch silicone rubber catheter using continuous 3-0 catgut (14.84). If the bulbospongiosus muscle can be found, it is approximated over the skin tube (14.85) and the skin is freed up and brought together

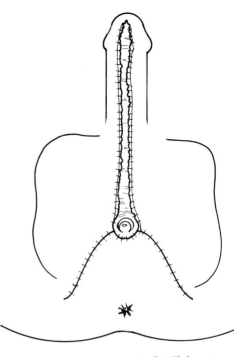

14.82. If the stricture goes the whole length of the urethra the strictured urethra is slit up and sewn to the skin all the way along.

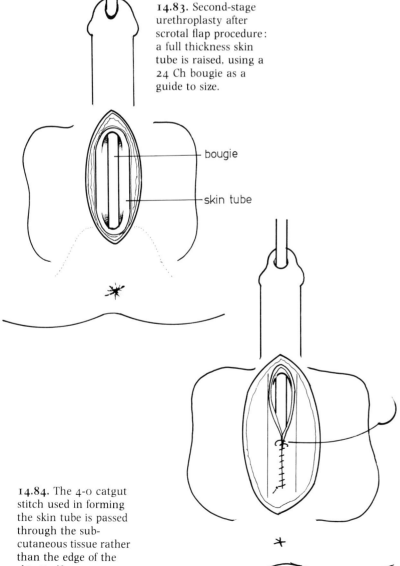

14.83. Second-stage urethroplasty after scrotal flap procedure: a full thickness skin tube is raised, using a 24 Ch bougie as a guide to size.

bougie

skin tube

14.84. The 4-0 catgut stitch used in forming the skin tube is passed through the sub-cutaneous tissue rather than the edge of the skin itself.

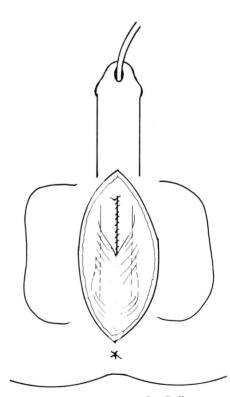

14.85. Bulbospongiosus muscle is approximated over the new skin tube. A thin 14 Ch cather is left *in situ.*

with interrupted mattress sutures of 3-0 nylon (14.86).

Hazards of urethroplasty operations

No procedure for urethral stricture is perfect. Necrosis of the tip of the scrotal flap may occur whether it is continuous or provided with a dartos myocutaneous pedicle. The advantage of the two-stage operation is that this necrosis can be detected and the flap revised within a few days of operation (14.87).

Reactionary haemorrhage is today largely prevented by meticulous haemostasis to the cut edge of the corpus spongiosum. Infection and haematoma still occur, but not with untoward frequency.

Since in many patients where there is a very high stricture the incision through the narrowed area seems to cross the external sphincter, incontinence may occur if the internal sphincter has been damaged. But, contrary to what might be expected, even when the patient has had to undergo prostatectomy, continence is not always threatened (Edwards *et al.* 1972; Colapinto & McCallum 1976). Impotence may follow any urological operation: it was noted in one of my patients, and may have gone unreported by others. Hair continues to grow, however carefully one attempts depilation between stages in the two-stage procedure. It appears to occur when the patch has become too baggy, and probably occurs only when there is some degree of stenosis at the downstream end of the patch.

High strictures of the membranous urethra

Although the initial management of the ruptured urethra should provide only short easy strictures that can be divided with the optical urethrotome, or that offer themselves to a one-stage island patch, it is still alas all too common for men to be referred with an unreduced fracture and an unreduced prostate. Separating the lower bulbar urethra from the upper prostatic urethra may be a thick mass of dense scar tissue, and these may be some of the most difficult strictures with which we have to deal.

Internal urethrotomy

When there has been little displacement, or when care has been taken to realign the disrupted urethra (page 214) there is usually an S-shaped bend (14.29). This may be cut with

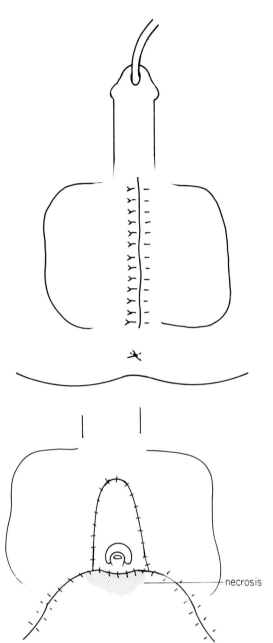

14.86. The scrotum is closed over the skin tube.

necrosis

14.87. Sloughing of the tip of the flap may occur; if unremedied, this leads to stenosis. The slough should be excised and the flap resutured in position.

the Storz–Sachse optical urethrotome, or failing this instrument, with a Collings knife or bee-sting electrode. Careful follow-up is needed in these patients, and one must be prepared to repeat the internal urethrotomy on several occasions (Chilton *et al.* 1983).

This procedure may still be successfully carried out even when the lumen has been entirely lost, and only a suprapubic tube has been used in the management of the disrupted urethra. A cystoscope or a flexible endoscope may be introduced through the suprapubic cystostomy, and its light used to guide the bee-sting electrode or Sachse knife (14.30).

Urethroplasty for difficult high strictures

Even with all these tricks it may still not be possible to find a way through the stricture.

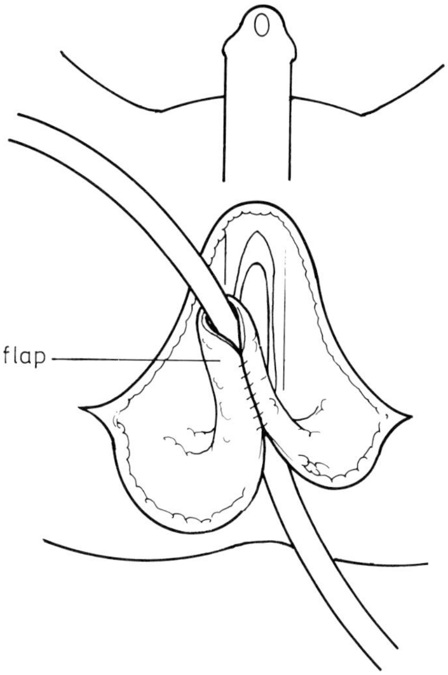

14.88. Forming skin tube from the scrotal flap and in the tubed flap modification urethroplasty.

tubed scrotal flap

channel for skin tube

retaining buttons

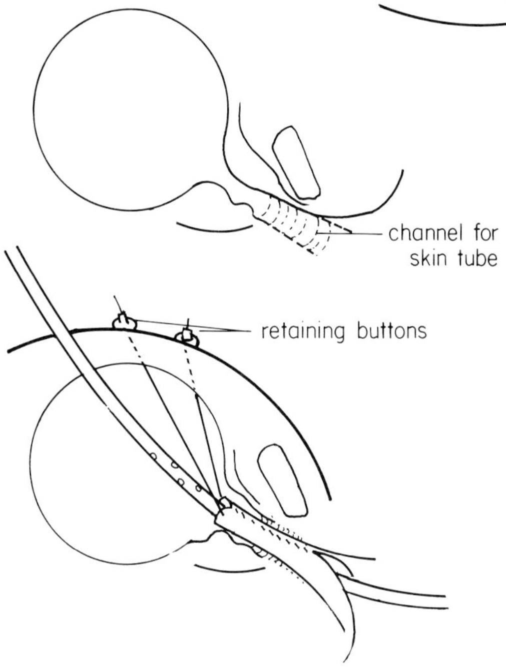

14.89. The catheter and tube are drawn up into the bladder and held there with a suprapubic button.

urethral bulb

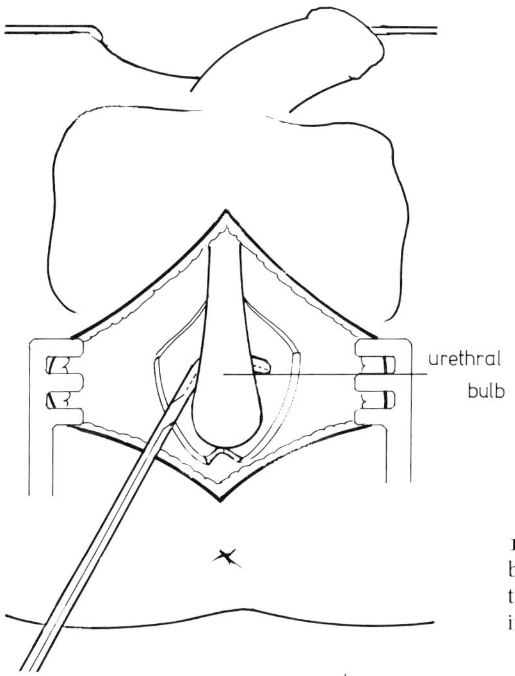

14.90. Mobilizing the bulbar urethra through the perineal incision.

After apparently successful urethrotomy some strictures return quickly, or there may be other complications such that urethroplasty is needed.

If the stricture is short, use the pedicled patch technique described above (page 221). If the stricture is very long and the fibrous tissue so dense as to be completely confusing, the scrotal flap may be adapted by forming it into a tube, skin side inside (14.88), attaching the tip of the tube to a stout nylon suture, and then, after carving a way through the scar tissue up into the bladder, pulling up the skin tube by means of the nylon into the bladder (14.89). After about three weeks, the nylon suture is removed and when the urethra is inspected, it will be seen that the skin tube has stuck to the raw abnormal part of the cavity, but where there is normal epithelium, for example the prostatic urethra and verumontanum, this is still visible and healthy. The second stage is carried out after six to eight weeks as described above (page 228).

Transpubic urethroplasty

A better procedure which is adaptable to the majority of these high membranous injuries is a modification of the transpubic urethroplasty described by Waterhouse *et al.* (1974). First, a midline perineal incision is made, and the bulbar urethra dissected out of its leaves of bulbospongiosus muscle. The bulbar urethra is separated by sharp dissection from the underneath of the corpora cavernosa, and followed upwards until it disappears into scar tissue at the site of rupture (14.90, 14.91).

14.91. The bulbar urethra is detached at the site of the stricture.

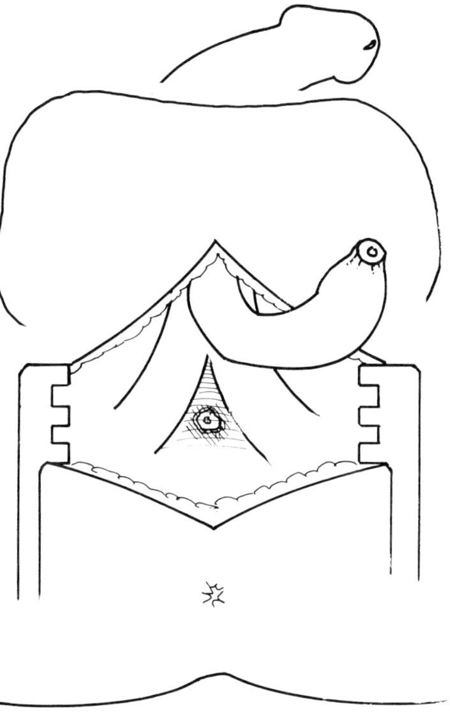

The two corpora cavernosa are now visible, diverging from the midline. One may dissect between them in the septum and separate them from each other (14.92). Small holes in the spongy tissue of the corpora must be carefully sutured with catgut to control bleeding. Retracting the two corpora allows access to the inferior edge of the symphysis pubis (14.93).

Through a separate Pfannenstiel incision, the bladder is opened and a bougie passed down from above. At this stage one may be able to feel the tip of the bougie peeping out just under the inferior edge of the symphysis, and one can incise down upon it without having to take away any of the bone of the symphysis (14.94). More often one must remove an arc or window from the inferior edge of the symphysis to get enough room to bring the bulbar urethra up to the prostatic urethra without tension.

To remove this window, first mark out a semicircle with the diathermy point on the periosteum and perichondrium of the symphysis (14.95). Take a periosteal elevator and scrape this layer away to lay the bone bare. Using an oscillating bone saw, cut along the semicircle (14.96). The oscillating action of the bone saw will allow you to cut only through

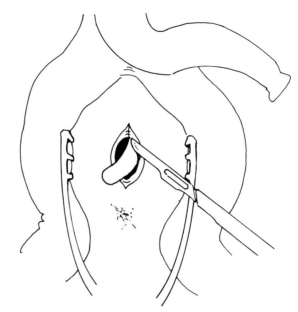

14.94. One may be able to feel the lower edge of the prostatic urethra by passing a bougie retrogradely.

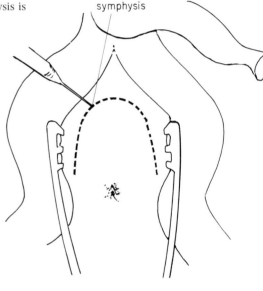

14.95. The periosteum over the symphysis is incised with the diathermy.

periosteum of symphysis

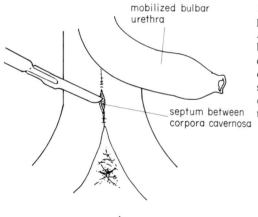

mobilized bulbar urethra

septum between corpora cavernosa

14.92. Modified transpubic urethroplasty. After mobilizing the bulbar urethra it is elevated, and the corpora cavernosa are separated from each other by dissecting in the midline.

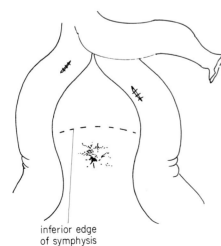

inferior edge of symphysis

14.93. Separating the corpora reveals the lower edge of the symphysis pubis.

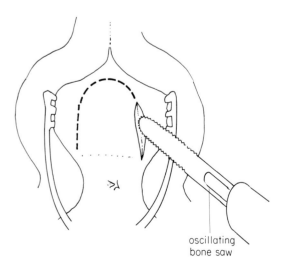

oscillating bone saw

14.96. An oscillating bone saw cuts out an arch.

bone; it will not damage soft tissue, so that it cannot injure the soft tissues of the pelvis. The free semi-circular piece of bone is now removed with bone-nibbling forceps, and you find yourself looking at the layer of periosteum on the inner aspect of the symphysis pubis (14.97). This must be deliberately incised before making the anastomosis. Feel again for the bougie that was passed down from the bladder. It may be easy to cut down upon it and make a generous elliptical window in the lower and anterior end of the prostatic urethra. In some patients it may be necessary to dissect the prostate off the back of the symphysis, and to deliberately cut out the window of periosteum before making this anastomosis; one must do whatever is most easy and provides the best access (14.98).

The bulbar urethra is now spatulated, led through the gap under the symphysis, and joined on to the prostatic urethra with a series of interrupted 3-0 chromic catgut sutures over an appropriate 16 Ch silicone rubber catheter (14.99).

The advantage of this modification of the transpubic operation is twofold: first, there is no disturbance of the integrity of the pelvic girdle and hence no interference with walking and running; second, the removal of a small window from the underside of the symphysis does not leave a large gap in the front of the pelvis into which the penis may fall—this may give rise to a most distressing deformity.

Urethrorectal fistula

Fistulae between urethra and rectum are fortunately rare. They occur after accidental injury during prostatectomy—especially an open prostatectomy done for cancer or stones in the prostate—after injury and after radiotherapy for cancer, usually of the uterus. Two methods for closing these fistulae were developed by Parks and they have superseded any other in my practice.

Low prostatorectal fistulae

A Parks' retractor is inserted into the anal canal. The fistula is circumcised, after infiltrating the submucosa with 1:200 000 adrenaline–saline, and an ellipse of the mucosa is

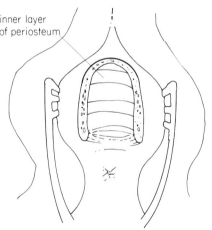

14.97. When the bony arch is removed, the inner layer of periosteum separates you from the prostate.

inner layer of periosteum

14.98. Incising the periosteum. It may be necessary to approach it through a retropubic dissection.

inner layer of periosteum of symphysis

urethra

14.99. The spatulated urethra is anastomosed to the lower end of the prostatic urethra.

removed (14.100) with scissors dissection, leaving the circular muscle of the anal canal exposed.

Then a full thickness flap of rectal wall is dissected off the posterior layer of Denonvilliers' fascia (14.101) for about 5 cm, freeing it up well above and to either side of the fistula track, which has been cut across.

No attempt is made to close the fistula, but the full thickness flap of rectal wall is now drawn down and sutured in two layers to the denuded circular muscle of the anal canal. One layer of sutures catches the muscle, the other the mucosa.

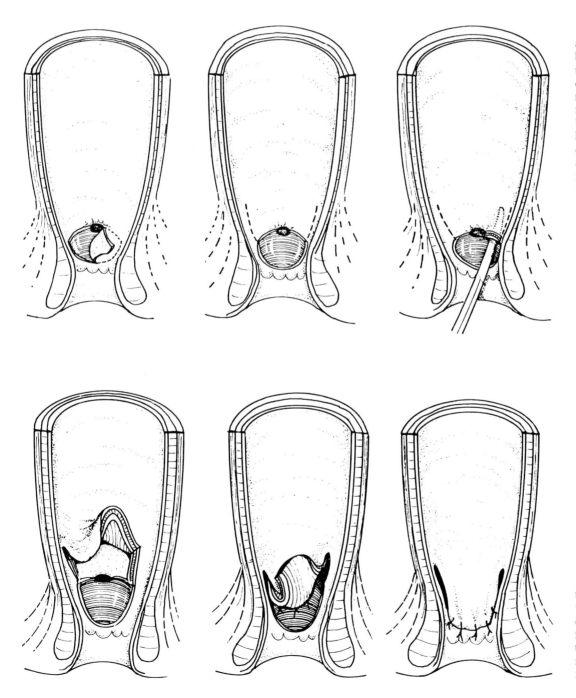

14.100. Parks' operation for fistula between prostatic urethra and anal canal. Via an anal retractor, an ellipse of mucosa is removed below the fistula, leaving the raw circular muscle. Then a full-thickness flap of rectal wall is elevated above the fistula.

14.101. The full-thickness flap of rectal wall is now drawn down to cover the fistula, and secured in two layers to the muscle and the mucosa.

14.102. The left colon is mobilized, if necessary, by dividing the splenic flexure.

High prostato- and vesicorectal fistulae

Again, the operation is preceded by a colostomy. The left colon is mobilized, if necessary by dividing the splenic flexure (14.102). The rectum is transected at a convenient distance above the fistula (14.103). Using 1:200 000 adrenaline–saline, the mucosa is lifted off the circular muscle of the rectum by injecting into the upper cut edge of transected rectum, as well as by a second assistant injecting through an anal rectractor (14.104). In this way the mucosa and muscularis mucosae are removed as a sleeve from the rectum from the point of transection down to the dentate line, leaving a raw inner surface. Again, the fistula

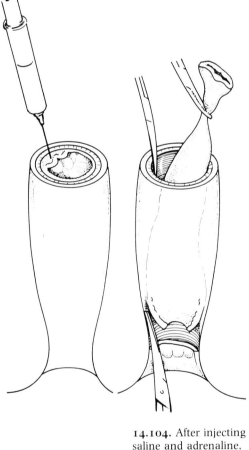

14.104. After injecting saline and adrenaline, the mucosa is separated from the circular muscle, leaving raw muscle to line the rectum.

14.103. The rectum is transected at a convenient distance above the fistula.

is cut across, but no attempt is made to close it (14.105).

Now the mobilized colon is drawn down through the sleeve of rectum and made to lie in such a way that the mesentery faces the fistula to lend extra thickness of tissue to the closure.

The full thickness of colon is now anastomosed to the edge of the anal mucosa, working through the anal retractor, and not everting the anal canal.

The advantage of these operations is that full thickness healthy rectal or colonic wall is made to close the defect, but at the same time the proprioceptive sensation and the control of continence in the bowel wall is not interfered with (14.106) (Tiptaft *et al.* 1983).

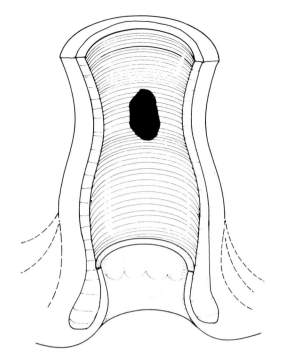

14.105. No attempt is made to close the fistula.

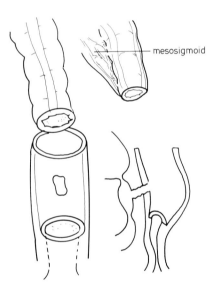

mesosigmoid

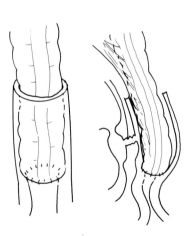

14.106. The mobilized sigmoid is brought through the raw sleeve of rectal muscle, which retains the sensation of fullness, and so preserves continence.

References

Al-Ali I.H. & Husain I. (1983) Disrupting injuries of the membranous urethra—the case for early surgery and catheter splinting. *Brit. J. Urol.* **55**, 716.

Attwater H.L. (1943) The history of urethral stricture. *Brit. J. Urol.* **15**, 39.

Blandy J.P. (1980) Urethral stricture. *Postgrad. Med. J.* **56**, 383.

Blandy J.P. & Singh M. (1975) The technique and results of One-stage Island Patch urethroplasty. *Brit. J. Urol.* **47**, 83.

Blandy J.P. & Tresidder G.C. (1967) Meatoplasty. *Brit. J. Urol.* **39**, 261.

Byars L.T. (1955) A technique for consistently satisfactory repair of hypospadias. *Surg. Gynec. Obstet.* **100**, 184.

Chilton C.F., Shah P.J.R., Fowler C.G., Tiptaft R.C. & Blandy J.P. (1983) The impact of optical urethrotomy on the management of urethral strictures in the context of the long-term follow-up of urethroplasty. *Brit. J. Urol.* **55**, 705.

Colapinto V. & McCallum R.W. (1976) Urinary continence after repair of membranous urethral stricture in prostatectomised patients. *J. Urol.* **115**, 392.

Duckett J.W. (1981) MAGPI (meatoplasty and glanuloplasty). A procedure for subcoronal hypospadias. *Urol. Clin. North Amer.* **8**, 513.

Eckstein H., Hohenfellner R. & Williams D.I. (eds.) (1977) *Surgical Pediatric Urology*. Thieme, Stuttgart.

Edwards L.E., Singh M., Notley R.G. & Whitaker R.H. (1972) Continence after scrotal flap urethroplasty. *Brit. J. Urol.* **44**, 23.

Flynn J.T., Johnston S.R. & Blandy J.P. (1980) Late sequelae of hypospadias repair. *Brit. J. Urol.* **52**, 555.

Glass R.E., Flynn J.T., King J.B. & Blandy J.P. (1978) Urethral injury and fractured pelvis. *Brit. J. Urol.* **50**, 578.

Hayes E.E., Sandler C.M. & Corriere J.N. (1983) Management of the ruptured bladder secondary to blunt abdominal trauma. *J. Urol.* **129**, 946.

Hodgson N.B. (1970) A one-stage hypospadias repair. *J. Urol.* **104**, 281.

Kinn A.C. & Fritjofsson A. (1983) Experience with two-stage scrotal flap urethroplasty for stricture. *Brit. J. Urol.* **55**, 57.

Patterson D.E., Barrett D.M., Myers R.P., DeWeerd J.H., Hall B.B. & Benson R.C. (1983) Primary management of posterior urethral injuries. *J. Urol.* **129**, 573.

Szemat-Nikolajenko R. & Cukier J. (1978) *Valves et Diaphragmes Congenitaux de l'uretre chez l'homme adulte. (Memoire pour le titre d'Assistant Etranger)*. University of Paris, Faculty of Medicine, Necker.

Tiptaft R.C., Motson R.W., Costello A.J., Paris A.M.I. & Blandy J.P. (1983) Fistulae involving rectum and urethra: the place of Parks' operations. *Brit. J. Urol.* **55**, 711.

Vijayan P. & Sundin T. (1983) Island patch urethroplasty: effects on urinary flow and ejaculation. *Brit. J. Urol.* **55**, 69.

Waterhouse K., Abrahams J.I., Caponegro P., Hackett R.E., Patil U.B. & Peng B.K. (1974) The transpubic repair of membranous urethral strictures. *J. Urol.* **111**, 118.

Chapter 15
Surgery of the testicle

Approach to the testicle through a scrotal incision

Many operations on the testicle, however trivial, are done through the scrotal approach but for years this has been dogged by the complication of haematoma. This can be avoided by following the technique taught to me by Howard Hanley (1963). Holding the testicle firmly, stroke the knife through all layers one by one, diathermizing even the most trivial of vessels, until the parietal layer of the tunica vaginalis is seen (15.1). Strip the skin and dartos off the testis in a single layer, until the testicle emerges through the incision by the pressure of your hand (15.2). As it emerges, continue to wipe away all the layers of covering tissue with a gauze swab.

When the operation is over, make sure that each little bleeding vessel has been sealed with the diathermy. Place an Allis forceps on each end of the incision to seize the dartos. The testis falls back into position. Begin the closure with a 4-0 catgut suture which takes up the dartos and all the underlying connective tissue (15.3). This is a haemostatic suture and must be firmly held up, its short end caught in a forceps (15.4). Using neat, closely set stitches, bring the dartos layer together and continue the same stitch back again in the subcuticular layer of the skin (15.5) until it can be tied to the free end of the catgut, allowing the knot

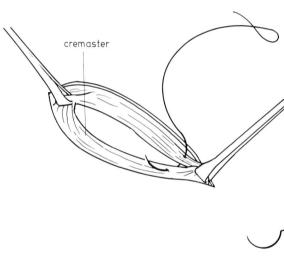

15.3. Closing the scrotal incision: a running 4-0 chromic catgut suture includes all the layers of tissue (which were reflected as one) in a continuous haemostatic stitch.

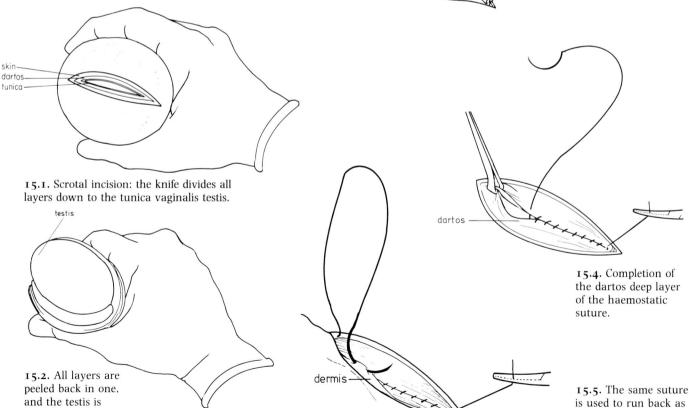

15.1. Scrotal incision: the knife divides all layers down to the tunica vaginalis testis.

15.2. All layers are peeled back in one, and the testis is delivered.

15.4. Completion of the dartos deep layer of the haemostatic suture.

15.5. The same suture is used to run back as a subcuticular stitch.

to fall back under the skin (15.6). This method leaves an inconspicuous scar, avoids the need to remove sutures, and provides excellent haemostasis.

Incisions in the scrotum should be placed transversely whenever possible, to follow the natural creases in the skin. After any operation, the scrotum should be elevated: the easiest method is to strap it up against the abdominal wall with strips of Micropore tape (15.7). Note that a drain is not only unnecessary but useless in the scrotum.

Biopsy of the testis

Indications

Biopsy of the testis may be useful when determining whether a patient whose semen contains no sperms at all has a block in the delivery system, or a failure of formation of sperms. It is probably not necessary if there is an elevation of the FSH and LH levels (when the outlook is hopeless) or when the patient has Klinefelter's syndrome, as detected in a buccal smear (Pryor *et al.* 1978).

Anaesthesia

General.

Position

Supine.

Steps of the operation

After cleaning the scrotum with betadine solution, the testis is held firmly in the hand. An incision is made down on to the tunica vaginalis, long enough to allow one to see it clearly (15.8). After incising the parietal layer, make a short stab incision into the visceral layer, to allow testicular tubules to bulge out (15.9). Snip off a tuft of tubules cleanly with

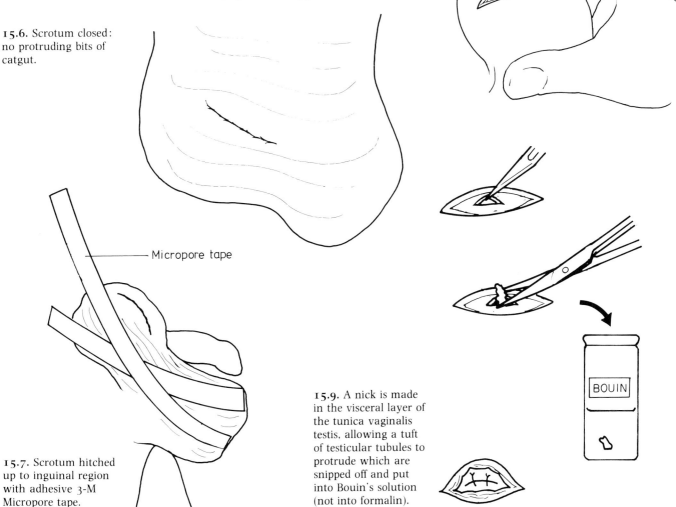

15.8. Testicular biopsy: a short incision is made over the testis.

15.6. Scrotum closed: no protruding bits of catgut.

Micropore tape

15.7. Scrotum hitched up to inguinal region with adhesive 3-M Micropore tape.

15.9. A nick is made in the visceral layer of the tunica vaginalis testis, allowing a tuft of testicular tubules to protrude which are snipped off and put into Bouin's solution (not into formalin).

BOUIN

fine sharp scissors (to avoid artifacts). Plunge scissors and biopsy at once into a specimen pot containing Bouin's solution (formaldehyde distorts the histological appearance of the testis). Close the incisions in the tunica with 4-0 catgut sutures, and close the scrotal skin in the way described above.

Epididymovasostomy

Indications

In infertile men whose semen show no sperms, whose FSH and LH levels are normal and whose testicular biopsy shows spermatogenesis, one must presume that there is a block somewhere in the delivery system. A vasogram should be performed to demonstrate that there is no blockage in the vas deferens or ejaculatory duct. If this has been ruled out, then one should aspirate fluid from the epididymis to confirm that sperms are present there, and finally proceed to bypass the blockage, presumed to be in the lower part of the epididymis, by anastomosing the distended upper epididymis to the normal vas deferens (Hendry et al. 1983).

Steps of the operation

Having exposed the testicle in the usual way, make a small incision into the vas deferens at the level of the caput epididymis, where you will (later on) make the anastomosis. Fine infant scalp vein cannulae fit the lumen of the vas (15.10). Inject 1 ml of water-soluble contrast medium towards the bladder and expose an X-ray film. This will show the contrast filling the vesicles and emerging in the urethra if the system is patent. One may attempt an epididymogram by injecting contrast medium towards the testis but my experience suggests that this investigation is futile. It is more useful to make sure that sperms are present in the congested upper third of the epididymis by aspirating some of the fluid, using a very fine intradermal needle and a tuberculin syringe. Examine the drop of fluid at once under a microscope, and do not be surprised if none of the sperms are motile. If sperms are present, go ahead and perform an epididymovasostomy.

Mobilize enough of the vas deferens to allow it to be brought without any tension against the caput epididymis. Secure it in this position with a few 4-0 catgut sutures that catch its adventitia without kinking it or entering its lumen.

Cut along the vas, to enlarge the opening that was made for the vasogram, and then make a long elliptical anastomosis between the wall of the vas deferens and the thin fascia that covers the epididymis, from which a window has been excised (15.11). 7-0 prolene or nylon is used for the anastomosis, and it helps me if I use a binocular loupe. No splint is necessary. Exact haemostasis is obtained, the testis carefully replaced and the scrotum closed in the way described above.

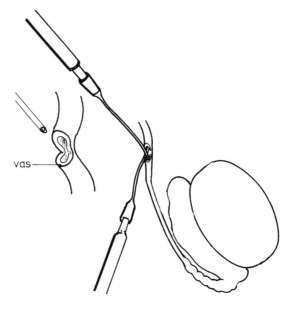

15.10. Vasography: fine Intracath cannulae just fit the lumen of the vas.

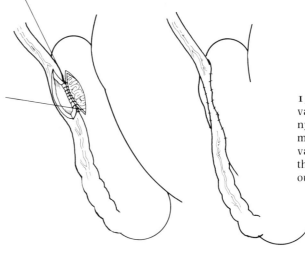

15.11. Epididymovasostomy: a 7-0 nylon suture approximates the edge of the vas to the covering of the epididymis without a splint.

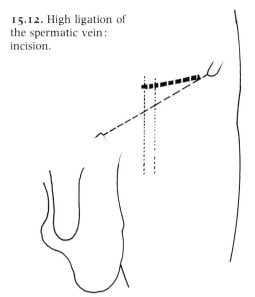

15.12. High ligation of the spermatic vein: incision.

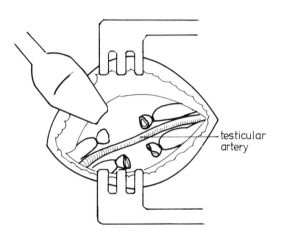

15.13. The testicular veins are divided between ligatures and the testicular artery spared.

— testicular artery

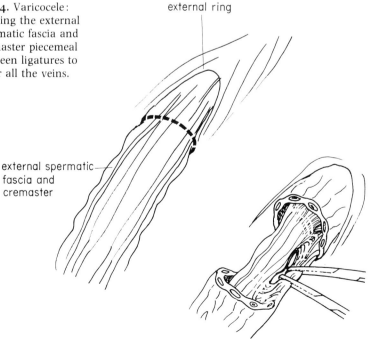

15.14. Varicocele: dividing the external spermatic fascia and cremaster piecemeal between ligatures to sever all the veins.

external ring

external spermatic fascia and cremaster

Varicocele

Indications

There are some sensible men who have very large and unsightly varicoceles that not only look ugly, but give pain that persists in spite of wearing supporting underpants or a jock-strap. Be careful, however, not to be trapped into operating on an introspective and neurotic sportsman: whatever the result, he will be disappointed.

Infertility and its relationship to varicocele have been the subject of fierce debate. There is, understandably, a reluctance on the part of surgeons to accept the evidence of those controlled trials which show that varicocelectomy is no better than doing nothing when it comes to treating infertility associated with oligozoospermia. I am of the opinion (at present) that there is no sound evidence at all to support the current practice of operating on varicoceles for infertility (Nilsson *et al.* 1979; Turner 1983). Two operations are in vogue: high and low ligation.

High ligation for varicocele

With the patient supine, under general anaesthesia with a little head-up tilt to the table, make a short crease incision above and parallel with the inguinal ligament lateral to the mid-inguinal point (15.12). After opening the external oblique aponeurosis, split the internal oblique and transversus muscles in the line of their fibres to enter the extra-peritoneal fat. Retracting the fat exposes the testicular vessels, which are easily identified before they curl around the inferior epigastric vessels. Gently separate them from the back of the peritoneum to which they adhere. Dissect the veins carefully away from the testicular artery, and divide them between 3-0 catgut ligatures (15.13). Close the wound with catgut. The patient may have a little post-operative swelling and discomfort in the scrotum and should wear a scrotal support for a week.

Low ligation

Through a short crease incision over the pubic tubercle, identify the spermatic cord and lift it up. Divide the cremaster muscle and all the associated veins that lie between the internal and the external spermatic fascia, catching them up between pairs of mosquito forceps and ligating them with 4-0 catgut (15.14).

Injury of the testicle

Every injury which results in a swelling of the testicle should be explored without delay. The testical is at risk from compression by a haematoma that is not evacuated and the best chance of preserving fertility is ensured by early intervention (Cass 1983).

Expose the testicle through a scrotal incision, and open the parietal tunica vaginalis. Evacuate the clot. The tear in the visceral layer of the tunica is identified and repaired with interrupted 3-0 chromic catgut. The scrotum is closed in the usual way.

When the injury is of long standing, there is always a possibility that the swelling may be a tumour that has been made to bleed. When your suspicion is thus aroused, explore the testicle through an inguinal incision.

Orchidopexy for undescended testicle

Indications

After the age of one year, there is little evidence that a testicle which has not reached the scrotum will ever do so. By the age of one year, there is clear histological evidence that the germinal epithelium of the inguinal testis is threatened. If detected, the undescended testis ought to be brought down into the scrotum by the age of two. From then onwards, the only matter for doubt is whether or not the testis is truly undescended, or merely retractile. Nothing is gained by waiting until puberty, and there is never any place for precipitating premature puberty by giving gonadotrophins merely to make clear the distinction between a high and low retractile testicle (Fonkalsrud & Mengel 1981).

Position on the table

Supine.

Anaesthesia

Full relaxation is needed to permit an extensive mobilization of the testicular vessels behind the peritoneum.

Incision

Make a crease incision with its centre over the internal ring (15.15).

Steps of the operation

Open the external oblique sufficiently to display the cord and the margins of the internal ring (15.16). Open the sleeve of the cremaster. Pick up the processus vaginalis (15.17), which is nearly always prominent and usually complete in young boys. Open it and separate it from the cord (which it may invest almost

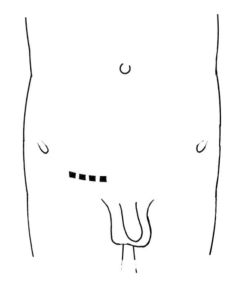

15.15. Orchidopexy: a crease incision is made overlying the internal ring.

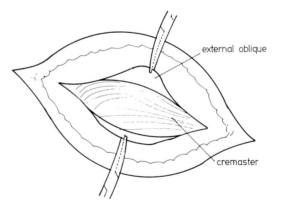

external oblique

cremaster

15.16. The external oblique aponeurosis is divided revealing the internal oblique and cremaster.

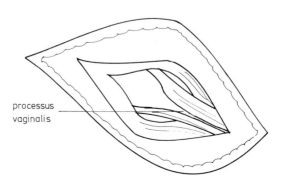

processus vaginalis

15.17. The cremaster is split in the direction of its fibres to show the sac of the processus vaginalis on the anterior aspect of the cord.

completely) by careful dissection (15.18). Dissect it upwards towards the peritoneum until the vessels of the cord are seen to bear off in one direction and the vas disappears down towards the bladder round the inferior epigastric vessels (15.19).

Lift up the peritoneum and pull down the vessels of the cord. They are tethered to the back of the peritoneum by thin tough bands of fascia which must be divided (15.20) to free the spermatic vessels as high as a finger can reach (15.21). Displace the spermatic vessels medially in order to straighten their retroperitoneal course.

Now turn your attention to the testicle. It will probably be lying in the inguinal canal or just outside it. Taking care to preserve the vas, which may loop down towards the scrotum, free the testicle until it is attached only by its

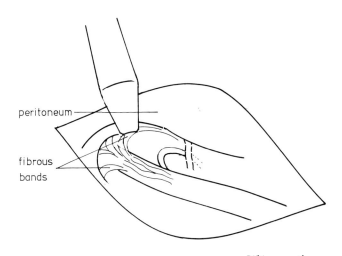

15.20. Lifting up the peritoneum off the testicular vessels to reveal the crescentic bands of fibrous tissue which anchor the vessels. These are divided to give length to the testicular vessels.

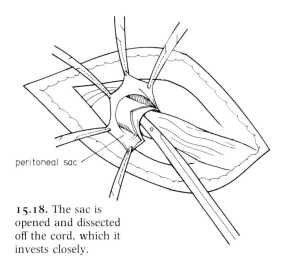

15.18. The sac is opened and dissected off the cord, which it invests closely.

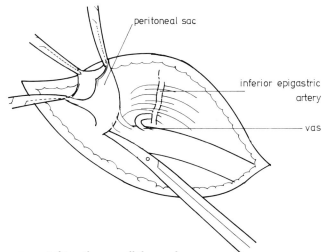

15.19. Lifting the sac off the cord progressively reveals the vas, turning off to pass behind the inferior epigastric artery, and the testicular vessels going up in the direction of the posterior abdominal wall.

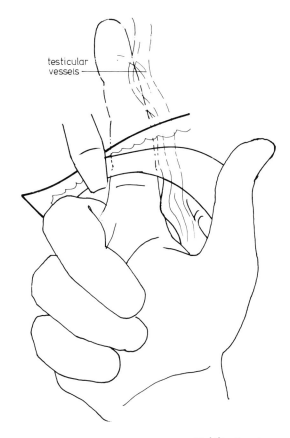

15.21. Mobilization is assisted by a finger which displaces the testicular vessels medially to straighten their course.

spermatic vessels and the vas (15.22).

A pocket is now made for the testicle in the scrotum. First pushing a finger down to tent up the scrotal skin (15.23), cut down just through the skin but not through the dartos. Develop the plane between dermis and dartos with scissors until a pocket is made big enough for the testicle to sit in easily (15.24). Make a tiny hole in the dartos, just big enough for the testicle to be pushed through (15.25), and lay the testicle in its subcutaneous pocket (15.26). The hole in the dartos may need to be narrowed if it has been made too large.

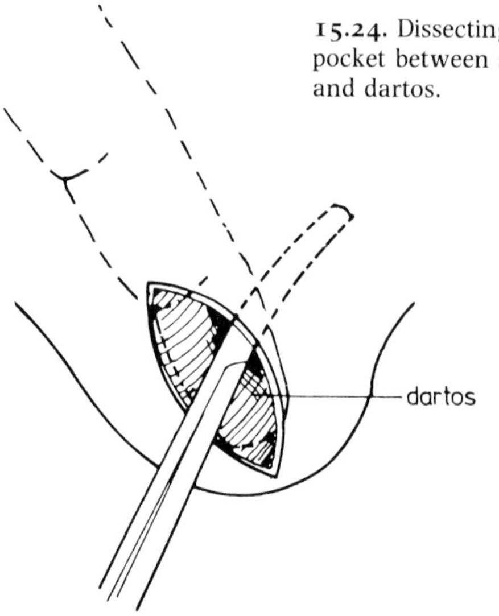

15.24. Dissecting a pocket between skin and dartos.

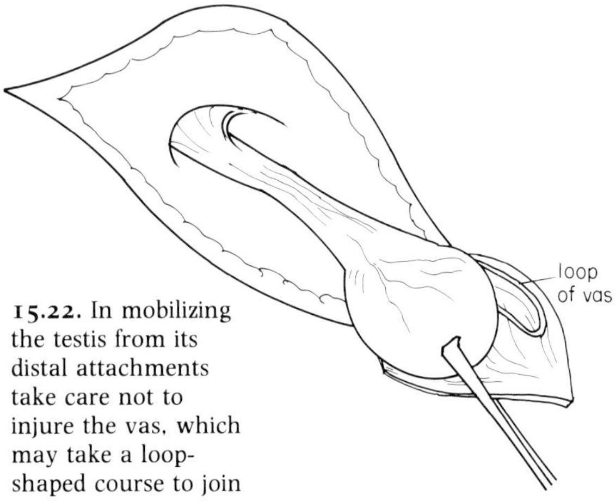

dartos

15.22. In mobilizing the testis from its distal attachments take care not to injure the vas, which may take a loop-shaped course to join the testis.

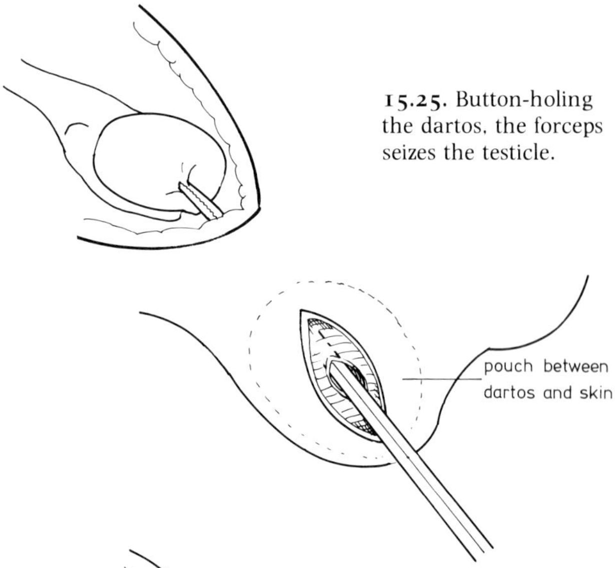

loop of vas

15.25. Button-holing the dartos, the forceps seizes the testicle.

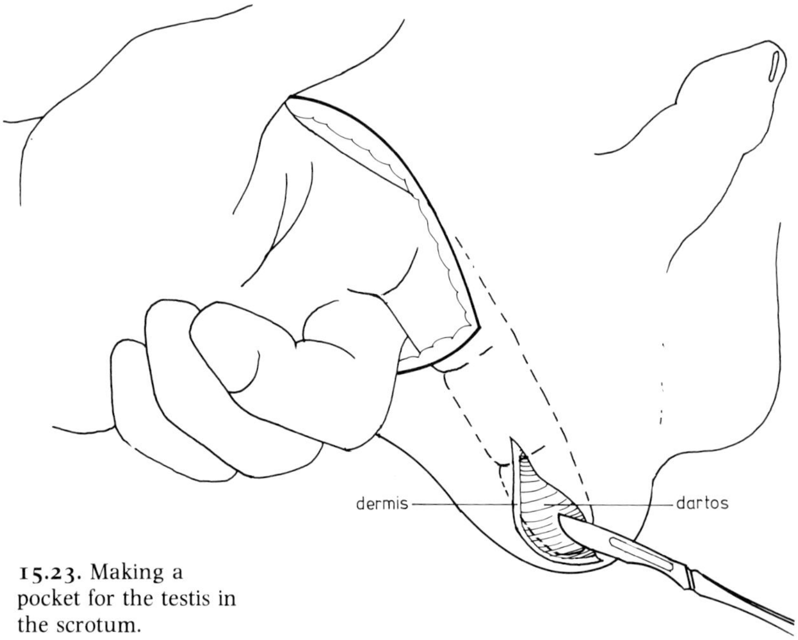

pouch between dartos and skin

15.23. Making a pocket for the testis in the scrotum.

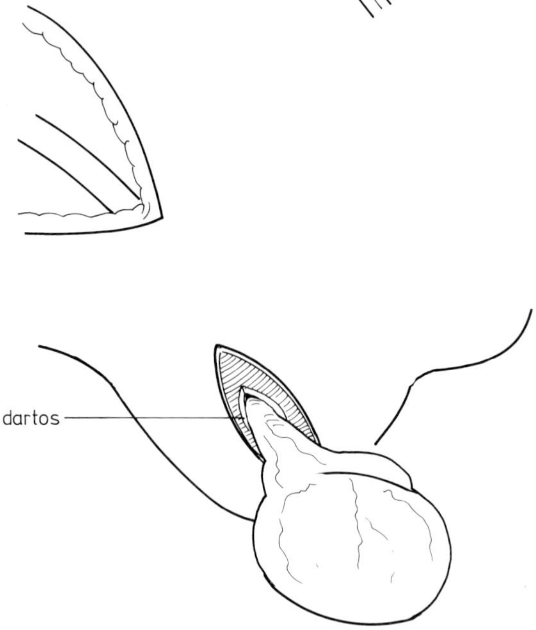

dermis   dartos

15.26. The testicle is brought out through the button-hole in the dartos.

dartos

The testicle may be secured in its pocket by catching it up in the fine interrupted mattress sutures that are now used to close the skin (15.27). After ligating the peritoneal sac, the inguinal canal is closed with 3-0 chromic catgut. A subcuticular suture leaves a painless and inconspicuous scar for the boy.

15.27. Closing the skin of the scrotum: the sutures just catch up the testis.

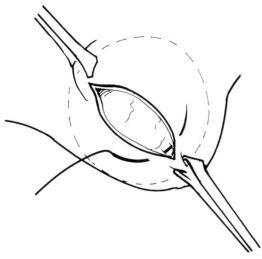

Hazards of the operation

If the testicle is only seen after opening the peritoneum, where it lies just inside the internal ring, it may be difficult to get down further than the external ring. It is better to be content with this small achievement, and plan to re-explore the groin one or two years later when, at a second operation, it is surprisingly easy to complete the procedure, as if with time the testicular vessels have grown longer.

Hydrocele

In children hydroceles may be left alone until the age of eighteen months. If persistent past this age, a tiny incision is made over the internal ring: the processus vaginalis is found, divided, its proximal end tied off and the distal end left open. The hydrocele will then disappear. There is no need to meddle with the testis.

In young males who come up with a hydrocele, always suspect that there is a testicular tumour underlying it. If the testis cannot be clearly felt, and a tumour excluded, then it is my practice to admit the patient without delay to explore the testicle as much to exclude cancer as to deal with the hydrocele.

Most hydroceles appear in middle age, when tumours are rare, so most hydroceles are entirely innocent. Always consider the choice of aspiration or operation. Many an elderly man is perfectly happily served by occasional aspiration of a hydrocele when it is troubling him. If it fills up very often, then offer him a radical cure. If there is difficulty in feeling the underlying testicle, it had better be aspirated to make sure.

Today ultrasound examination of the testis is a useful ancillary diagnostic measure. It enables one to be fairly sure in a hydrocele that the underlying testis is or is not of uniform consistence (Tiptaft et al. 1982).

Aspiration of a hydrocele

The patient is supine. In a darkened room, shine a torch through the hydrocele to identify large superficial veins so that they may be avoided. Clean the skin with cetrimide and instil a bleb of 1% lignocaine into the dermis (15.28). Inject more local anaesthetic through this bleb down to the wall of the hydrocele, aspirating and injecting alternately, until the needle aspirates hydrocele fluid. Take an IV cannula attached to a three-way tap and syringe: thrust the cannula firmly into the hydrocele, withdraw the stylet, and advance the plastic sheath. Attach the syringe and tap, and empty the hydrocele (15.29). Never use a syringe and needle to tap

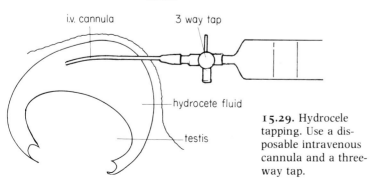

15.29. Hydrocele tapping. Use a disposable intravenous cannula and a three-way tap.

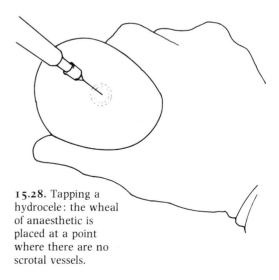

15.28. Tapping a hydrocele: the wheal of anaesthetic is placed at a point where there are no scrotal vessels.

a hydrocele: it is very easy to lacerate the visceral layer of the tunica vaginalis and give rise to a haematocele. After the sac is emptied, compress the edges of the puncture and apply a drop of sterile sealing fluid. In former days haematomas were common, and easily became infected, leading to a very unpleasant infection that often resulted in 'fungus testis' and loss of the organ. Always warn your patients to report if there is pain or persistent swelling after tapping a hydrocele.

Radical cure of a hydrocele

Lord's operation

In a thin flaccid hydrocele, a scrotal incision is made down to the parietal layer of the tunica, which is seized with two pairs of forceps and incised. After the fluid has been removed, make the testicle emerge, and then insert a series of 4-0 catgut sutures to bunch up the frill of tunica vaginalis all round the testis (15.30). Then replace the testis and close the scrotum with care to prevent a haematoma in the method described above (15.31) (Lord 1964).

Thick old hydroceles

Deliver the testicle completely and open the tunica. Excise the thick sac all round, taking care not to trespass upon the epididymis, but leave a frill of tunica all the way around (15.32). Oversew the frill with 4-0 catgut for haemostasis (15.33). Make very sure that every other minute vessel has been ligated or sealed with diathermy and restore the testicle to the scrotum, closing the scrotum haemostatically as described above.

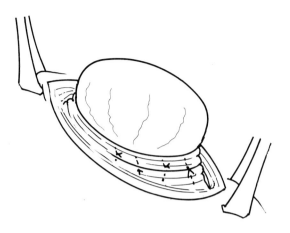

15.31. The testicle is replaced in the scrotum.

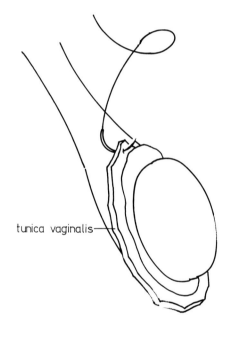

tunica vaginalis

15.32. Excision of the thick-walled tunica of an old hydrocele leaves a vascular rim which must be over-sewn for haemostasis.

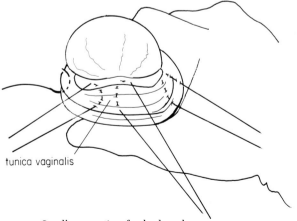

tunica vaginalis

15.30. Lord's operation for hydrocele: a series of catgut sutures is inserted to bunch up the surplus hydrocele sac into a frill around the testicles.

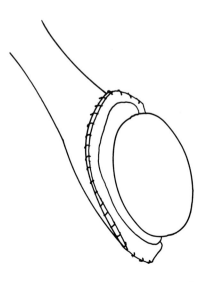

15.33. The edge of the hydrocele sac oversewn with 4-0 catgut for haemostasis.

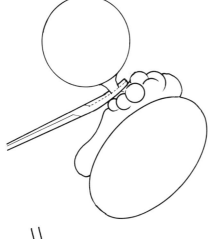

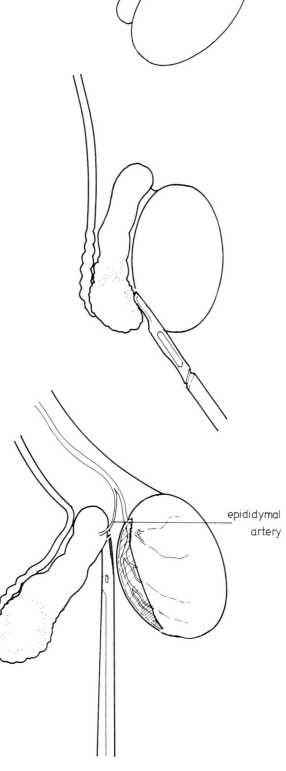

epididymal
artery

Cysts of the epididymis

Indications

Cysts of the epididymis hardly ever need anything doing to them at all, and certainly must never be meddled with in young men before they have finished having their family, for removal of an epididymal cyst (which is essentially a diverticulum of one of the vasa efferentia testis) may sterilize that gonad. They should not be aspirated: it hurts, and because they are multilocular, it is usually unsatisfactory.

Steps of the operation

After delivering the testicle through a scrotal incision each cyst is carefully dissected through the thin layers that invest it. Shell each cyst out towards its attachment, and there ligate it and cut it off (15.34). There is no need to remove the whole of the wall of the cyst, and when they are multilocular, it is enough to uncap the smaller ones.

Epididymectomy

Indications

This is rarely indicated today except in neglected seminal tuberculosis, and in some instances where the epididymis is involved in a chronic painful seminal granuloma.

Steps of the operation

Exposing the testicle through the scrotum, dissect between the testis and epididymis, beginning at the lower end where the lump is often biggest, and work towards the upper pole (15.35) where the main testicular artery gives off a branch to the head of the epididymis, which can sometimes be seen and diathermized. It is usually very small and to avoid damage to the main artery of the gonad, it is safer to cut at the expense of the epididymis (15.36).

Torsion of the testicle

Indications

Except for the rare extravaginal torsion of the testicle said to occur in new-born infants, when the testicle twists it is always inside the tunica vaginalis, and it twists because the tunica is large and invests the epididymis completely to provide the gonad with a kind of mesentery. It should be an absolute rule to explore every testicle which seems inflamed, unless it is clear that the epididymis alone is inflamed and quite distinct from the testicle. Torsion ought to be diagnosed more often at an early stage, for previous incomplete episodes of torsion are very common, and should call for prophylactic fixation of the testis (Chapman & Walton 1972; Cattolica *et al.* 1982).

Incision

In all obvious cases the testicle is explored through the scrotum but in late neglected instances, the woody mass is indistinguishable from a cancer and should be explored through the groin.

Steps of the operation

Deliver the testicle. Open the tunica vaginalis. Aspirate the bloody fluid that has collected there. Untwist the testicle on its stalk—often rotated through several complete turns (15.37)—and then decide whether or not to try to save the testis. It is sometimes difficult to know whether the testis is or is not dead. Incise it and if it bleeds, conserve it (Blandy 1957). Since the other testis is likely to have a similar arrangement of the tunica vaginalis, it should also be explored and the testicle fixed preferably there and then, unless there is doubt about infection.

Orchidectomy

Indications

Today there are two main indications for orchidectomy: cancer of the prostate, and cancer of the testicle. For cancer of the prostate, orchidectomy avoids the cardiovascular side effects of oestrogen therapy. One may perform a subcapsular orchidectomy or remove both testicles completely: temper the wind to the shorn lamb when you advise the patient. There is a theoretical advantage in removing the entire testicle, but much to be said for sparing the patient's feelings (McDonald & Calams 1959).

Subcapsular orchidectomy

Make a short transverse scrotal incision. Squeeze out one testicle first, open the visceral layer of the tunica vaginalis, and wipe out all the testicular tissue with gauze on your finger. The hilum will bleed. Insert a 3-0 catgut suture from the outside of the tunica and having knotted it, run along the hilum to seal off the bleeding vessels. Then bring the same suture along the tunica to close it tightly. Do the same the other side, and make sure that you have achieved perfect haemostasis before closing the scrotum (15.38).

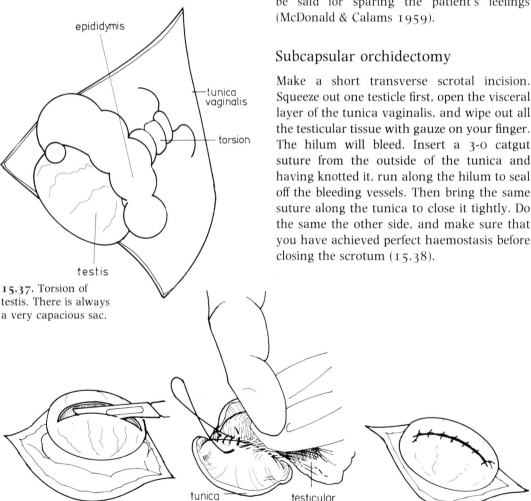

15.37. Torsion of testis. There is always a very capacious sac.

15.38. Subcapsular orchidectomy.

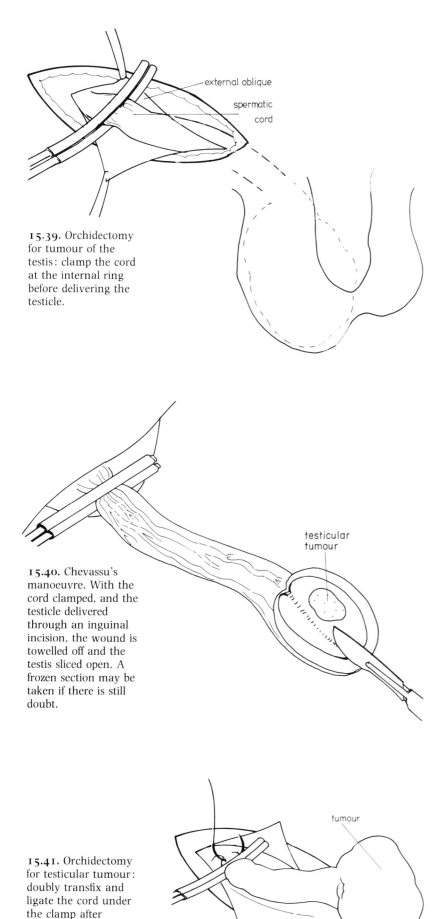

15.39. Orchidectomy for tumour of the testis: clamp the cord at the internal ring before delivering the testicle.

external oblique

spermatic cord

15.40. Chevassu's manoeuvre. With the cord clamped, and the testicle delivered through an inguinal incision, the wound is towelled off and the testis sliced open. A frozen section may be taken if there is still doubt.

testicular tumour

15.41. Orchidectomy for testicular tumour: doubly transfix and ligate the cord under the clamp after verifying that the swelling is a tumour.

tumour

In younger patients, consider whether your patient would not prefer a pair of silicone rubber prosthetic testicles. If so, remove both gonads completely but suture-ligature the entire cord, and insert the prostheses, one into each scrotal sac before closing the scrotum.

Orchidectomy for testicular cancer

The first step in the management of known or suspected testicular tumour is to remove the testicle. In view of the well-documented risk of opening up the inguinal lymphatics and scrotal tissues to implantation of cancer, the exploration should be performed through an inguinal rather than a scrotal incision (Blandy *et al.* 1976, 1977).

Steps of the operation

Through a crease incision over the internal ring, slit up the external oblique in the line of its fibres. Pick up the cord and clamp it with a Doyen's clamp to prevent squeezing cancer cells up the spermatic veins (15.39).

Deliver the testicle from the scrotum with a little counter pressure. Avoid carrying the incision into the scrotum whever possible, although this may be needed when a tumour is unusually large.

As soon as the testicle is in the wound, the diagnosis is nearly always obvious, for there is a large, hard, irregular mass in the testis. Occasionally you may be in difficulty, for example with the young man who has already lost one testis from injury or cryptorchidism. It is absolutely essential to get the diagnosis right. Here one may towel off the wound and perform Chevassu's manoeuvre. Take a large knife blade and slice the testis along the border opposite to the epididymis (15.40). Have a frozen section taken if you discover anything suspicious. If the testis is normal, the tunica can be closed up with continuous 3-0 catgut, and it will be impossible to distinguish the operated from the normal side six months later.

If, as is more usual, the diagnosis is obvious, doubly transfix and ligate the entire cord, well proximal to the Doyen's clamp, and cut it off (15.41). Take extra care with haemostasis when closing the wound in layers—haematoma may defer radiotherapy and sepsis may postpone giving chemotherapy.

Retroperitoneal node dissection for testicular cancer

Indications

The old debate between the proponents of radical node dissection versus radiotherapy for early cases of non-seminomatous germ cell tumours of the testis is, today, stale and irrelevant. In its place the rapid advance of chemotherapy has confronted the urologist with a new challenge—salvage node dissection. Young men who are first diagnosed when there are large bulky para-aortic masses of secondary tumour are today given chemotherapy with the result that gigantic masses of secondary cancer disappear as if by magic. In some however a problem remains: CAT scanning continues to show persistent abnormal masses of tissue, or the tumour markers (AFP or HCG) remain elevated. One is obliged to remove the suspicious tissue (Donohue *et al.* 1980; Hendry *et al.* 1981; Oliver *et al.* 1983).

Preparations

Although with care to preserve the last two lumbar sympathetic ganglia many of these young men are able to retain ejaculation, most are made infertile from paralysis of the seminal vesicles. This must be explained and discussed (Proctor & Howards 1983).

In salvage node dissection one is never quite certain how bad things are going to be when the abdomen is opened. Tumour masses may be adherent to the aorta and vena cava, the ureter and colon may be part and parcel of the white cheesy material that represents all that is left of massive metastases. Bowel should be prepared, and arrangements made with one's vascular surgical colleagues to patch or replace the aorta or cava should this be necessary.

Blood loss may be considerable, and six units should be available.

Position on the table

Supine.

Anaesthesia

General, with full relaxation and monitoring of all vital functions.

Incision

From xiphisternum to pubic symphysis.

Steps of the operation

On entering the abdomen, spend enough time dividing omental and small bowel adhesions so that the bowel may be safely delivered onto the chest. Run scissors along the ascending colon and round the caecum up the mesentery so that all the gut supplied by the superior mesenteric trunk can be lifted up and out of the abdomen, to be carefully protected between wet packs in a plastic bag (15.42).

Dividing the inferior mesenteric vein between ligatures allows the left renal vein to be

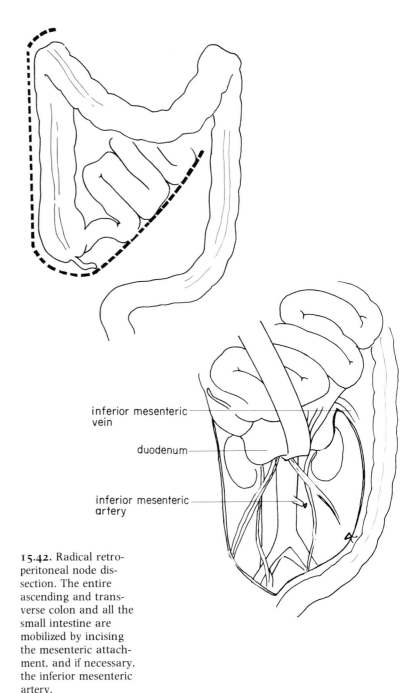

inferior mesenteric vein

duodenum

inferior mesenteric artery

15.42. Radical retroperitoneal node dissection. The entire ascending and transverse colon and all the small intestine are mobilized by incising the mesenteric attachment, and if necessary, the inferior mesenteric artery.

seen clearly, and dividing the inferior mesenteric artery gives access to the left side of the aorta (15.43).

Removing the mass of nodes from the retroperitoneal space is performed in four steps (15.44). Beginning at the level of the renal arteries and running down along the anterior surface of the vena cava, the vena cava is dissected clean, taking all the tissue along its front and lateral aspect from the renal arteries and renal veins downwards *en bloc*. If the tumour was on the right side, this will include the testicular artery and vein on the right side, and the specimen lays bare the entire vena cava, psoas, ureter and right common iliac vessels down to the division of the internal iliac artery. This portion is removed at the internal ring, where the stump of the testicular vessels was originally tied off (15.45).

On the left side, a similar dissection runs down the front of the aorta, and includes all the tissue on the lateral aspect and front of the aorta out to the ureter (15.46).

A wedge-shaped collection of tissue now

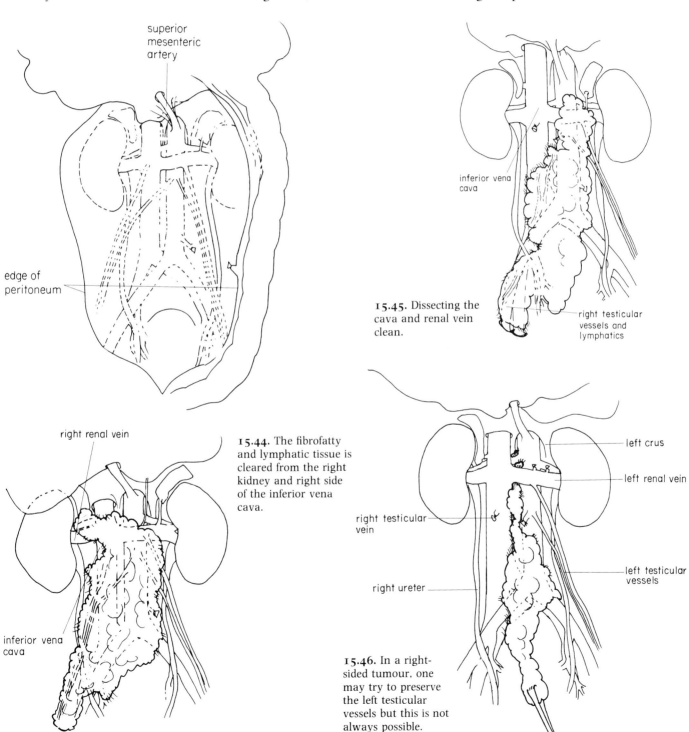

15.43. The structures to be dissected clear are concealed by lymph nodes and fibrofatty tissue.

superior mesenteric artery

edge of peritoneum

15.44. The fibrofatty and lymphatic tissue is cleared from the right kidney and right side of the inferior vena cava.

right renal vein

inferior vena cava

15.45. Dissecting the cava and renal vein clean.

inferior vena cava

right testicular vessels and lymphatics

15.46. In a right-sided tumour, one may try to preserve the left testicular vessels but this is not always possible.

left crus

left renal vein

left testicular vessels

right testicular vein

right ureter

lies anteriorly between vena cava and aorta. This is dissected carefully from under the left renal vein downwards, leaving the cava and aorta naked (15.47).

Finally the fourth wedge of tissue is taken from behind, between cava and aorta. It does not seem (to me) justified to divide the lumbar veins or arteries in this dissection, but any fibrous or lymphatic tissue must be meticulously dissected out (15.48).

At the conclusion of the dissection the aorta and the cava and their branches should resemble an anatomical drawing. The only difficulty in this operation arises when the white cheesy material actually invades the wall of the great vessels or the bowel. It is for this reason that the dissection must be taken slowly, using great care, and always being prepared to tape the aorta and cava before either is breached.

Closure of the wound includes every known precaution against wound dehiscence. A few days ileus is the rule, but these fit young men usually recover with remarkably little disturbance (Donohue & Rowland 1981; Babaian *et al.* 1981).

Vasectomy

Indications

Vasectomy is occasionally indicated for recurrent epididymitis but is usually performed nowadays for voluntary sterilization. The ethical and legal precautions surrounding this procedure should be carefully studied by any surgeon embarking upon this operation: few operations in surgery are attended by so many medico-legal difficulties.

It is essential that husband and wife understand that the operation is difficult to reverse and reversal can never be guaranteed successful (Howard 1982). They must know that sufficient time must be allowed for the storage system to empty out, and that there is a faint (perhaps 1%) chance of spontaneous recanalization, whatever technique is used for division of the vasa. They should be warned about the hazard of haematoma, and that in a proportion of men an uncomfortable thickening of the epididymis is found afterwards, probably caused by inflammation around extravasated sperm.

Most patients may be vasectomized under local anaesthetic, but the very nervous, and those who have undergone previous hernia surgery or orchidopexy, will need a general anaesthetic. Always examine the patient care-

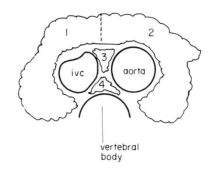

15.47. The tissue all around the cava and aorta are removed in four parts.

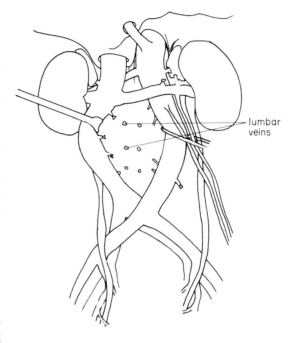

15.48. To remove the last part of the lymphatic tissue the lumbar veins are divided, and often several of the lumbar arteries.

fully first, and avoid attempting vasectomy under local anaesthetic when the patient is grossly apprehensive or has a thick, tight scrotum.

Position

Supine. The scrotum should have been shaved.

Steps of the operation

Infiltrate the skin with 1% lignocaine and 1:1000 adrenaline. My preference is for a single midline incision (15.49); others use one incision over each vas. After infiltrating and incising the skin, feel for the vas, pick it up gently between finger and thumb, infiltrate more anaesthetic, and then seize the vas gently but firmly with an Allis forceps. Incise its connective tissue sheath; infiltrate again right down onto the vas, and give time for the local to work before pulling on the vas. Having incised the sheath of the vas longitudinally, grasp the vas deferens itself and lift it out of its

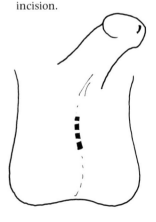

15.49. Vasectomy: midline scrotal incision.

sheath. Unless you have taken trouble to infiltrate the sheath well this may be painful: if it hurts, stop and put in more local (15.50).

Lift out a loop of vas deferens about 3 cm long. Tie off the testicular end with 3-0 chromic catgut, remove 1 cm of vas (for

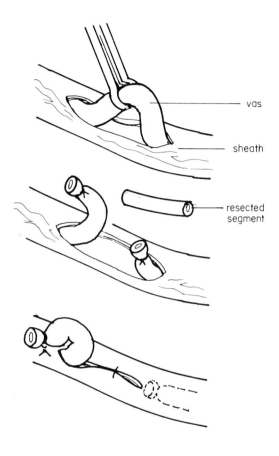

15.50. Vasectomy: after resecting 1 cm of vas, one end is turned back and sewn outside the vas sheath.

vas

sheath

resected segment

histological confirmation that the operation has been done right), turn the vas upon itself and ligate the bladder end twice so that the end is turned back. Finally close the sheath of the vas to bury the testicular cut end. Close the skin and dartos with two or three 4-0 chromic catgut sutures. Check that there is complete haemostasis, and to protect yourself against a charge of negligence, make a careful note that haemostasis was checked.

After-care

The patient wears a scrotal support for the first forty-eight hours. Complications include haematoma (the most common), cellulitis, and pain. Appell (1977) showed that patients who developed post-operative infections in the wounds had organisms growing in their semen, of which, of course, the surgeons had no knowledge. For this reason every patient ought to be instructed to report any untoward inflammatory features, as well as any un-

toward swelling. A haematoma should probably be treated by evacuation of the clot, antibiotics, and a period of rest in hospital.

Late spontaneous reunion is well documented, and occurs, whatever method has been used for the division of the vasa, in about 1% of cases. It is most important that the patient and his medical advisers know this fact, for much is made of it in the courts, and no doctor should ever promise his patient that the operation will guarantee sterility.

Very great care must be taken to make sure that two consecutive semen specimens are shown to be without sperm. There is some doubt now as to whether or not it is safe to accept the finding of a few motionless sperms in the centrifuged specimen as being safe: an Eosin-Nigrosin stain will show that the sperms are motionless, and such a patient can reasonably be assured that he is sterile.

Reanastomosis after vasectomy

Many an unfortunate man loses his wife and family in an accident, or from divorce, after vasectomy and would like to start another family. Unfortunately vasectomy seems sometimes to raise antibodies to the man's own sperm, which may render him infertile. The chance of losing these antibodies is increased if both vasa are reunited. It seems from most surgeons' experience that about 80% of reconstituted vasa give motile sperms in the ejaculate, but only about 50% of these patients achieve fatherhood (Amelar & Dubin 1979).

Anaesthesia

General.

Steps of the operation

Through a generous scrotal incision deliver the testicle, identify the site of division of the vas first on one side, and then on the other (15.51). Dissect the vas proximal and distal to

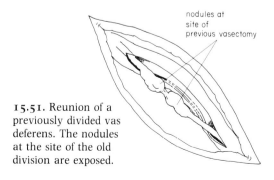

nodules at site of previous vasectomy

15.51. Reunion of a previously divided vas deferens. The nodules at the site of the old division are exposed.

the knob that marks the site of division, and trim away the scar tissue until semen flows from the testicular end, and an obvious lumen is visible in the bladder end of the vas. Spatulate each cut end of the vas and make an elliptical end-to-end anastomosis with the aid of a loupe and 7-0 nylon or prolene. No splint is needed (15.52).

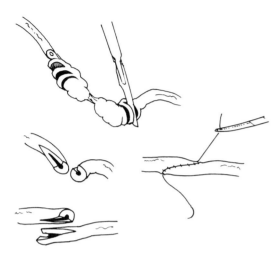

15.52. Slice back each nodule until healthy vas is seen. Spatulate the ends, and anastomose them with 7-0 non-absorbable suture.

After-care

One may start to examine the semen for sperms after about six weeks. Thereafter the sperm density mounts rapidly. There is sound theoretical and experimental evidence that both sides should be rejoined to give the best chance of avoiding auto-immune infertility. If the operation fails, it is worth doing again.

References

Amelar R.D. & Dubin L. (1979) Vasectomy reversal. *J. Urol.* **121**, 547.

Appell R. (1977) Personal communication.

Babaian R.J., Bracken R.B. & Johnson D.E. (1981) Complications of transabdominal retroperitoneal lymphadenectomy. *Urology*, **17**, 126.

Blandy J.P. (1957) Three cases of torsion of the testis. *Brit. Med. J.* **1**, 807.

Blandy J.P. (1976) Testicular neoplasms. *Urology*, (ed. by Blandy J.P.), p. 1203. Blackwell Scientific Publications, Oxford.

Blandy J.P. (1977) Testicular tumours. *Recent advances in Surgery*, (ed. by Taylor S.). Churchill Livingstone, Edinburgh.

Cass A.S. (1983) Testicular Trauma. *J. Urol.* **129**, 299.

Cattolica E.V., Karol J.B., Rankin K.N. & Klein R.S. (1982) High testicular salvage rate in torsion of the spermatic cord. *J. Urol.* **128**, 66.

Chapman R.H. & Walton A.J. (1972) Torsion of the testis and its appendages. *Brit. Med. J.* **1**, 164.

Donohue J.P., Einhorn L.H. & Williams S.D. (1980) Cytoreductive surgery for metastatic testis cancer: considerations of timing and extent. *J. Urol.* **123**, 876.

Donohue J.P. & Rowland R.G. (1981) Complications of retroperitoneal lymph node dissection. *J. Urol.* **125**, 338.

Fonkalsrud E.W. & Mengel W. (1981) *The Undescended Testis.* Year Book Publishers Inc. Chicago, London.

Hendry W.F., Parslow J.M. & Stedronska J. (1983) Exploratory scrototomy in 145 azoospermic males: operative findings, serum antisperm antibodies, reconstructive techniques and results. *Brit. J. Urol.* **55**, 785–91.

Hendry W.F., Goldstraw P., Husband J.E., Barrett A., McElwain T.J. & Peckham M.J. (1981) Elective delayed excision of bulky para-aortic lymph node metastases in advanced non-seminoma germ cell tumours of testis. *Brit. J. Urol.* **53**, 648.

Howard G. (1982) Who asks for vasectomy reversal and why. *Brit. Med. J.* **285**, 490.

Lord P.H. (1964) A bloodless operation for the radical cure of idiopathic hydrocele. *Brit. J. Surg.* **51**, 914.

McDonald J.H. & Calams J.A. (1959) Extraperitoneal Leydig-like cells; observations following subcapsular orchietomy. *J. Urol.* **82**, 145.

Nilsson S., Edvinsson A. & Nilsson B. (1979) Improvement of semen and pregnancy rate after ligation and division of the internal spermatic vein: fact or fiction? *Brit. J. Urol.* **51**, 591.

Oliver R.T.D., Blandy J.P., Hendry W.F. & Pryor J.P. (1983) Post-treatment surgical staging in management of metastatic germ cell tumours. *Brit. J. Urol.* **55**,

Pavone Macaluso M., Smith P.H. & Bradshaw M.A. (1985) Testicular Cancer and other Tumours of the Urinary Tract, p. 403–9 Plaenum Press, New York and London.

Proctor K.G. & Howards S.S. (1983) The effect of sympathomimetic drugs on post-lymphadenectomy aspermia. *J. Urol.* **129**, 837.

Pryor J.P., Cameron K.M., Collins W.P., Hirsh A.V., Mahony J.D.H., Pugh R.C.B. & Fitzpatrick J.M. (1978) Indications for testicular biopsy or exploration in azoospermia. *Brit. J. Urol.* **50**, 591.

Tiptaft R.C., Nicholls B.M., Hately W. & Blandy J.P. (1982) The diagnosis of testicular swellings using water-path ultrasound. *Brit. J. Urol.* **54**, 759.

Turner T.T. (1983) Varicocele: still an enigma. *J. Urol.* **129**, 695.

Index